Nelson Yuan-sheng Liang

ADVANCES IN NEUROLOGY
Volume 42

Advances in Neurology

Advances in Neurology

Volume 42

Progress in Aphasiology

Editor

F. Clifford Rose, F.R.C.P.

Physician in Charge
Department of Neurology
Charing Cross Hospital
London, England

Raven Press ■ New York

Raven Press, 1140 Avenue of the Americas, New York, New York 10036

Made in the United States of America

Library of Congress Cataloging in Publication Data
Main entry under title:

Progress in aphasiology.

(Advances in neurology; v. 42)
"Based on a Mansell Bequest Symposium of the Medical Society of London held in the summer of 1983"—Pref.
Includes bibliographies and index.
1. Aphasia—Congresses. I. Rose, F. Clifford (Frank Clifford) II. Mansell Bequest Symposium (1983 : London, England) III. Medical Society of London. IV. Series. [DNLM: 1. Aphasia—congress. W1 AD684H v. 42 / WL 340.5 P964 1983]
RC321.A276 vol. 42 616.8 s [616.85'52] 84-15979
[RC425]
ISBN 0-88167-023-5

The material contained in this volume was submitted as previously unpublished material, except in the instances in which credit has been given to the source from which some of the illustrative material was derived

Great care has been taken to maintain the accuracy of the information contained in the volume. However, Raven Press cannot be held responsible for errors or for any consequences arising from the use of the information contained herein.

Advances in Neurology Series

Vol. 42: Progress in Aphasiology
F. Clifford Rose, editor. 384 pp., 1984.

Vol. 41: The Olivopontocerebellar Atrophies
R. C. Duvoisin and A. Plaitakis, editors. 304 pp., 1984.

Vol. 40: Parkinson-Specific Motor and Mental Disorders, Role of the Pallidum: Pathophysiological, Biochemical, and Therapeutic Aspects
R. G. Hassler and J. F. Christ, editors. 601 pp., 1984.

Vol. 39: Motor Control Mechanisms in Health and Disease
J. E. Desmedt, editor. 1,224 pp., 1983.

Vol. 38: The Dementias
R. Mayeux and W. G. Rosen, editors. 288 pp., 1983.

Vol. 37: Experimental Therapeutics of Movement Disorders
S. Fahn, D. B. Calne, and I. Shoulson, editors. 339 pp., 1983.

Vol. 36: Human Motor Neuron Diseases
L. P. Rowland, editor. 592 pp., 1982.

Vol. 35: Gilles de la Tourette Syndrome
A. J. Friedhoff and T. N. Chase, editors. 476 pp., 1982.

Vol. 34: Status Epilepticus: Mechanisms of Brain Damage and Treatment
A. V. Delgado-Escueta, C. G. Wasterlain, D. M. Treiman, and R. J. Porter, editors. 579 pp., 1983.

Vol. 33: Headache: Physiopathological and Clinical Concepts
M. Critchley, A. Friedman, S. Gorini, and F. Sicuteri, editors. 417 pp., 1982.

Vol. 32: Clinical Applications of Evoked Potentials in Neurology
J. Courjon, F. Mauguiere, and M. Revol, editors. 592 pp., 1982.

Vol. 31: Demyelinating Diseases: Basic and Clinical Electrophysiology
S. Waxman and J. Murdoch Ritchie, editors. 544 pp., 1981.

Vol. 30: Diagnosis and Treatment of Brain Ischemia
A. L. Carney and E. M. Anderson, editors. 424 pp., 1981.

Vol. 29: Neurofibromatosis
V. M. Riccardi and J. J. Mulvihill, editors. 288 pp., 1981.

Vol. 28: Brain Edema
J. Cervós-Navarro and R. Ferszt, editors. 539 pp., 1980.

Vol. 27: Antiepileptic Drugs: Mechanisms of Action
G.H. Glaser, J.K. Penry, and D.M. Woodbury, editors. 728 pp., 1980.

Vol. 26: Cerebral Hypoxia and Its Consequences
S. Fahn, J.N. Davis, and L.P. Rowland, editors. 454 pp., 1979.

Vol. 25: Cerebrovascular Disorders and Stroke
M. Goldstein, L. Bolis, C. Fieschi, S. Gorini, and C.H. Millikan, editors. 412 pp., 1979.

Vol. 24: The Extrapyramidal System and Its Disorders
L.J. Poirier, T.L. Sourkes, and P. Bédard, editors. 552 pp., 1979.

Vol. 23: Huntington's Chorea
T.N. Chase, N.S. Wexler, and A. Barbeau, editors. 864 pp., 1979.

Vol. 22: Complications of Nervous System Trauma
R.A. Thompson and J.R. Green, editors. 454 pp., 1979.

Vol. 21: The Inherited Ataxias: Biochemical, Viral, and Pathological Studies
R.A. Kark, R. Rosenberg, and L. Schut, editors. 450 pp., 1978.

Vol. 20: Pathology of Cerebrospinal Microcirculation
J. Cervós-Navarro, E. Betz, G. Ebhardt, R. Ferszt, and R. Wüllenweber, editors. 636 pp., 1978.

Vol. 19: Neurological Epidemiology: Principles and Clinical Applications
Bruce S. Schoenberg, editor. 672 pp., 1978.

Vol. 18: Hemi-Inattention and Hemisphere Specialization
E.A. Weinstein and R.P. Friedland, editors. 176 pp., 1977.

Vol. 17: Treatment of Neuromuscular Diseases
R.C. Griggs and R.T. Moxley, editors. 370 pp., 1977.

Vol. 16: Stroke
R.A. Thompson and J.R. Green, editors. 250 pp., 1977.

Vol. 15: Neoplasia in the Central Nervous System
R.A. Thompson and J.R. Green, editors. 393 pp., 1976.

Vol. 14: Dystonia
R. Eldridge and S. Fahn, editors. 509 pp., 1976.

Vol. 13: Current Reviews
W.J. Friedlander, editor. 400 pp., 1975.

Vol. 12: Physiology and Pathology of Dendrites
G.W. Kreutzberg, editor. 524 pp. 1975.

Preface

Despite the tragic consequences of aphasia—for patient, relatives, and community—our ability to help has not greatly advanced in the past century. This explains, in part, why few neurologists actively pursue research in this field. Neurologic contributions in the past were seminal, interest being engendered largely because of the localization value of aphasia. With the advent of modern neuroimaging techniques, some of these anatomicoclinical concepts have been shown to be inaccurate. Perhaps yet another reason for the lack of interest has been the inherent difficulties of applying scientific methods to psychologic and behavioral abnormalities.

Speech is peculiar to man, and its disorders provide the greatest challenge to our understanding of how the human brain works. This volume, based on a Mansell Bequest Symposium of the Medical Society of London held in the summer of 1983, attempts to give some indication of recent developments. If it encourages others to take up that challenge, its purpose will be well served.

London 1984 F. Clifford Rose

Contents

Contributors

Renee Beland
Laboratoire Theophile-Alajonanine
Centre de Recherche
Centre Hospitalier Cote des Neiges
4565 Chenin de la Reine-Marie
Quebec, Canada H3W 1W5

Ria de Bleser
Department of Neurology
RWTH Aachen
Pauwelstrasse
D-5100 Aachen, West Germany

David Caplan
Faculty of Medicine
McGill University and Montreal Neurological Institute
Montreal, Canada

Macdonald Critchley
National Hospital for Nervous Diseases
Queen Square
London WC1 3BG, England

David Crystal
Department of Linguistic Science
University of Reading
Whiteknights
Reading RG6 2AA, England

Gerard Deloche
Unite INSERM u 84
Hopital de la Salpetriere
47 Bd de l'Hopital
75013 Paris, France

Gill Edelman
Hammersmith Hospital
Ducane Road
London W12 OHS, England

Susan Fowler
University Laboratory of Physiology
University of Oxford
Parks Road
Oxford, England

Susan Franklin
Speech Therapy Department
St. Mary Abbott's Hospital
Marloes Road
Kensington
London W8, England

U. Hadar
Department of Neurology
Charing Cross Hospital
Fulham Palace Road
London W6 8RF, England

Frances M. Hatfield
MRC Applied Psychology Unit
15 Chaucer Road
Cambridge CB2 2EF, England

David Howard
Speech Therapy Department
Regional Neurological Unit
Eastern Hospital
Homerton Grove
London E9 6BY, England; and
Psychology Department
University College Hospital
Gower Street
London WC1E 6AU, England

Walter Huber
Department of Neurology
RWTH Aachen
Goethestrasse 27-29
D-5100 Aachen, West Germany

Yves Joanette
CRMC and Chercheur Adjoint
Faculte de Medicine
Universite de Montreal
Montreal, Canada

Eirian V. Jones
The City University
Centre for Clinical Communication Studies
86 Blackfriars Road
London SE1, England

Robert J. Joynt
Department of Neurology
University of Rochester
School of Medicine and Dentistry
601 Elmwood Avenue
Rochester, New York 14642

Andrew Kertesz
Department of Clinical Neurological Sciences
University of Western Ontario
St. Joseph's Hospital
London, Ontario, Canada N6A 4V2

Diedrich Graf von Keyserlingk
Department of Neurology
RWTH Aachen
Pauwelstrasse
D-5100 Aachen, West Germany

Leonard L. LaPointe
Department of Speech and Hearing Science
Arizona State University
Tempe, Arizona 85287

Andre Roch Lecours
Faculte de Medicine
Universite de Montreal
Montreal, Canada

Ruth Lesser
Department of Speech
The University
Newcastle-upon-Tyne NE1 7RU, England

Francois Lhermitte
Clinique de Neurologie et de Neuropsychologie
Unite de Recherches Neuropsychologiques
U84 INSERM
Hopital de la Salpetriere
47 Bd de l'Hopital
75013 Paris, France

I. C. McManus
Department of Psychology
Bedford Hospital
Kempston Road
Bedford, England; and
Department of Psychiatry
St. Mary's Hospital
London W2, England

John C. Marshall
Neuropsychology Unit
Neuroscience Group
The Radcliffe Infirmary
Woodstock Road
Oxford OX2 6HE, England

Jean-Luc Nespoulous
Department de Linguistique et Philologie
Universite de Montreal
Montreal, Canada

Freda Newcombe
Neuropsychology Unit
Neuroscience Group
The Radcliffe Infirmary
Woodstock Road
Oxford OX2 6HE, England

Virginia Orchard-Lisle
Speech Therapy Department
Regional Neurological Unit
Eastern Hospital
Homerton Grove
London E9 6BY, England

John M. Oxbury
Department of Neurology
Radcliffe Infirmary
Woodstock Road
Oxford OX2, 6HE, England

Susan M. Oxbury
Department of Neurology
Radcliffe Infirmary
Woodstock Road
Oxford OX2 6HE, England

Karalyn E. Patterson
MRC Applied Psychology Unit
15 Chaucer Road
Cambridge CB2 2EF, England

Klaus Poeck
Department of Neurology
RWTH Aachen
Pauwelstrasse
D-5100 Aachen, West Germany

Ivar Reinvang
Sunnaas Sykehus
1450 Nesoddtangen, Norway

F. Clifford Rose
Department of Neurology
Charing Cross Hospital
Fulham Palace Road
London W6 8RF, England

John Rosenbek
Wm. S. Middleton Memorial VA Hospital
Madison, Wisconsin 53705

Xavier Seron
Neuropsychologie Experimentale de l'Adulte (NEXA)
Cliniques Universitaires St. Luc
Hippocrate Avenue
B-1200 Brussels, Belgium

J. F. Stein
University Laboratory of Physiology
University of Oxford
Parks Road
Oxford, England

T. J. Steiner
Department of Neurology
Charing Cross Hospital
Fulham Palace Road
London W6 8RF, England

Christine M. Temple
Neuropsychology Unit
Neuroscience Group
The Radcliffe Infirmary
Woodstock Road
Oxford OX2 6HE, England

Rita Twiston-Davies
Department of Neurology
Charing Cross Hospital
Fulham Palace Road
London W6 8RF, England

L. A. Vignolo
Department of Neurology
University of Milan
20122 Milan, Italy

Dorothea Weniger
Department of Neurology
University of Zurich
8091 Zurich, Switzerland

Klause Willmes
Department of Neurology
RWTH Aachen
Goethestrasse 27-29
D-5100 Aachen, West Germany

Advances in Neurology, Vol. 42: Progress in Aphasiology, edited by F. C. Rose.
Raven Press, New York © 1984.

Introduction

F. Clifford Rose

Department of Neurology, Charing Cross Hospital, London W6 8RF, England

HISTORIC

Probably the earliest case of aphasia is recorded in the Gospel according to Luke (1:20–22; 62–64), where Zacharias is struck dumb but still could write. During Roman times, it is recorded that in A.D. 30, Valerius Maximus lost his memory for letters after being struck by a stone. The word *aphasia* was used in a philosophic rather than its modern medical sense by Sextus Empericus (A.D. 200). Inability to read (alexia) and the disorderly, roundabout way of saying something was first described by Johann Schmidt (1624–1690). Many different disciplines were involved in the earliest reports: the great botanist Linnaeus (1707–1778) described a case of aphasia; the retention of the power to sing in expressive aphasia was noted by Dolin (1708–1763); the anatomist Morgagni (1682–1771) pointed out that aphasia occurred with left cerebral lesions but drew no conclusions; Goethe (1749–1832), in his novel *Wilhelm Meister*, portrayed motor aphasia; and Heberden (1816), the great English clinician who described angina and gout, made several observations on aphasics.

The first attempt at localization of function in the brain came from Franz Joseph Gall (1807). The founder of phrenology, the study of relating the shape of the skull to the characteristics of its owner, he thought speech resided in the inferior frontal lobes and described six varieties of memory (e.g., for names, verbs, grammar). Bouillaud (1825) distinguished dysphasia from dysarthria and emphasized that the brain contains a special center for speech. In 1836, Marc Dax of Montpelier noted the association of a right hemiplegia with a speech disturbance; since these observations were not published until 1864 (by his son Gustave Dax), the credit for the first description of a speech center is often accorded to Broca.

In February 1861, at a meeting in Paris of the Société d'Anthropologie, Gratiolet read a paper discussing the significance of the volume of the skull and its relationship to intelligence, a concept opposed by Auburtin (who was Bouillaud's son-in-law). Broca, secretary to this society, joined in the discussion and asked Auburtin to see a patient at the Bicêtre hospital. The following week, the patient died; at post-mortem examination, there was a cavity the size of a hen's egg in the posterior third of the left second and third frontal convolutions (now Brodmann area 44). By chance, 1 month later, another patient was seen by Broca with a speech disorder, called by him aphemia (but previously termed alalia); it was Trousseau who reintroduced the word *aphasia* in 1864.

Much has been written about the early history of our knowledge regarding aphasia. British contributions have included those by Hughlings Jackson, Ogle, Broadbent, Bastian, Henry Head, and more recently, Russell Brain and Macdonald Critchley. Throughout this history, there has been debate between the localizationist diagram makers and the holistic antilocalizationists (Table 1).

Hughlings Jackson was a Yorkshireman who originally wanted to study philosophy and became a friend of Spencer. He studied medicine and became a member of the staff of the London Hospital and the National Hospital. His approach was clinical; he regarded aphasia as a psychologic disorder. Speaking is making propositions, and aphasia and agraphia were secondary to a breakdown in this ability. Jackson pointed out that a speechless man was not necessarily wordless, because he may still have emotional language and could copywrite. Although he wrote little about sensory aphasia, he considered that the right hemisphere played a part in language. It is to Jackson that we owe our concepts of automatic speech, the relationship between language and thinking; he was the first to describe the related disorders of apraxia and agnosia. Hughlings Jackson also pointed out that "to locate the damage which destroys speech and to locate speech are two different things."

The inability to write was called agraphia by Ogle (1867), and the term jargon aphasia was introduced by Broadbent (1872). Bastian (1869) was one of the first to insist that we think in words; a believer in abiogenesis and an opponent of Pasteur, he was the first of the diagram makers, describing glossokinesthetic and cheirokinesthetic centers, i.e., centers for tongue and hand movements, respectively, and areas for visual and auditory function (1880). Wernicke (1874) pointed out that aphasia was a symptom complex and classified it into: (a) motor, (b) sensory, (c) conductive, and (d) total. Ferrier (1875), from his extirpation experiments on monkeys at King's College, London, localized the auditory center to the first temporal convolution and the visual association center to the supramarginal and angular gyri. Exner (1881) described a writing center in the posterior part of the third frontal convolution. The greatest of all French neurologists, Jean Pierre Charcot (1887), working at the Salpêtrière, classified aphasia into (a) auditory, (b) visual, (c) articulatory, and (d) graphic. One of his pupils, Sigmund Freud (1891),

TABLE 1. *Aphasiology*

Localizationist	Holistic
Broca, 1861	Hughlings Jackson, 1864
Wernicke, 1874	Freud, 1891
Lichtheim, 1885	Marie, 1906
Charcot, 1889	Head, 1926
Bastian, 1898	Kinner Wilson, 1926
Henschen, 1922	Pick, 1931
Kleist, 1934	Critchley, 1970

is best known as the founder of the psychoanalytic theory but began his professional career as a neurologist; he produced his own classification of aphasia into (a) verbal, (b) asymbolic, and (c) agnostic. Asymboly was described by the German school of localizationists (Finkelnberg, 1870; Kussmaul, 1885; and Lichtheim, 1885).

Another of Charcot's pupils, Pierre Marie, reexamined the brains of Broca's two patients and disagreed with Broca's concept of localization, maintaining that all patients showed both motor and sensory aphasia together with intellectual loss. Another successor to Charcot's chair at the Salpêtrière, Dejerine (1908), born in Switzerland of French parentage, took the orthodox localizationist view.

In more recent times, this view has been upheld by Henschen and Kleist. Henschen (1920–1925), while in retirement, analyzed 1,337 published cases of aphasia, brought back Broca's word *aphemia* for aphasia, and considered that the area for hearing was centered bilaterally in Heschl's transverse gyri. Kleist (1928–1959) based his views on patients injured in World War I and produced yet another classification:

1. Word deafness (equivalent to sensory aphasia)
2. Word sound deafness (more commonly called word deafness)
3. Name deafness
4. Sentence deafness (he invented the word *paragrammatism* to describe faulty sentence formation).

There were as many neurologists opposed to as there were for the idea of a speech center. Von Monakow (1914–1928), who introduced the word *diaschisis*, pointed out that there is no such thing as aphasia but only aphasics; i.e., each one differed from the other.

The clinical psychologist Arnold Pick (1905) considered that there were two forms of agrammatism, dependent on where the lesion was: (a) temporal lobe, where there was a confusion of prefixes and suffixes (Kleist's paragrammatism), and (b) frontal lobe, resulting in telegrammatism.

Another antilocalizationist was Goldstein (1924–1948). Despite his holistic approach, he suggested that there were background processes (so that in disease there was dedifferentiation). Henry Head (1920) pointed out that, as there were no centers for walking or eating, there need not be one for speech. He devised tests for "symbolic formulation and expression" and classified aphasia into four types:

1. Verbal, in which comprehension was normal
2. Syntactic, where articles and conjunctions were dropped and there was defective formation of words, giving jargon aphasia, temporal lobe agrammatism (Pick), and paragrammatism (Kleist)
3. Nominal, where there was a loss of power to employ words as names
4. Semantic, where there was difficulty in describing a picture because of failure to recognize the significance and intention of words and phrases. (The author thought that this type was associated with a lesion of the supramarginal gyrus and could be thought of as a moderate localizationist.)

The arguments against localization of speech may be summarized as follows:

1. Patients with similar lesions do not have the same defects.
2. The same defects may be associated with different lesions, as evidenced by postmortem examination and now computerized tomography (CT) scanning.
3. Other symptoms may be associated with the lesion.
4. The type and degree of aphasia depends on premorbid personality, and there are inconsistent psychologic deviations.
5. There is difficulty in differentiating specific areas of the brain; e.g., histologically, the cellular organization may be different in the same area, whereas the same type of neurons may have different functions, depending to some extent on training.

These seem strong arguments, but the fact still remains that in 95% of aphasics, the lesion is in the dominant hemisphere and involves the lower portion of the precentral convolution. In this regard, the work of the New York anatomist, Mettler, is interesting. In 1949, he reported two cases of patients who had Broca's area removed in both the right and left sides, and yet both patients were able to speak.

Perhaps our attitude to aphasia is too rigid. Alajouanine (1956)—yet another holder of Charcot's chair—spoke of "ensembles," equivalent to the Gestalt or holistic approach. He classified the symptoms into (a) agrammatism, (b) verbal stereotypies, (c) phonetic disorder, and (d) jargon aphasia.

Kinnier Wilson (1909, 1926) pointed out that aphasia is a psychologic disorder of a physiologic action based on an anatomic lesion. Brain (1961) emphasized that much of our present confused nomenclature, e.g., subcortical motor aphasia, is due to mixing anatomic (subcortical), physiologic (motor), and psychologic (aphasia) terms.

Critchley, who has added greatly to our knowledge of the language of gesture, tactile thought in the blind, and the content of aphasic utterance, subscribes to the holistic viewpoint.

DEFINITION

Aphasia can be defined as loss of expression or understanding of language caused by brain damage. Many disciplines are involved: psychologic subspecialties, e.g., developmental, experimental, and neuropsychology; linguistic subspecialties, e.g., in neurolinguistics and psycholinguistics; neuroscientists besides the clinical neurologist, e.g., neuroanatomists, neuropathologists, and neurochemists; psychiatrists; and, above all, speech pathologists and speech therapists.

Irrespective of discipline and any favored theory, the clinician treating the aphasic patient must be concerned with observed phenomena: how to best regard and standardize them as well as measure change, be it progress or deterioration. Testing a behavioral disorder, such as aphasia, requires validation as well as standardization. "Science is measurement"; if a parameter cannot be measured, it cannot be scientifically analyzed. (It is wrong to try and fit facts with theory; any theory should explain the facts.)

There is a fundamental difference between language, the communication of ideas and feelings, and speech, the expression of these using verbal symbols, a facility that is the prerogative of man. Aphasiology necessitates the study of cerebral dominance, the development and acquisition of language by children, and polyglot aphasia, each of which can shed light on different aspects of one of the most difficult subjects in medicine. Attempts have been made to correlate the development of speech in the child with different types of aphasia, but this is fanciful. Since speech is in evolutionary terms so recently acquired, it is not surprising that it is so easily disturbed, e.g., under stress.

ASSESSMENT OF APHASIA

There are three categories of tests for aphasia. In addition to clinical testing at the bedside (*klinikos* = bed), many different standardized aphasia test batteries, as well as experimental techniques, are used to discover how the brain functions in speech and language.

CLINICAL TESTING

Conversational Speech

Conversational speech is by far the oldest method, although it is neither exacting nor complete. The broad dichotomous division between fluent and nonfluent was described by Hughlings Jackson (1868), but these terms were first proposed by Wernicke (1908).

Nonfluent Aphasia

There is, as the name suggests, a decreased ability of word output in nonfluent aphasia. Standard speed for a shorthand secretary is 120 words per minute; less than 50 words would be nonfluent, although most dysphasics have an output lower than 10 words per minute. In addition to the lower output of words, the length of phrases is less; indeed, a response to a question may be a single word.

Output limited to a single word or syllable, but with variations in meaning, as in Broca's original patient who repeated the sound "tan-tan," is termed verbal stereotypy (although Hughlings Jackson originally called it recurring utterances). With this minimal output, there is obvious increased effort; the patient struggles in an attempt to communicate with facial grimacing and body movements.

Many dysphasic patients also have poor articulation, a dysarthria that is extremely difficult for the normal speaker to imitate. This dysrhythmic and unmelodic speech, named dysprosody by Monrad-Krohn (1947), is often the feature that most distinguishes nonfluent from fluent aphasia.

The words produced by the nonfluent aphasic convey as much information as a sentence, since they consist of nouns and verbs with an absence of syntactic words, to produce one-word sentences (telegrammatism); agrammatism is the term used to include errors in plurals and verb tenses (Table 2).

TABLE 2. *Aphasia subtypes*

Parameter	Fluent	Nonfluent
Output	Increased	Decreased
Phrase length	Normal	Decreased
Melodic features	Normal	Dysprosody
Effort	Normal	Increased
Articulation	Normal	Dysarthria
Syntactic features	Paragrammatism	Agrammatism
	Circumlocution	Verbal stereotypy
	Paraphasia	
	Jargon aphasia	

Fluent Aphasia

The features of fluent aphasia are the opposite of nonfluent aphasia; the verbal output is normal or above normal, with perhaps 200 words per minute (as opposed to the normal range of 100 to 150 words per minute). There is no extra effort, and the phrases are of normal length, that is, about five words per phrase, and there is no dysprosody. Characteristic abnormalities include frequent pauses, which are often distinctive, especially when the specific meaningful word is not readily available. For this reason, the patient may give a lengthy, meaningless description, circumlocution, or periphrasis, which has been facetiously described as a "circumlocutory cycle of oratorical sonority circumscribing an atom of ideality lost in verbal profundity." A fluent aphasic substitutes a generalization for the unavailable word, for example, "them, it," so that the verbal output conveys little information (so-called "empty speech"). There may also be errors of grammatical structures, known as paragrammatism (e.g., incorrect tenses).

Paraphasia is substitution of a letter (literal paraphasia), syllable (phonemic paraphasia), or word (verbal paraphasia), which may be a nonsensical, meaningless neologism. The incomprehensible speech of the fluent dysphasic with numerous paraphasic substitutions is termed jargon aphasia.

Repetition

An extremely useful test in distinguishing different types of aphasia is repetition, that is, the ability to exactly repeat words spoken by the examiner. This can be done by repeating digits (up to seven is normal) or frequently used words, increasing complexity to multisyllabic phrases with complicated syntactic relationships. Repeating the examiner's words (echolalia) may extend to whole sentences and can be the only words the patient can say. Many echolalics will complete a phrase with the correct word and can continue nursery rhymes or poems initiated by the examiner.

Comprehension

This may a difficult test to perform at the bedside, the usual method being to give commands and ascertain the ability to carry out movements. Failure does not necessarily mean lack of understanding and the response may be misinterpreted, for example, in patients with apraxia. Another technique is to ask the patient to point to named objects, increasing the complexity of the test but, because of associated paralysis, this too is not necessarily accurate. Some patients will understand common words but not those of low frequency.

Word Finding

Word finding is another test that is abnormal in nearly all aphasic individuals. The most common, anomia, is the inability to recall names. Word finding difficulty is not pathognomonic of aphasia, as it occurs in dementia and confusion. Asking the patient to choose the correct word in a selection of names is not a test of naming but of comprehension, and it is preferable to give some prompting (cues).

There are eight ways of testing word finding:

1. A defect in word production or an inability to retrieve the correct word
2. Naming objects seen visually
3. Naming objects felt
4. Naming sounds heard
5. Naming objects related to the illness
6. Naming objects from a description of their use
7. Response to prompting
8. Producing words in a given category (e.g., animals).

Reading

The loss of the ability to read, dyslexia, is easily tested (e.g., by giving the patient a newspaper and asking the meaning of a story). There are those who can read well but do not understand what they have read; it is this inability that signifies alexia. Another test is to ask the patient to recognize the word that the examiner spells out, which will distinguish between occipital alexia (where they can do this test) and parietotemporal alexia (when they cannot).

There are several varieties of difficulty with writing, dysgraphia, but this subdivision is not necessarily of clinical use. The patient may fail to write even his own name, but this is not sufficient for the diagnosis. Testing should include sentences, dictation, and commenting (for example, describing their job).

Further Tests

All these clinical tests can be performed in only a few minutes. Since they can be misleading, however, more formal tests are required, which include those of Wepman, Eisenson, Schuell, and Porch, the Boston, and the Western. Finally, there are research procedures that are used by either linguists, psychologists, or phonologists (Table 3). The relationship of these tests to intelligence is another debate, as is the relationship of aphasia to cerebral dominance.

TABLE 3. *Aphasiology: Standardized tests*

Test	Diagnosis	Therapy	Research
Eisenson, 1954	+	+	−
Schuell, 1957	++	++	+
NSCTA, 1960	++	−	++
Wepman, 1961	++	+	+
Porch (PICA), 1967	−	++	−
Taylor (FCP), 1968	−	++	−
Boston (BDAE), 1972	++	−	+

There is agreement that cerebral dominance for language exists, and that fluent dysphasia is due to a more posterior lesion (Wernicke's area) than nonfluent dysphasia (Broca's area). McFie and others attempted to take this further by indicating that the right hemisphere was more concerned with spatial concepts. Normal speech has a wide range, and premorbid ability may be more important than site, size, or progress of the responsible lesion.

EPIDEMIOLOGY

The vast majority of aphasic patients have had a stroke; since approximately 30% of stroke patients have aphasia, the annual incidence of aphasia is 1 in 200. Most stroke aphasias are nonfluent, in the proportion of 2:1 against fluent aphasias; the younger the patient, the higher this ratio becomes.

One-fourth of patients will make a complete recovery, usually within 3 months, whereas one-fourth will still be severely affected at the end of 1 year, after which little improvement is to be expected. Initial severity is highly predictive of eventual outcome.

There are two stages in recovery in stroke. In the first, which takes up to 3 weeks, there is absorption of edema. The explanation of the second stage, which can be more than 1 year, is more difficult. Theories have included axonal regrowth, collateral sprouting (both of which are unlikely in man), diaschisis, denervation hypersensitivity, and right hemisphere substitution.

One great advance in the past decade has been the CT scanner, which demonstrates the size of the lesion within minutes. Succeeding chapters in this volume prove that the relationship between the size of lesion and type of aphasia is not as great as was thought before the advent of newer neuroimaging techniques.

FURTHER READING

1. Benson, D. F. (1979): *Aphasia, Alexia and Agraphia*. Churchill Livingstone, New York.
2. Critchley, M. (1970): *Aphasiology, and Other Aspects of Language*. Arnold, London.
3. Espir, M. M. E., and Rose, F. C. (1983): *The Basic Neurology of Speech and Language*, third edition. Blackwell Scientific, Oxford.

Advances in Neurology, Vol. 42: Progress in Aphasiology, edited by F. C. Rose.
Raven Press, New York © 1984.

Aphasiology: Present Status and Trends

Macdonald Critchley

National Hospital for Nervous Diseases, Queen Square, London WC1 3BG, England

It was only 200 years ago that physicians realized that speech impairment is the result of a disorder of the brain and not a palsy of the tongue. The dawn of aphasiology broke with the unorthodox ideas of Gall, adopted and made respectable by such pioneers in France as Bouillaud, the all-powerful dean of the faculty, his son-in-law Auburtin, Andral, Belhomme, Durand-Fardel, Trousseau, and Dax, culminating in the chance findings of Broca in 1861.

Since then, the pace of research into the problems of language and language pathology has been rapid. As one might expect, the emerging opinions were highly controversial; F. Lhermitte describes how Pierre Marie and Dejerine almost came to blows.

Throughout the decades, there has been perpetual discord not only between localizers and nonlocalizers but also within the ranks of the localizationists themselves. Incessant dissatisfaction also attended all attempts to reach a logical classification of the many clinical variants of aphasia. Even today, this question remains unsolved.

Forty or fifty years ago, while I was bemoaning the lack of interest on the part of professional linguists in the problem of aphasia, I predicted that cooperation in this field might be highly rewarding. Since then, we have witnessed a liaison with related disciplines that has resulted in the birth and development of psycholinguistics. The product of that relationship has brought about a considerable expansion in our knowledge of the phenomenology of aphasia.

The other and more recent event has been the invention of the computerized axial tomography (CAT) scan. In a few minutes, a technician can now demonstrate the site of the lesion in an aphasic patient, something that previously taxed all the skill and finesse of an experienced diagnostician.

One unfortunate outcome of these two important occurrences is that fewer neurologists are now dedicating themselves to a serious study of aphasia. This is most regrettable, for it is all too obvious that psycholinguistics alone is not enough. As F. L. Lucas said:

> A research student may turn his life into a concentration camp; he may amass in his own field a staggering erudition; but he cannot write. And where the words are so muddled, I suspect that the mind is muddled too.

The cooperation of the disciplined, up-to-date neuroscientist is still needed. Furthermore, in a way, the brain scan alone has done an actual disservice to neurology. It has merely demonstrated the emplacement within the anfranctuosities of the brain of a clump of dead cells. Dead cells, however, have no function. As Hughlings Jackson said, they are no more than "dirt in the brain"; they represent merely the hole in the doughnut. How then do we explain the nature of the fragmentary speech remnants of our patients? Why are some of them relatively fluent but barely understandable? Why are others laconic, being restricted to a solitary repetitious word or phrase? And what ordains the structure of the verbal stereotypy? Why does this patient say nothing but "yes" and that one "no," while the third patient is limited to the unlikely remark, such as "ace of spades"? T. Alajouanine described the recurring utterance as "an insignificant spar remaining from the shipwreck of speech." To Jackson, it represented a "stillborn proposition." An uncontrolled activity of the brain tissues adjacent to the dead cells may play a role, as indeed may the intact nondominant hemisphere. Such matters remain mysterious and puzzling. The novelist Leslie Thomas got the idea when he wrote *Virgin Soldiers:*

> The poor sod is incapable of getting the next words out. He knows what it should be—he knows all right—but he can't say it. So he's stuck there. Like a bleeding goldfish.

Before turning our attention to an analysis of speech remnants, the linguistic rubble of aphasia, let us bear in mind that even in normal circumstances, speech as a means of communication is far from ideal. No wonder it is so vulnerable, and that the picture of aphasia is so complicated.

Language—the specific endowment of *Homo sapiens*—is a slowly built-in aspect of the Ego comprising personality and cognition. No two persons possess an identical treasury of words. The idiolect is as specific as the fingerprint.

As units of meaning, words are seriously inadequate. They are imprecise and loaded with mental and emotional associations and complex overtones. Often they cannot be satisfactorily translated from one language to another. How fickle, mischievous, potentially dangerous they may be. They are deadly weapons of propaganda, the bread and butter of the lawyer and the sales promoter.

The first of several perplexing matters in aphasiology is classification, a subject that aroused the sarcasm and wit of Hughlings Jackson. Most will surely agree that no wholly satisfactory classification of the aphasias exists. Eponyms are parochial, inexact, and are best discarded, as are terms like central aphasia, the conduction aphasias, both afferent and efferent, and others. We are invited to accept at least a dozen varieties of dyslexia, as well as distinctions between coding, encoding, decoding, and transcoding. We are reminded of entomologists who recognize 5,200 varieties of what ordinary people call "flies." Have we so soon forgotten what Gowers pointed out, namely, that nature is prone to ignore our divisions and to blend that which we distinguish? No wonder that some of our wisest aphasiologists shun all attempts to classify, and, like Jackson, merely speak of disorders of expression or, simply, the aphasias.

The second matter concerns what has been called the law of language specificity. It is axiomatic that no two aphasic subjects are identical. This statement calls for closer study. Years ago, neurologists were discussing what was called "the four factors of the insanities," something we now would call highest level nervous dysfunction, including, of course, the aphasias. The first three factors comprised the site of the lesion, its size, and its rate of growth. The fourth was the type of brain as it was throughout the premorbid period. This may be the most significant agent of all in determining the pattern of the speech debris and also the prognosis. This aspect has been sadly neglected.

An individual's word bank (the vogue term, I believe, is logogen) reflects the size of his vocabularies, of which there are two: the one that is available, and the smaller one that is in constant use. These reflect the intellectual and, more particularly, the educational status. Bilingualism and polyglottism play an important role here. Most tenuous of all is that sensitive appreciation of the aesthetic properties of the shape and sound of words. Some persons are enslaved by the sheer beauty of words, both written and spoken, scrupulously selecting and matching them as though they were precious stones. Here are the poets, the stylists in prose, the spellbinding orators. Intrigued by the euphony and the allusive properties of their medium, they are fortunate indeed, but only so long as this endowment is intact. I fear, however, that such an exquisite sensitivity may prove to be a handicap when injury or disease supervenes. This subject should be studied in depth by neurologists with access to the premorbid circumstances of their patients. The results might prove depressing. I cannot forget the poet Baudelaire, whose aphasia was massive, limiting him to the coarse and truncated interjection *"Cré nom."* His friend Nadar wrote, after visiting him in the hospital:

> Those two solitary words that would escape those lips from which had sprung immortal lamentations. Oh the horror of that distressful and appalling cruelty of Him who had destroyed the speech of that gem-setter of rubies—Baudelaire, just as He had deprived Beethoven of his hearing and Michelangelo of his sight!

To date, most of our evidence is anecdotal, and I remind you of the severity of the aphasia of the writer and lexicographer H. L. Menken. The last days of Lenin, whose oratory changed the face of the world and toppled empires, were marked by the recurrent utterance *"chort,"* which means devil.

The third unsolved problem regards the thinking of our aphasic patients. How far does an impairment of speech connote an impairment of intelligence? Although this subject has been debated for more than a century, no satisfactory answer has yet emerged. Aphasiologists have frankly hedged in their proclamations when indeed they have not brushed the subject under the carpet. Does the severity of the speech loss correspond with the seriousness of the affront to the processes of thought? When psychologists and physicians are in doubt, they should not overlook the masters of literature, for professional writers are often shrewder and more accurate observers of the human comedy than we. Zola knew about aphasia, and he described Madame Raquin's:

> Walled-in intelligence, still alive yet imprisoned in dead flesh . . . she could see, hear, and doubtless she could reason quite clearly. Yet she had no movement or speech to express her thoughts to the outside world. Maybe her thoughts choked her. . . . Her mind was like one of those people who are, by some mischance, buried alive and who wake up in the middle of the night with five or six feet of earth on top of them.

Perhaps that was an extreme example, and milder aphasics may seem normal in their mentation. We cannot take too seriously the comments of those patients who have become cured. In retrospect, they often minimize any change in their intellectual powers during their period of illness. Such remarks are not wholly credible; as clinicians realize, the common unawareness or forgetfulness of past handicaps that are cerebral in origin minimize the defects they overcame.

Thus far, the comments of neurologists and psychologists have been cautious, evasive, even quibbling in character. What we do not realize is that at any moment, the hair-splitting would be halted when suddenly confronted by the practical problem of an aphasic who wants to make a will, alter an existing will, or continue to attend to his intricate business affairs. What down-to-earth advice can we, as philosophers of language, put before the Courts of Law in such cases, advice that would stand up to the cold logic of the legal profession as opposed to our less demanding colleagues and students? In such circumstances, how much weight would a Judge be seriously expected to place on the jargon and indecisiveness, or perhaps the overconfidence, of the so-called expert witness? Very little, I can assure you, and rightly so.

This chapter has merely skimmed the surface of a deep and unexplored pool. In conclusion, I realize I have been guilty of all the faults a seventeenth century Law Lord had detected in an official sermon:

> The Bishop was learned, but he did play with his Text as a Jack-an-apes does who takes up one thing and tosses and plays with it, and then he takes up another and plays a little with it. Here's a pretty thing, and there's a pretty thing.

Advances in Neurology, Vol. 42: Progress in Aphasiology, edited by F. C. Rose.
Raven Press, New York © 1984.

The Natural History of Aphasia

Ivar Reinvang

Sunnaas Sykehus, 1450 Nesoddtangen, Norway

The natural history of a phenomenon or disease concerns its rate of occurrence, associated phenomena, and variations exhibited. When a disease is studied, the alterations with time are of particular interest, especially the rate and extent of spontaneous recovery. It has been pointed out (44) that knowledge of the natural course of recovery is a prerequisite for determining the efficacy of treatment, so that a study of natural history is undertaken usually to form a basis for testing specific hypotheses with experimental methods. A concern with natural history thus may reflect the highly imperfect state of our knowledge of aphasia, but includes inherently complex phenomena that can be studied appropriately only in a biologically relevant context. The study of a phenomenon in a "natural" condition, therefore, is not inherently inferior to an experimental study.

The Nature of Language

With the dominating position of structural and transformational linguistics in the study of language in the last decades comes the view that a special logical structure is characteristic of human language. A disturbance of this structure, as revealed in faulty syntactic or semantic operations with language, is characteristic of aphasia and defines it as a linguistic disturbance (9). This replaces or changes the emphasis of the older view that aphasia is a defect in the "instrumentalities" of language (15), i.e., the interface of abstract (inner) language with sensory and motor schemata. (A schema is a complex information structure, which is triggered as a unit by specific stimuli.) Both these views are structuralistic in viewing language (and aphasia) as a property of the information-processing capacities of specialized areas of the brain.

The structuralist emphasis has determined what phenomena should count as aphasic, i.e., among disorders of communication, only those disturbances that show an impairment in the structure of language. It has also determined the context in which aphasia is studied by underplaying or disregarding the communicative interchange of information that is the normal context of language acts.

Modules of the Communication Process

Among the broad spectrum of neurologically based disturbances of communication, the demarcation lines between sensorimotor disturbances, language disturbances, and disturbances of cognition are conceptually clear; in clinical groups, however, the disorders overlap. The language disturbance that is not the exclusive or even major cause of communicative malfunction is still a clinical problem. Although we may be well advised not to speak of the disorder of communication in diffuse afflictions of the brain as "aphasia," a more open attitude to comparative study of language behavior in different neurologic diseases would be fruitful. An increased interest in language behavior in aging and dementia as well as in closed head injury (CHI) has been recently documented (27,37).

INCIDENCE OF APHASIA

According to Broman et al. (6), each year 0.6% of the population of Gothenburg, Sweden, become aphasic. Among the aphasics, 85% are stroke (CVA) patients, a figure based on hospital admissions. The Department of Neurology at the Sahlgren Hospital of Gothenburg is well suited for epidemiologic studies, because it serves a well-defined and representative population; practically all acute cases are admitted.

Diagnosis

With CVA, the incidence of aphasia after the first stroke was given as 21% by Brust et al. (8) and 33% by Marquardsen (33). The discrepancy probably reflects difficulties with setting criteria for the presence of aphasia in acute stroke.

Penetrating head injuries and aphasia have been studied in victims of wartime injuries. The development in weapons technology makes comparisons of epidemiologic data between different major wars difficult. Russell and Espir (43) gave the incidence of aphasia from World War II as 31% in penetrating injuries; Taylor and Jablon (53) reported 22% with speech abnormalities among casualties of the Korean war; and Mohr et al. (36) noted the incidence in casualties from Vietnam as 24%.

Language disturbances in CHI are receiving increasing attention. On the basis of aphasia testing of a series of consecutively admitted patients, Levin et al. (28) found a high incidence of language deficit. Clinical examination concluded that 16% of patients showed signs of aphasia, whereas testing showed that close to 50% had clinical or subclinical deficits. In survivors of CHI who are referred for rehabilitation, Sarno (45) found 32% with classic symptoms of aphasia, but another 30% had more subtle verbal deficits on testing.

Age

There is no strong evidence that the incidence of aphasia varies with age. In children with acquired aphasia of mixed origin, Guttmann (17) and Hécaen (19) both considered that the same types of lesions that produce aphasia in adults do so in children. In their critical review of the literature, Satz and Bullard-Bates (50) concluded: "The risk of aphasia or language impairment is approximately the same in right-handed children and adults if the left hemisphere is damaged" (p. 421).

Sex

Many reported populations of aphasics show a disproportionately high incidence of males, which has led to speculation about differences in brain organization between males and females (see ref. 34 for review). Kertesz and Sheppard (25) suggested that the observed disproportion can be explained by variations in age-specific incidence of stroke. Men between the ages of 50 and 60 years have a considerably higher risk of stroke than do women, whereas this is not true for either younger or older individuals. These differences are reflected in the aphasic population, and selection criteria favoring middle-aged individuals tend to increase the proportion of males.

Handedness

Studies of left-handed individuals show conflicting results, since these subjects probably are a mixed group within which those with a family history of left handedness comprise a distinctive subgroup with evidence of less extreme cerebral lateralization of function than right-handed people (21). Russell and Espir (43), in their series of penetrating head injuries, gave the incidence of aphasia with lateralized injury as 37% for right handers and 27% for left handers, in contrast to other reports (52), which concluded that aphasia after lateralized injuries is more frequent in left handers. The results are sensitive to sampling variations and criteria of handedness, and the matter remains unresolved. From the hypothesis of higher degree of language representation in the right hemisphere for left handers, it follows that the risk of aphasia with right hemisphere injuries is higher in left handers; this is confirmed by Russell and Espir (43), who gave the incidence as 17%, compared to 1% in right handers.

TYPE AND SEVERITY OF APHASIA

Aphasia varies in both type and severity, and several classification systems have been proposed to systematize this variation (22). The most accepted classification system is based on fluency of speech and on severity of deficit in comprehension and repetition.

In CVA, aphasics with reduced fluency of speech are more common than those who are fluent. According to Brust et al. (8), 68% are nonfluent, and 32% are fluent in the acute stage after stroke. A severe aphasia with nonfluent speech is a sign of severe neurologic injury, with a corresponding rise in morbidity risk.

Russell and Espir (43) report aphasias with nonfluent speech to be the most common types after penetrating head injury, with Broca's (motor) aphasia accounting for 12% of cases with aphasia. In CHI, forms of aphasia with preserved fluency of speech are the most common, anomia being the most frequent aphasic symptom. While there is no doubt that the language disturbance in some cases is connected with a general reduction in neuropsychologic function, it is also clear that in many cases [about 30% in the study by Levin et al. (29)], deficit is behaviorally "focal."

TABLE 1. *Factors influencing incidence or type of aphasia*[a]

Factor	Incidence	Type/severity
Diagnosis	+	+
Age	−	+
Sex	−	−
Handedness	(+)	(+)

[a]+, Definite relationship between factors; −, lack of relationship; ( ), uncertainty of the nature of the relationship (+ or − is added if any indications can be found).

A systematic variation of fluency with age has been reported by Alajouanine and Lhermitte (1), Obler et al. (38), and Brown (7). Aphasias with preserved fluency are uncommon in children and relatively less frequent in younger than in older adults. Both in American and other populations of aphasics, as reviewed by Obler and Albert (37), the mean age of Wernicke's aphasia is higher than that of Broca's, which we have confirmed in Norwegian aphasics (41). There is no strong evidence that type of aphasia is related to handedness or sex, but it may be less severe in left handers than right-handers with left hemisphere lesions (20). A relationship between sex and severity or aphasia type was not found by Kertesz and Sheppard (25) or in the Norwegian aphasia population.

A further complexity only briefly touched upon is the possibility of interactions between factors. Thus, for example, males of a certain age and diagnosis may have an elevated incidence of aphasia. Since the possibilities are so many, any specific combination of factors is only likely to be checked if it is crucial to the testing of specific hypotheses (Table 1).

RECOVERY

What is the natural context for the evolution of language behavior? The anecdotal account of the misguided experiment by the medieval emperor Frederik II, who deprived a group of infants of language stimulation from birth to observe what language they would "naturally" develop, is pertinent to the discussion of recovery from aphasia. Although it is highly desirable to study untreated control groups, it is important to specify the condition of "untreated" as distinct from "unstimulated." Reinvang and Engvik (42) have suggested that the condition of untreated is satisfied even when there is evidence of supportive social environment and of insight into the aphasic condition by persons in this environment who play an active part in facilitating communicative interchange. An overview of published studies with untreated groups is given in Table 2. Limiting further discussion to data from untreated groups is unnecessary when studies indicate that there is no effect of treatment on the variable in question.

TABLE 2. *Published studies of untreated aphasiacs and follow-up data*

Reference	No. of subjects	Comparison with treated
Vignolo (54)	27	Yes, significant effect
Basso et al. (2)	94	Yes, significant effect
Basso et al. (3)	119	Yes, significant effect
Kertesz and McCabe (23)	83	Yes, no effect
Lomas and Kertesz (31)	31	No
Sarno and Levita (46)	14	No
Sarno et al. (49)	8	Yes, no effect
Culton (10)	21	No
Brust et al. (8)	177	No
Hagen (18)	10	Yes, significant effect
Levita (30)	18	Yes, no effect
David et al. (12)	78	Yes, no effect[a]

[a]In this study, the control group is simulated by nonprofessional volunteers.

Rate of Recovery

Some acutely aphasic individuals recover completely; in the rest, an improvement usually is observed. The rate of complete recovery in survivors of stroke can be calculated as 25% on the basis of data given by Brust et al. (8) and was reported as 21% by Kertesz and McCabe (23). Complete recovery after acute injuries usually takes place in the first 8 to 12 weeks. A cardinal feature of the improvement over time in both recovered and unrecovered patients is that it shows a decelerating rate. Estimates of the length of the improvement period vary with the criteria used. From the data of Basso et al. (Tables 5 and 6 in ref. 3), few untreated aphasics show significant improvement beyond 6 months; the authors used a dichotomous scale of improved versus not improved. When a continuum of graded test scores was used, Kertesz and McCabe (23) found improvement up to 1 year after onset in both treated and untreated patients. From the data of Brust et al. (8), the proportion of moderate or severe cases at the end of a 3-month follow-up of surviving aphasics can be calculated as 36%. Kertesz and McCabe (23) found, at the end of 1 year, that 25% remain severe, as defined by scoring below the 25th percentile on the aphasia test.

Recovery Pattern

In considering aphasia in the time perspective, most authors have concentrated on the question of rate of recovery, but the change in the characteristic patterns of deficit in aphasic syndromes was discussed by Leischner (26) and stressed by Kertesz (22; and *this volume*). The currently used classification schematas for aphasia are detailed, counting at least nine major syndromes and additional rare types. These syndromes may not be independent but interrelated, as shown by the regular change of one into another in the course of recovery. Mohr et al. (35) have suggested that global and Broca's aphasia is one syndrome with a common pathologic substrate but different levels of severity. The same assertion could be made for conduction and Wernicke's aphasia, since the former may evolve into the latter (5,40).

Geschwind (13) found anomic aphasia and transcortical sensory aphasia closely related in respect to both symptomatology and pathology. Anomic aphasia is a term sometimes used to describe a slight aphasic disturbance having evolved from various other aphasic syndromes (16). Both Kertesz and McCabe (23) and Reinvang and Engvik (40,42) report repeated classifications of patients studied over time. The latter conclude that stability of syndromes is present in a statistical sense, but some aphasia syndromes clearly are related. Lomas and Kertesz (31) found the best recovery of comprehension in untreated patients, while others found it in treated cases (39,48).

Summary

The following general conclusions can be drawn: (a) about 20 to 25% of acute stroke cases with aphasia recover fully and spontaneously; (b) improvement takes place at a decelerating rate over a time period of about 1 year; (c) comprehension improves more than speech; and (d) aphasia syndromes show stability over time, although decreasing severity sometimes is associated with a change in classification. The question of prognosis is taken in this context to mean that knowledge of factors (in addition to the patient being aphasic) would lead to modification of any of the above-mentioned points.

PROGNOSTIC FACTORS

The percentage of complete recoveries seems higher in penetrating head injuries than in strokes. In Table 3, the data from the two largest reported samples of stroke patients (8,23) are compared with data from the two largest samples of head injuries (36,43). The chi-square value of 17.10 ($p<0.001$) shows a significant relationship. The same patterns of deficit are found in strokes and head injuries, and there are no indications of differences in the course of recovery (23,36).

Levin et al. (29) found full recovery in nine of 21 initially aphasic patients with CHI, but the numbers are too small for statistical inferences.

TABLE 3. *Complete recovery in head injuries and stroke*

Diagnosis	Unrecovered	Recovered
Head injury	243	161
Stroke	172	53

Age

The relationship between age and prognosis in adults is a weak one, giving a statistically significant result in some studies but not in others (11,23,40,46). The prognosis is better in children than in adults, although the presence of inferior scholastic achievement in children with a history of aphasia should temper optimism (1).

Sex and Handedness

There is no strong evidence for differential prognosis or pattern of recovery in males and females. Reinvang (40) found no influence of sex on prognosis; this is in accordance with findings by Kertesz and McCabe (23). Better prognosis in left handers is reported by Subirana (52) and Gloning et al. (14). Luria (32) reports that even right handers with left handedness among close relatives recover better than right handers without such a family history.

Aphasia Type, Severity, and Associated Symptoms

The published reports are consistent with the notion that improvement over time is a constant but diminishing addition to the initial state (3,40). Since performance profile and severity of language deficit are confounded in present classification systems, the existing reports on varying prognoses for different aphasia syndromes may support the statement that outcome is a function of initial severity. Present reports are confusing. For example, Kertesz and McCabe (23) report a more favorable prognosis in Broca's aphasia; Mohr et al. (36) agree with this in their study of penetrating injuries. On the other hand, Brust et al. (8) report a favorable outcome in fluent aphasics, while Basso et al. (3) find no difference between fluent and nonfluent syndromes.

Even when initial severity is controlled, it is still true that some aphasics make virtually no improvement, regardless of treatment program. The issue of prognosis in the very severe (i.e., global) aphasics has been a source of controversy. Sarno et al. (49) reported a poor prognosis despite treatment; poor outcome also was found by Kertesz and McCabe (23). Smith et al. (51) brought another aspect into the discussion by reporting that the presence of associated symptoms influenced the recovery rate negatively. A negative influence of presence of hemiparesis on recovery is reported by Brust et al. (8) and can also be inferred from Mohr et al. (36). From the latter study, it appears that hemiparesis stabilizes before aphasia. Reinvang (40) finds that nonverbal test results are correlated with extent of recovery when initial severity of defect is controlled; but the author finds no influence of hemiparesis. Global aphasics usually have large lesions (24), with a high incidence of hemiparesis and nonverbal neuropsychologic disorders. When the distinction is made between global aphasics with severe associated symptoms and "alert" global aphasics, Sarno and Levita (48) find limited recovery of language function in the latter group.

TABLE 4. *Factors influencing recovery*[a]

Prognostic factor	Recovery rate	Recovery pattern
Time	+	−
Diagnosis	+	(−)
Age	(+)	( )
Sex	(−)	(−)
Handedness	(+)	( )
Aphasia type/severity	+	(+)
Associated symptoms	+	(−)
Treatment	(+)	−

[a]For explanation of symbols, see footnote to Table 1.

There are few suggestions of different recovery curves for different aphasia types. An interesting finding by Sarno and Levita (47) is that fluent aphasics conform to the expected pattern of most rapid recovery in the first 6 months after stroke, whereas nonfluent aphasics recover more than fluent aphasics in the 6 to 12 month period.

Treatment

The difficult issue of effect of treatment is unresolved. The intricacies of defining "treatment" and "no treatment" are considerable, as are the practical difficulties of designing studies and the ethical difficulties of performing them (4).

A case can be made for the effect of treatment on the degree of improvement in language behavior for chronic aphasics (see Table 2), but there is no evidence that functional treatment can increase the proportion of cases with complete recovery or change the time course or overall pattern of the recovery process.

Summary

The discussion on recovery can be summarized as in Table 4. Again, the question of interaction of factors has only briefly been discussed, but the most important one is the interaction of treatment with time since injury, aphasia severity, aphasia type, and associated symptoms.

CONCLUSION: THE FIXEDNESS OF NATURE

An important lesson to be learned from the study of the natural history of recovery is that the state of the nervous system does not stabilize for a considerable time after injury, and that presently known intervention methods interact with underlying time-dependent processes. The lack of significant age effects indicates that these processes are not closely dependent on normal age-related biologic changes but are special mechanisms responding to injury. Conceptually, the problems of research in this area are similar to those in developmental biology, and a fruitful interdisciplinary exchange might take place at the level of conceptual and methodologic models.

REFERENCES

1. Alajouanine, T., and Lhermitte, F. (1965): Acquired aphasia in children, *Brain*, 88:653–662.
2. Basso, A., Faglioni, P., and Vignolo, L. A. (1975): Etude controllée de la rééducation du langage dans l'aphasie: Comparaison entre aphasiques traités et non-traités. *Rev. Neurol.*, 131:607–614.
3. Basso, A., Capitani, E., and Vignolo, L. A. (1979): Influence of rehabilitation on language skills in aphasia patients. A controlled study. *Arch. Neurol.*, 36:190–196.
4. Benson, D. F. (1979): Editorial: Aphasia rehabilitation. *Arch. Neurol.*, 36:187–189.
5. Benson, D. F., Sheremata, W. A., Buchard, R., Segarra, J., Price, D., and Geschwind, N. (1973): Conduction aphasia. A clinicopathological study. *Arch. Neurol.*, 28:339–346.
6. Broman, T., Lindholm, A., and Melin, B. (1967): Rehabilitering av afasipasienter. *Läkartidningen*, 64:4595–4600.
7. Brown, J. W. (1979): Language representation in the brain. In: *Neurobiology of Social Communication in Primates*, edited by H. Steklis and M. Raleigh. Academic Press, New York.
8. Brust, J. C. M., Schafer, S., Richter, R., and Brunn, B. (1976): Aphasia in acute stroke. *Stroke*, 7:167–174.
9. Caramazza, A., and Berndt, R. S. (1978): Semantic and syntactic processes in aphasia: A review of the literature. *Psychol. Bull.*, 85:898–918.
10. Culton, G. L. (1969): Spontaneous recovery from aphasia. *J. Speech Hear. Res.*, 12:825–832.
11. Culton, G. (1971): Reaction to age as a factor in chronic aphasia in stroke patients. *J. Speech Hear. Disord.*, 36:563–564.
12. David, R., Enderby, P., and Bainton, D. (1981): Treatment of acquired aphasia: Speech therapy and volunteer attention compared. Paper presented at 4th International Neuropsychological Society, Bergen, Norway.
13. Geschwind, N. (1965): Disconnection syndromes in animals and man. *Brain*, 88:234–294; 585–644.
14. Gloning, I., Gloning, K., Haub, G., and Quatember, R. (1969): Comparison of verbal behavior in right-handed and non-right handed patients with anatomically verified lesions of one hemisphere. *Cortex*, 5:43–52.
15. Goldstein, K. (1948): *Language and Language Disturbances*. Grune & Stratton, New York.
16. Goodglass, H., and Kaplan, E. (1972): *The Assessment of Aphasia*. Lea & Febiger, Philadelphia.
17. Guttmann, E. (1942): Aphasia in children. *Brain*, 65:205–219.
18. Hagen, C. (1973): Communication abilities in hemiplegia: Effect of speech therapy. *Arch. Phys. Med. Rehabil.*, 54:454–463.
19. Hécaen, H. (1976): Acquired aphasia in children and the ontogenesis of hemispheric functional specialization. *Brain Lang.*, 3:114–134.
20. Hécaen, H., and de Ajuriaguerra, J. (1964): *Left Handedness: Manual Superiority and Cerebral Dominance*. Grune & Stratton, New York.
21. Hécaen, H., and Sauguet, J. (1971): Cerebral dominance in left-handed subjects. *Cortex*, 7:19–48.
22. Kertesz, A. (1979): *Aphasia and Associated Disorders*. Grune & Stratton, New York.
23. Kertesz, A., and McCabe, P. (1977): Recovery patterns and prognosis in aphasia. *Brain*, 100:1–18.
24. Kertesz, A., Harlock, W., and Coates, R. (1979): Computer tomographic localization, lesion size, and prognosis in aphasia and non-verbal impairment. *Brain Lang.*, 8:34–50.
25. Kertesz, A., and Sheppard, A. (1981): The epidemiology of aphasic and cognitive impairment in stroke. *Brain*, 104:117–128.
26. Leischner, A. (1972): Über den Verlauf und die Einteilung der aphasischen Syndrome. *Arch. Psychiatr. Nervenkr.*, 216:219–231.
27. Levin, H. S. (1982): Aphasia in closed head injury. In: *Acquired Aphasia*, edited by M. T. Sarno, Academic Press, New York.
28. Levin, H. S., Grossman, R. G., and Kelly, P. S. (1976): Aphasic disorder in patients with closed head injury. *J. Neurol. Neurosurg. Psychiatry*, 39:1062–1070.
29. Levin, H. S., Grossman, R. G., Sarwar, M., and Meyers, C. A. (1981): Linguistic recovery after closed head injury. *Brain Lang.*, 12:360–374.

30. Levita, E. (1978): Effects of speech therapy on aphasics' responses to the Functional Communication Profile. *Percept. Mot. Skills*, 47:151–154.
31. Lomas, J., and Kertesz, A. (1978): Patterns of spontaneous recovery in aphasic groups: A study of adult stroke patients. *Brain Lang.*, 5:388–401.
32. Luria, A. R. (1970): *Traumatic Aphasia*. Monton, The Hague.
33. Marquardsen, J. (1969): *The Natural History of Acute Cerebrovascular Disease*. Munksgaard, Copenhagen.
34. McGlone, J. (1980): Sex differences in cerebral asymmetry: A critical survey. *Behav. Brain Sci.*, 3:215–263.
35. Mohr, J. P., Pessin, M., Finkelstein, S., Funkenstein, H., Duncan, G., and Davis, K. (1978): Broca aphasia. Pathological and clinical aspects. *Neurology*, 28:311–324.
36. Mohr, J. P., Weiss, G. H., Caveness, W. F., Dillon, J., Kistler, J., Meirowsky, A., and Rish, B. (1980): Language and motor disorders after penetrating head injury in Viet Nam. *Neurology*, 30:1273–1279.
37. Obler, L. K., and Albert, M. L. (1982): Language in the elderly aphasic and in the dementing patient. In: *Acquired Aphasia*, edited by M. T. Sarno. Academic Press, New York.
38. Obler, L. K., Albert, M. L., Goodglass, H., and Benson, D. F. (1978): Aphasia type and aging. *Brain Lang.*, 6:318–322.
39. Prins, R., Snow, C., and Wagenaar, E. (1978): Recovery from aphasia: Spontaneous speech versus language comprehension. *Brain Lang.*, 5:192–211.
40. Reinvang, I. (1981): Patterns of restitution in aphasia. Paper presented at the 4th International Neuropsychological Society, Bergen, Norway.
41. Reinvang, I. (1983): *Aphasia and Brain Organization*. University of Oslo, Oslo.
42. Reinvang, I., and Engvik, H. (1980): Language recovery in aphasia from 3 to 6 months after stroke. In: *Aphasia, Assessment and Treatment*, edited by M. T. Sarno and O. Höök. Almqvist & Wiksell, Stockholm.
43. Russell, W. R., and Espir, M. L. E. (1961): *Traumatic Aphasia*. Oxford University Press, London.
44. Sarno, M. T. (1976): The status of research in recovery from aphasia. In: *Recovery in Aphasics*, edited by Y. Lebrun and R. Hoops. Swets and Zeitlinger, Amsterdam.
45. Sarno, M. T. (1980): The nature of verbal impairment after closed head injury. *J. Nerv. Ment. Dis.*, 168:685–692.
46. Sarno, M. T., and Levita, E. (1971): Natural course of recovery in severe aphasia. *Arch. Phys. Med. Rehabil.*, 52:175–179.
47. Sarno, M. T., and Levita, E. (1979): Recovery in treated aphasia in the first year post-stroke. *Stroke*, 10:663–670.
48. Sarno, M. T., and Levita, E. (1981): Some observations on the nature of recovery in global aphasia. *Brain Lang.*, 13:1–12.
49. Sarno, M. T., Silverman, M., and Sands, E. (1970): Speech therapy and recovery in severe aphasia. *J. Speech Hear. Res.*, 13:607–623.
50. Satz, P., and Bullard-Bates, C. (1982): Acquired aphasia in children. In: *Acquired Aphasia*, edited by M. T. Sarno. Academic Press, New York.
51. Smith, A., Champoux, R., Levi, J., London, R., and Muraski, A. (1972): *Diagnosis, Intelligence and Rehabilitation of Chronic Aphasics*. University of Michigan, Ann Arbor.
52. Subirana, A. (1969): Handedness and cerebral dominance. In: *Handbook of Clinical Neurology, Vol. 4*, edited by P. Vinken and G. Bruyn. Elsevier, New York.
53. Taylor, A. R., and Jablon, S. (1970): *Posttraumatic Symptoms in Head Injured Veterans of the Korean Campaign*. Report to the National Institute of Neurological Diseases and Stroke.
54. Vignolo, L. A. (1964): Evolution of aphasia and language rehabilitation: A retrospective exploratory study. *Cortex*, 1:344–367.

Advances in Neurology, Vol. 42: Progress in Aphasiology, edited by F. C. Rose.
Raven Press, New York © 1984.

Recovery from Aphasia

Andrew Kertesz

Department of Clinical Neurological Sciences, University of Western Ontario, St. Joseph's Hospital, London, Ontario, Canada N6A 4V2

Recovery from aphasia has interested clinicians mainly in the rehabilitation specialties. The patterns of clinical recovery are important from the scientific point of view and provide a model to study the organization of the brain after various lesions, such as stroke or trauma. Most of this chapter is related to recovery from stroke. Recovery patterns are specific for different etiologies, so that recovery from trauma is quite different from that from stroke, and it is important to separate them in any study.

STAGES OF RECOVERY

There are two basic stages of recovery. The initial stage is related to the absorption of edema and cellular exudative phenomena around the infarct. In about 2 or 3 weeks, the effects of edema and hemorrhage usually subside. Whatever recovery occurs after is called the second stage, which is more difficult to explain pathologically. Many experimental studies in animals suggest that axonal regrowth and collateral sprouting are operative not only in the peripheral nervous system but also in the central nervous system and probably also in man. It is unlikely, however, that the recovery seen in aphasia is related to local axonal regrowth or collateral sprouting.

DIASCHISIS

Von Monakow (31) introduced the concept of diaschisis to explain the substantial initial deficit that recovers after a sudden insult to the brain. This implies that damage to the nervous system would affect areas that are functionally connected to or neighboring the area of damage. This central "shock" effect then wears off; subsequently, the unaffected structures regain their function by acquiring innervation from elsewhere. Collateral sprouting, of course, could be one of the mechanisms in diaschisis. Recently, other physiologic concepts, such as denervation hypersensitivity, were invoked to explain diaschisis. In fact, denervation hypersensitivity is used to provide an explanation for recovery in two ways. The first states simply that the denervated tissue becomes more sensitive to the regrowth of axons or collateral sprouting even at a distance, and the remaining neurons become more responsive to the available neural transmitters, even though they are reduced in quantity and availability. The other explanation is that denervation hypersensitivity introduces an initial inhibition (similar to the diaschisis of von Monakow) by rendering the denervated tissue more sensitive to inhibitory influences; whenever these tissues regain innervation, there is less hypersensitivity to inhibitory systems, and function recovers.

SUBSTITUTION-REORGANIZATION

Aphasia is often viewed as a static disturbance. Most classic studies paid little attention to recovery, with a few notable exceptions. Wernicke (42) thought that recovery from comprehension and aphasic disturbances was related to the right hemisphere taking over the same function. Right hemisphere substitution was a prevalent idea at the end of the 19th century, following unilateral ablation studies for various physiologic mechanisms, such as locomotion, but some of the predictions of permanent paralysis from bilateral lesions were not confirmed. In other words, when the other side was removed as well, the animals continued to recover from the second operation, indicating that instead of homologous areas in the right hemisphere, structures in the same hemisphere or in the brain would be responsible for substitution. The idea of hierarchical representation of the brain was espoused by Hughlings Jackson (17), who based his neurologic theory on the Spencerian doctrine of hierarchical evolution.

ETIOLOGIC DIFFERENCES

Another interesting early comment on the effect of the nature of the lesion on outcome was made by Dax (8), who observed that slowly progressive lesions in the left hemisphere did not necessarily cause language disturbance, unlike the sudden large lesions that cause initial deficit much greater than that seen in slowly growing tumors. This was subsequently confirmed experimentally in animals and became an important principle, called the "serial lesion effect" (1). This explains why some slowly growing tumors will produce different neurologic deficits, even though a large area of the brain is destroyed or compressed, compared to the initial deficit produced by a lesion of similar size caused by a stroke.

LONGITUDINAL STUDIES

Studies of spontaneous recovery from aphasia are few, although the importance of the changing picture in aphasia was recognized by von Monakow (31), who often observed the considerable discrepancies between lesion size and location and the resulting deficit. Unfortunately, this is often neglected in recent literature, when studies compare chronic with acute stroke lesions in the same area without clearly distinguishing them, claiming that the lesion caused the deficit in one instance but not in another. This lack of attention to the temporal changes in the clinical symptomatology of aphasia results in considerable confusion with respect to localization.

Systematic studies of recovery are difficult to carry out. Most involved post-traumatic war veteran populations that were largely uncontrolled for treatment (4,41); a few studies used untreated patients as controls or studied them independently (2,5,15,23,35,40). There are several criticisms of the early studies, the most obvious being the mixing of etiologies and the lack of established numerical measures to follow change. Initial studies did not distinguish between treated and nontreated patients, the ones quoted above being chosen because they controlled for this factor.

In 1977, we published a 5-year longitudinal study of 91 aphasics, 83 of whom were untreated (23), using a comprehensive aphasia examination, the Western Aphasia Battery (WAB) (20), which looks at all modalities with a combined neurologic and psycholinguistic approach developed in Boston. It is a practical examination which can be carried out within 1 hr for the oral and written language tests and another 30 min for the praxis, construction, calculation, and other supplementary tests; more severely affected patients may take longer. The baseline test is administered in the acute stage, 2 to 6 weeks poststroke, with follow-up tests at 3, 6, and 12 months.

RATE OF RECOVERY

The results of this study indicated that recovery rates were greatest for the initial 0 to 3 months, which is in agreement with other studies (5,34,40), and plateau at 1 year. Follow-up examinations after the 1-year period showed little or no change in function, similar to the finding of Culton (5) but different from those of Schuell et al. (36), Marks et al. (29), and Smith (38). Among the aphasia types, Broca's and conduction aphasics showed the most recovery. Anomic aphasics, although they reached the highest levels, also start high, so that the difference between the beginning and the outcome was not as great; this is the "ceiling effect" operative in milder patients.

FINAL OUTCOME

Outcome measures are different from recovery rates. As a rule, the more mildly affected the patient is at the beginning, the better the outcome, even though the extent of recovery itself is slight. In the context of the previously mentioned study (23), we measured final outcome in those patients in whom follow-up was carried out through 1 year. Sixty-seven patients were included in this group, which was divided into various aphasic categories (Table 1). Final outcome was categorized as poor, fair, good, and excellent, depending on the quartile of the aphasia quotient (AQ) the patient achieved at 1 year. It is evident that global aphasics remained in the poor category, with the exception of one patient who recovered very well. Broca's and Wernicke's aphasics are fairly widely distributed with respect to outcome; and conduction, transcortical, and anomic aphasics have a generally good outlook. If a more general view of the total aphasic population is taken, it appears that just about an equal number of patients will remain in the poor category and

TABLE 1. *Aphasia outcome in stroke*

Aphasic type initially	*N*	Poor 0–25	Fair 25–50	Good 50–75	Excellent 75–100
Global	12	10 (12)	2		
Broca's	12	(4)	5 (4)	3 (4)	4
Conduction	4		(1)	1 (2)	3 (1)
Wernicke's	7	3 (4)	1 (2)	2 (1)	1
Transcortical and isolation	3		1 (1)[a]	(2)	2
Anomic	9			(2)	9 (7)
Total	47	13 (28%)	9 (19%)	6 (13%)	19 (40%)

[a]Isolation syndrome.
From Kertesz and McCabe (23), with permission.

recover well, with an equal number distributed in between. Initial severity is highly predictive of outcome (13,14,23,33,35,36).

EVOLUTION OF SYNDROMES

The evolution of aphasic syndromes is of considerable interest. The data presented in Table 2 incorporate patients from subsequent studies as well (19): the initial aphasia types are listed with their numbers on the left and the evolution of these types to subsequent diagnostic categories on the right. Initially, we thought that global aphasics had a poor prognosis and did not usually change, an opinion prevalent in other studies (35); but subsequent patients we looked at showed a more optimistic picture. In fact, although many recovered toward Broca's aphasia and remained severely handicapped, at least their comprehension recovered significantly. Some of these patients, which we classify as severe, persisting Broca's aphasics, would be labeled "mixed anterior," "big Broca's," or even global aphasics in some other classifications.

Broca's aphasics often recover toward anomic aphasia when their fluency and agrammatism improves, even though speech output is still stumbling and a phonetic-articulatory disturbance remains. Wernicke's aphasics tend to recover toward anomic or conduction aphasia; in fact, all the chronic conduction aphasics initially were Wernicke's type. A further linguistic and behavioral study of recovery from Wernicke's aphasia dealing with the complexities of the changing pattern is discussed below. Anomic aphasia and conduction aphasia, as well as the transcortical aphasias, with the exception of the isolation syndrome, have an excellent prognosis and recover completely or become anomic only.

There is no general agreement as to what constitutes complete recovery. We decided to take a mean AQ of the clinically nonaphasic but brain-damaged control group as a conservative cutoff score of 93.8, which is more strict than the right hemisphere lesion control group, with an AQ of 97.1. This conservative cutoff point results in a higher false positive rate, indicating that the AQ alone cannot be

TABLE 2. *Evolution of aphasic syndromes (0 to 12 months)*

Acute syndromes	*n*	Chronic syndromes at 1 year							
		Global	Broca's	Transcortical motor	Conduction	Transcortical sensory	Wernicke's	Anomic	Recovered
Global	21	6	12	2				1	
Broca's	17		2					15	
Isolation	1			1					
Conduction	9							6	3
Transcortical motor	2								2
Transcortical sensory	3							2	1
Wernicke's	9				3		4	2	
Anomic	29							10	19
Total	91								

From Kertesz (19), with permission by Aspen Systems Corporation.

used to label whether a brain-damaged patient is aphasic. It can be used as a cutoff point, however, between aphasic patients and normals, because none of the latter score below this level, and most right hemisphere patients remain above it. The normal control group showed a mean AQ of 99.6, with only a few errors in the naming and repetition tasks, indicating that the WAB is easy for normal subjects and has a high specificity for aphasia.

The evolution of linguistic and behavioral characteristics in Wernicke's aphasia, illustrated in Table 3, indicates the various pathways from the most severe neologistic jargon to anomic aphasia. This includes most fluent aphasics, which are interrelated, such as conduction aphasia and semantic jargon, the "original" Wernicke's aphasia, and the so-called pure word deafness. The various cognitive processes are indicated, as is a differential diagnostic table of impaired modalities. The linguistic characteristics of output are major contributing factors in clinically classifying these entities. The evolution follows a regular pattern from neologistic substitutions of most substantives to only occasional phonemic and semantic errors or the disappearance of neologisms and the relative persistence of semantic substitutions or phonemic paraphasias. The end stage of most of these entities is impaired word finding and circumlocution in spontaneous speech but good comprehension, although the occasional patient shows pure word deafness with impaired comprehension only (19).

The pattern of evolution of these syndromes has practical relevance for the clinician. A reversal of this pattern, for instance, a patient who changes from anomic toward Wernicke's aphasia or from conduction toward a nonfluent, more severe aphasia, suggests neoplasm or degenerative disease or repeated vascular insults rather than a single stroke or trauma. A consideration of the evolution of syndromes can also account for the discrepancies of observations in localization, i.e., why the same lesion can produce different degrees and patterns of impairment. When studying recovery, recurrent brain damage results in a substantially different recovery pattern and should be treated separately from single strokes.

The evolution of aphasic groups, specifically in stroke, was further examined by an objective statistical method called numerical taxonomy (24). The method of minimum variance clustering selects the individual patients who are closest to each other according to test scores. The clusters are formed at an arbitrarily chosen level (relatively low percentage of total) of variance. Acute aphasics had testing in the first 6 weeks after stroke and chronic aphasics beyond 330 days, usually around 1 year post stroke. Mean ages and sex ratios were similar in both groups. Fifty-eight of these patients had testing both in the acute and chronic stages, and their evolution followed separately.

In both acute and chronic groups, the first cluster established by the computer consisted mostly of global aphasics but appeared to be much larger in the acute group, indicating that many of these patients recover. Similarly, the large Wernicke's group, or second cluster, almost disappears in the chronic population; however, a new group consisting of the mild, chronic Wernicke's group mixed with conduction aphasics appears. We considered this group to be distinct enough clinically and

TABLE 3. *Evolution of Wernicke's aphasia*

Stages	Neologistic jargon	Conduction aphasia	Semantic jargon	Paraphasic word deafness	Pure word deafness	Anomic aphasia
Impaired processes	Phonemic and semantic selectors Comprehension Naming Repetition	Phonemic selector Repetition	Semantic selector Comprehension Naming Repetition	Phonemic and semantic selector Comprehension Naming Repetition	Comprehension Repetition	Naming
Linguistic characteristics of output	Neologistic substitutions of substantives	Phonemic paraphasias and anticipation	Semantic substitutions, circumlocution	Occasional phonemic and semantic errors	Normal	Impaired word finding, circumlocution

From Kertesz (19), with permission by Aspen Systems Corporation.

taxonomically to deserve the term "afferent" conduction aphasia, being characterized by a slight comprehension difficulty, more than usually seen in conduction patients. Broca's aphasia is substantially represented in the acute population, but the chronic Broca's cluster is small.

There are two new chronic clusters related to recovery from Broca's aphasia. One consists of milder Broca's aphasics mixed with conduction aphasics, a group we called "efferent" conduction aphasia; this is a fairly large group of chronic patients with relatively lower fluency and mildly impaired repetition and naming. Although labeled anomic in our classification, they resemble Broca's and transcortical motor aphasics in their lower fluency. The second cluster comprises severe nonfluent aphasics but with relatively good comprehension, representing chronic Broca's aphasia persisting in a severe form. The great increase in the anomic clusters in the chronic populations indicates that recovering patients often become reclassified as anomics; i.e., anomic aphasia seems to be an end stage in the evolution of many aphasia syndromes. There is an acute anomic cluster which was different from other anomic groups in the impairment of sentence comprehension; this group comes close to what Head (16) called "semantic aphasia." Finally, another cluster contains mostly recovered patients.

RECOVERY OF LANGUAGE COMPONENTS VERSUS APHASIC TYPES

In our next study, we looked at the recovery of various parameters in groups that were defined by percentile ranking rather than classic aphasia types (28). Because initial severity was such an important factor in recovery, we used this factor to covary in the analysis and did not include the parameters analyzed in the factors to be used to type the patients. The best recovering component appeared to be comprehension; the least was word fluency. The relatively low scores in the word fluency task combined with the analysis of covariance results in a negative value (Fig. 1).

The best recovery is observed in the low fluency, high comprehension group, the majority of whom were in fact Broca's aphasics. The next best recovery is seen in the high fluency, low comprehension group, which approaches Wernicke's aphasics; the least amount of recovery is seen in the low fluency, low comprehension group, the majority of whom were global aphasics (Fig. 2).

The recovery of different parameters in each of the four groups is also instructive, especially in the first group, in which comprehension was low at the start but was the most significant recovering factor, especially using the "yes–no" comprehension subtest. Unless this particular subtest is examined in aphasics, this important factor in recovery can be missed. Many of the severe global aphasics recover considerably; if only the difficult comprehension tasks are used, however, they may continue to be considered global. When "yes–no" questions are administered, especially those that are relevant to the personal information and needs of the patient, a considerable amount of comprehension can be detected by 3 months post onset.

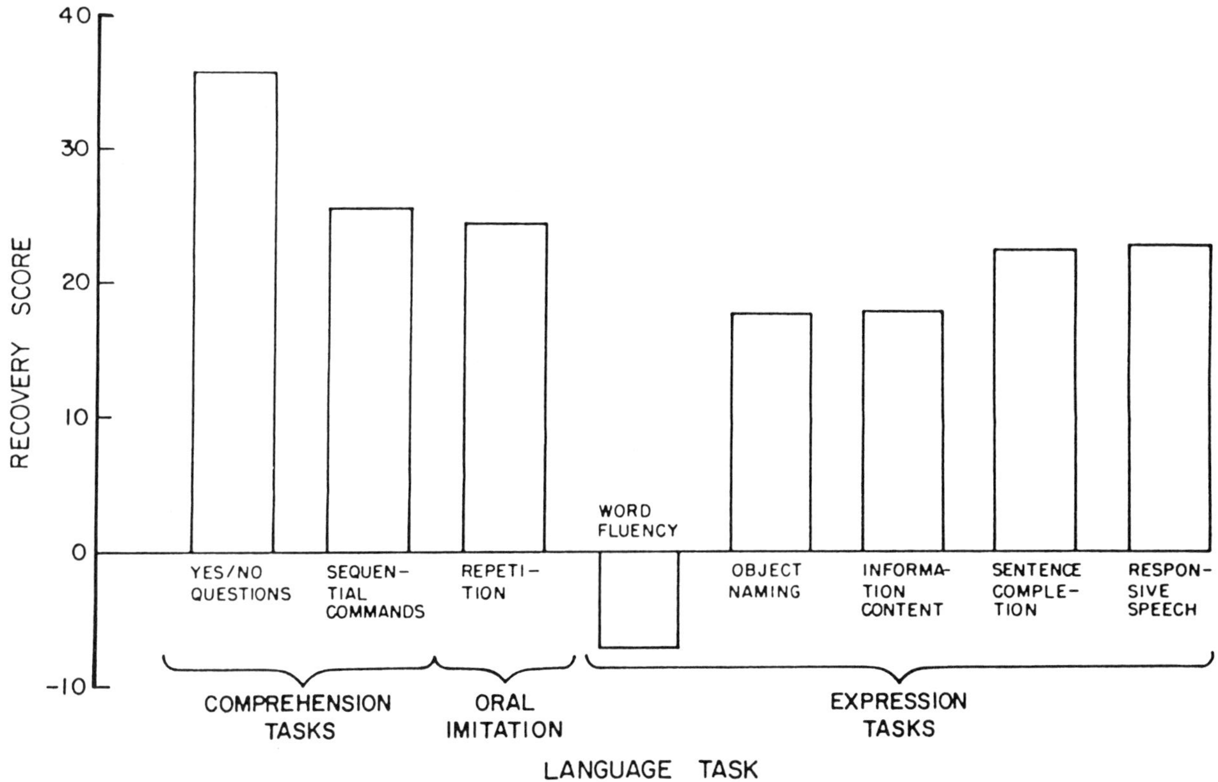

FIG. 1. Overall recovery of each aphasic group. The recovery score is the score at 3-month testing minus the score at initial testing with covariate adjustment for the effects of differing initial severities. (From Lomas and Kertesz, ref. 28, with permission.)

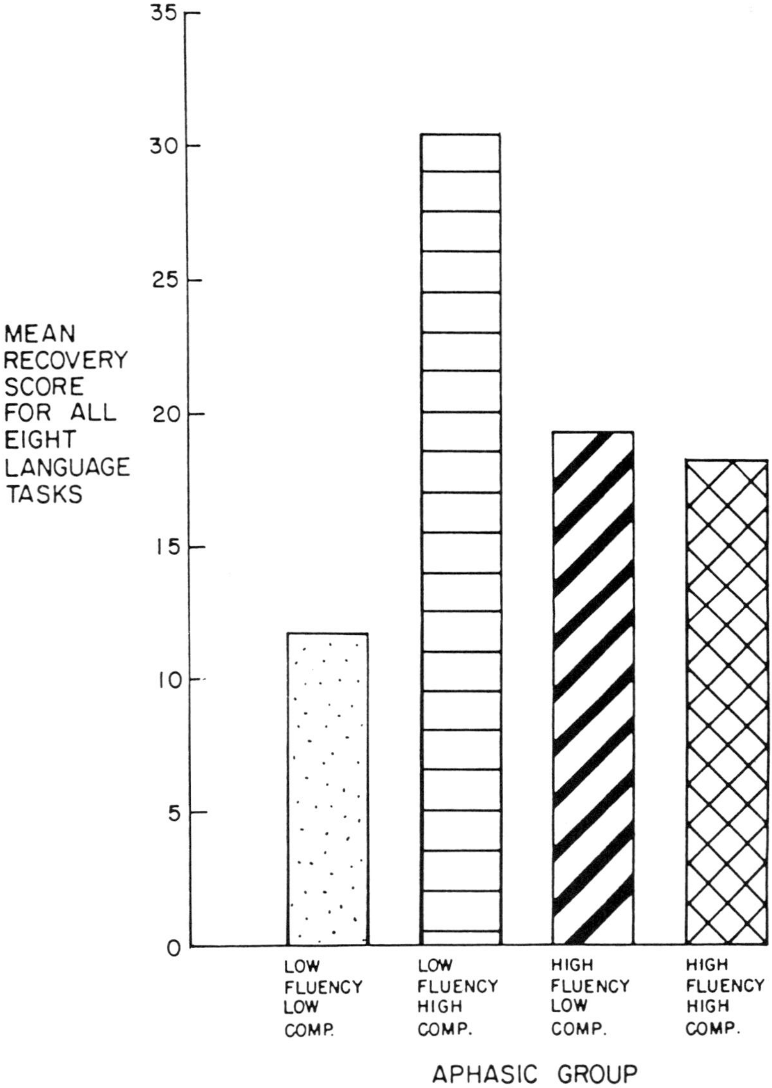

FIG. 2. Recovery scores on the eight language tasks for all 31 patients regardless of aphasic group. (From Lomas and Kertesz, ref. 28, with permission.)

The recovery curves from a more recent 3-year study following 100 patients confirm the rather steep recovery in the first 3 months and a considerable plateauing in the 3- to 6- and 6- to 12-month periods for the overall group (26). The global group showed a similar curve but at a lower level. Broca's aphasics seem to show more continuing recovery in the 6 to 12 months, but this is based on a much smaller number of patients; the same applies to Wernicke's aphasics. Conduction aphasia appeared to show a continuous recovery throughout the study. Anomic aphasics showed some decline; the more severe ones remained in the last group, and recovered patients tended to leave the study earlier, which also accounts for the dip in the recovery curve of Wernicke's aphasics. The parameters were again examined individually, and spontaneous speech and fluency showed a great deal of initial recovery with further improvement in Broca's and conduction aphasics but less improvement in the global, Wernicke's, and anomic groups. The latter two groups are fluent to begin with, so that much recovery from that high level cannot be expected (the ceiling effect). On the other hand, information content of spontaneous speech shows great gain in the Wernicke's group during the last period. Similarly, Broca's aphasics can convey more information at 1 year than at any of the previous stages. This also occurs in the recovery of auditory comprehension, although most gains are seen with the more severely affected groups, especially global, Wernicke's, and Broca's aphasics. Naming does not recover as well as comprehension in global aphasics. Broca's, conduction, and Wernicke's aphasics all improve in naming throughout the course of recovery.

READING, WRITING, AND CALCULATION

Reading and writing were separately examined. Recovery rates in writing appeared to be greater than in reading, but writing also appears to be more impaired at the beginning. Especially interesting is the impairment in the anomic groups, which is more in writing than in any of the other parameters examined. An exception was seen in global aphasics, who were different from the other groups because their writing and reading did not improve as much as the other parameters. Generally, writing scores are lower at all intervals in all groups, reflecting the usually severe impairment of writing in aphasia. The recovery of calculation parallels that of reading.

In the collapsed aphasic group following those patients who had all four tests up to 1 year, recovery curves appeared to be more parallel, except for calculation, where the initial curve was not as steep and more recovery was seen at 3 to 6 months than in the other parameters.

RECOVERY OF PRAXIS

We studied recovery from apraxia by following 50 aphasics with a standardized apraxia battery. The test consisted of 20 movements elicited by commands, imitation, or providing an object for performance. The actual movements selected were transitive, intransitive, buccofacial, and complex. Recovery of praxis was similar to language function in all aphasic groups, except in global aphasics, in whom praxis recovered better in the initial interval, as did comprehension. In Broca's aphasics, praxis difficulty seemed to persist longer. Wernicke's aphasics have recovery rates of praxis similar to those of Broca's aphasics, even though the patterns of language recovery are substantially different. Transcortical sensory and anomic aphasics show relatively little recovery in praxis, but they have relatively high starting levels. Although this is often not reflected in group statistics, the recovery of praxis can be substantially better initially, resulting in the not uncommon situation of a patient with substantial language problems but no apraxia. Apart from these dissociations, praxis recovery closely followed recovery of language and comprehension.

HEMIPLEGIA AND RECOVERY FROM APHASIA

The extent of hemiplegia was examined as a possible factor in influencing recovery. Clinically, a great deal of dissociation can be observed. In other words, there are many aphasics who are not hemiplegics initially, and recovery from hemiplegia does not parallel recovery from aphasia in every instance. Few quantitative studies are available. Boone (3) examined the recovery of aphasia and hemiplegia and did not find a significant correlation. In our prospective study, we collected data on the extent of hemiplegia as a factor in recovery. When we compared the groups, namely severe, moderate, mild, and no hemiplegia, there was no difference in the extent of recovery from aphasia, except in word fluency. Severe hemiplegics showed little recovery from impaired word fluency.

RECOVERY OF VISUOSPATIAL/NONVERBAL FUNCTION

The recovery of visuospatial nonverbal function in aphasic stroke patients was studied using the Raven's Coloured Progressive Matrices (RCPM), the block design subtest of the Wechsler Adult Intelligence Scale (WAIS), and the drawing subtest consisting of presenting the patient with an image for 10 sec and then asking for a drawing of the item, which is also named for the patient. The items include a circle, square, Christmas tree, cube, clock, house, and person. Finally, a line bisection task is used to rate neglect. Although these functions are variably affected in aphasia (22), they tend to recover considerably, along with verbal parameters.

Global aphasics showed better recovery in RCPM than language performance in the first 3 months and continued to improve in the 3 to 6 months poststroke, even though language recovery tended to fall off. Drawing and block design recovered more in later intervals but not quite to the same extent as RCPM. Broca's aphasics showed considerable language recovery, but they started higher in the RCPM performance and show a more modest recovery. Drawing and block design recovery rates are higher in the first 3 months. Wernicke's aphasics have relatively poor recovery of RCPM and block design as compared to language function. Conduction aphasics also showed more recovery in language than in the RCPM. The relatively low recovery rate in these groups indicates a ceiling effect, because they started at a higher level. The same applies to anomic aphasia, except that anomic aphasics also showed the ceiling effect for language recovery. Those aphasics who had all four tests showed nearly the same rise of scores in RCPM as in language, except in the first 3 months, when recovery rate appeared to be slower than language recovery. On the other hand, recovery from visuospatial impairment continued, even in the 6 to 12 months poststroke, and these rates were significant at all intervals using repeated measures *t*-test. The correlation of the recovery of visuospatial function with language parameters are more significant in the 0- to 3-month period. Sentence comprehension, object naming, responsive speech, and reading are correlated more significantly; AQ, sentence completion, repetition, drawing, and praxis correlate at a lower level (18).

AGE

The clinical impression that younger patients recover better has produced a widespread impression of age being an important factor. Such a trend, however, has not been found to be statistically significant in our studies (23,37), even when we excluded the posttraumatic group, which had a mean age well below that of the infarct group. There was a negative correlation between age and initial recovery rates, but this just missed being significant statistically. This was also the case in the studies of Culton (6), Sarno and Levita (34), and Smith (38). We observed remarkedly good recovery in elderly patients, whereas some of the young will remain severely disabled.

SEX DIFFERENCES

In our initial study, we did not find a significant sex difference in recovery, even though there is a recently popularized concept that females may have less language impairment after brain damage because of more bilaterally or diffuse representation of language. Our recent studies of the epidemiology of aphasia in stroke indicated that the higher incidence of aphasia in males is related to their higher incidence of strokes (25). When the actual severity of impairment is compared, there is no significant sex difference, and some of our more recent data in recovery showed no sex differences in rate of recovery (37). The combined results of the two studies show no significant sex difference for the total aphasic population (Table 4).

HANDEDNESS

Most of our data are related to right handers; few studies were able to collect enough left handers to draw significant conclusions. In fact, we found a smaller than expected number of left handers in our population of aphasics (25), which may be related to the more bilateral cerebral organization of left handers. Some data, which are not entirely quantitative (12,39), indicated that left handers recover better from aphasia than right handers. Gloning et al. (12) suggested that left handers are likely to become aphasic regardless of which hemisphere is damaged, which is contrary to our experience, because in that case, a higher incidence of aphasia would be expected in left handers. According to Geschwind (10), right handers with a history of left handedness among parents, siblings, or children recover better than right handers without such family history, but reliable quantitative data are lacking to support this contention.

TABLE 4. *Mean recovery scores 3 months postonset for males and females*[a]

Group	Sex	*N*	Mean	SD	*t*	*p*
Content	M	89	1.9	2.2		
	F	69	1.8	2.4	0.07	>0.1
Fluency	M	89	1.3	1.6		
	F	69	1.3	1.9	0.20	>0.1
AQ	M	89	17.4	15.6		
	F	69	16.4	16.8	0.38	>0.1
Comprehension	M	89	1.7	1.8		
	F	69	1.5	1.6	1.02	>0.1
Repetition	M	89	2.0	2.5		
	F	69	1.7	1.7	1.00	>0.1
Naming	M	89	1.9	1.8		
	F	69	2.3	2.0	1.30	>0.1

[a]Values computed are the differences at 0 and 3 months for content, fluency, AQ, comprehension, repetition, and naming. Groups comprise Broca's, Wernicke's, anomic, global, and conduction aphasics.

ANATOMIC ASYMMETRIES

Asymmetries in the planum temporale (11) and probably in Broca's area (9) provide an anatomic basis for the well-known functional asymmetry. Various neuroradiologic asymmetries also were noted, the more recent one being the observation of LeMay (27), who suggested that skull asymmetries may be correlated with cerebral dominance. In right handers, there is a left occipital prominence balanced by a less obvious prominence of the right frontal lobe. Such asymmetries may be reversed in left handers. Pieniadz et al. (32) suggested that the atypical pattern may be associated with better recovery after left hemispheric lesions. Individual variations between the degree of asymmetry could account for some degree of the variation between recovery rates.

LESION SIZE AND LOCATION

The extent of recovery was correlated with lesion size and location for the total language score as well as for various components of language (21). Negative correlation was found between the recovery rates of AQ (total score), fluency, repetition, and naming. This indicated that, with larger lesions, less recovery occurs in total language deficit. The exception to this rule is comprehension, where positive correlation was found, which can best be explained if one considers that the comprehension deficit caused by large lesions has a considerable potential to recover. Small lesions, however, often cause aphasia with little if any comprehension deficit, and the extent of the recovery is small.

The correlation of lesion size with outcome provides different results; this points out the importance of not confusing outcome data with recovery rates. Yarnell et al. (44) had 16 cases in which lesion size on computerized tomography correlated negatively with outcome in aphasia. In our study (21), the results were similar in all language components and total score. In other words, the size of the lesion is an excellent prognostic sign for eventual outcome, but it should be remembered that strategically placed small lesions in Wernicke's and Broca's areas produce more severe and persisting deficits. In cases of Broca's aphasia, the area is the posterior portion of the third frontal gyrus, the precental gyrus, and some of the parietal operculum. Recovery from jargon aphasia will occur if the lesion is small and does not involve the posterior end of the temporal and parietal operculum together. In persistent jargon aphasia, both these lesions are necessary (19).

TREATMENT

The effect of treatment on recovery from aphasia is difficult to quantitate because of the paucity of controlled studies in the literature. Vignolo (40) studied treated and untreated patients and did not find a significant difference between these groups. Sarno et al. (35), comparing two forms of therapy with no treatment in global aphasics, did not find any effect. Hagen (15) used small treated and untreated groups and found a significantly better recovery in language formulation, speech production, reading comprehension, spelling, and arithmetic in the treated group but no difference in recovery of auditory comprehension, reading, and visuomotor abilities. Basso et al. (2) had a large number of controls, but these were not randomized. Unfortunately, all aphasics were lumped into two categories; this possibly allowed more global aphasics or severe jargon aphasics to be included in the untreated sample. Instead of controlling the time of inclusion after onset, the investigators examined this variable in a factor analysis; this provided an opportunity to include more treated patients in the early group, in which more recovery is likely to occur. Examination of the data distribution indicates that because initial severity was not controlled, the untreated group had a higher number of more severely affected patients.

In a recent cooperative study of aphasia therapy (42), no significant differences were found in individual stimulation therapy or social interaction group therapy. We have conducted a longitudinal study in which three randomized groups of language-oriented stimulation therapy and untrained therapists were compared; no significant differences were found (37). Several British studies comparing the effect of speech therapy by volunteers and qualified speech therapists indicated no significant difference between the two (7,30).

ACKNOWLEDGMENT

Some of the research presented here was done in collaboration with Patricia McCabe, Dr. Daniel Bub, Jonathan Lomas, and Dr. Cynthia Shewan.

REFERENCES

1. Ades, H. W., and Raab, D. H. (1946): Recovery of motor function after two-stage extirpation of Area 4 in monkeys. *J. Neurophysiol.*, 9:55–60.
2. Basso, A., Capitani, E., and Vignolo, L. A. (1979): Influence of rehabilitation on language skills in aphasic patients. A controlled study. *Arch. Neurol.*, 36:190–196.
3. Boone, D. R. (1961): Relationship to progress in speech therapy to progress in physical therapy. *Arch. Phys. Med. Rehabil.*, 42:30–32.
4. Butfield, E., and Zangwill, O. L. (1946): Re-education in aphasia: A review of 70 cases. *J. Neurol. Neurosurg. Psychiatry*, 9:75–79.
5. Culton, G. L. (1969): Spontaneous recovery from aphasia. *J. Speech Hear. Res.*, 12:825–832.
6. Culton, G. L. (1971): Reaction to age as a factor in chronic aphasia in stroke patients. *J. Speech Hear. Dis.*, 36:563–564.
7. David, R., Enderby, P., and Bainton, D. (1982): Treatment of acquired aphasia: Speech therapists and volunteers compared. *J. Neurol. Neurosurg. Psychiatry*, 45:957–961.
8. Dax, M. (1865): Lesions de la moitie gauche de l'encephale coincidant avec l'oubli des signes de la pensee. *Gazette Hebdomadaire de Medicine et de Chirurgie*, Paris.
9. Galaburda, A. M., and Mesulam, M. M. (1983): Neuroanatomical aspects of cerebral localization. In: *Localization in Neuropsychology*, edited by A. Kertesz, pp. 21–61. Academic Press, New York.
10. Geschwind, N. (1974): Late changes in the nervous system: An overview. In: *Plasticity and Recovery of Function in the Central Nervous System*, edited by D. G. Stein, J. J. Rosen, and N. Butlers. Academic Press, New York.
11. Geschwind, N., and Levitsky, W. (1968): Human brain: Left-right asymmetries in temporal speech regions. *Science*, 161:186–187.
12. Gloning, I., Gloning, K., Haub, G., and Quatember, R. (1969): Comparison of verbal behavior in right-handed and non-right-handed patients with anatomically verified lesions of one hemisphere. *Cortex*, 5:43–52
13. Gloning, K., Trappl, R., Heiss, W. D., and Quatember, R. (1976): Prognosis and speech therapy in aphasia. In: *Neurolinguistics, 4, Recovery in Aphasics*, edited by Y. Lebrun and R. Hoops. Swets & Zeitlinger, Amsterdam.
14. Godfrey, C. M., and Douglass, E. (1959): The recovery process in aphasia. *Can. Med. Assoc. J.*, 80:618–624.
15. Hagen, C. (1973): Communication abilities in hemiplegia: Effect of speech therapy. *Arch. Phys. Med. Rehabil.*, 54:454–463.
16. Head, H. (1926): *Aphasia and Kindred Disorders of Speech*. Cambridge University Press, Cambridge.
17. Jackson, H. (1873): On the anatomical and physiological localization of movements in the brain. *Lancet*, 1:84–85; 162–164; 232–234.
18. Kertesz, A. (1979): *Aphasia and Associated Disorders*. Grune & Stratton, New York.
19. Kertesz, A. (1981): Evolution of aphasic syndromes. *Top. Lang. Disord.*, 1(4):15–27.
20. Kertesz, A. (1982): *The Western Aphasia Battery*. Grune & Stratton, New York.
21. Kertesz, A., Harlock, W., and Coates, R. (1979): Computer tomographic localization, lesion size and prognosis in aphasia. *Brain Lang.*, 8:34–50.
22. Kertesz, A., and McCabe, P. (1975): Intelligence and aphasia. *Brain Lang.*, 2:387–397.
23. Kertesz, A., and McCabe, P. (1977): Recovery patterns and prognosis in aphasia. *Brain*, 100:1–18.
24. Kertesz, A., and Phipps, J. (1980): The numerical taxonomy of acute and chronic aphasic syndromes. *Psychol. Res.*, 41:179–198.
25. Kertesz, A., and Sheppard, A. (1981): The epidemiology of cognitive and aphasic impairment in stroke. *Brain*, 104:117–128.
26. Kertesz, A., and Shewan, C. M. (1984): The recovery of aphasic syndromes and their language components in stroke. *(In preparation.)*
27. LeMay, M. (1977): Asymmetries of the skull and handedness. *J. Neurol. Sci.*, 32:243–253.
28. Lomas, J., and Kertesz, A. (1978): Patterns of spontaneous recovery in aphasic groups: A study of adult stroke patients. *Brain Lang.*, 5:388–401.
29. Marks, M. M., Taylor, M. L., and Rusk, L. A. (1957): Rehabilitation of the aphasic patients: A survey of three years' experience in a rehabilitation setting. *Neurology*, 7:837–843.

30. Meikle, M., Wechsler, E., Tupper, A., Benenson, M., Butler, J., Mulhall, D., and Stern, G. (1979): Comparative trial of volunteer and professional treatments of dysphasia after stroke. *Br. Med. J.*, 2:87–89.
31. Monakow, C. von (1914): Die Lokalisation. *Grosshirn und der Abbau der Funktionen durch corticale Herde*. Bergmann, Wiesbaden.
32. Pieniadz, J. M., Naeser, M. A., Koff, E., and Levine, H. L. (1979): CT scan cerebral hemispheric asymmetry measurements in stroke cases with global aphasia: Atypical asymmetries associated with improved recovery. *Cortex*, 19:371–391.
33. Sands, E., Sarno, M. T., and Shankweiler, D. (1969): Long-term assessment of language function in aphasia due to stroke. *Arch. Phys. Med. Rehabil.*, 50:202–207.
34. Sarno, M. T., and Levita, E. (1971): Natural course of recovery in severe aphasia. *Arch. Phys. Med. Rehabil.*, 52:175–179.
35. Sarno, M. T., Silverman, M., and Sands, E. (1970): Speech fluency and language recovery in severe aphasia. *J. Speech Hear. Res.*, 13:607–623.
36. Schuell, H., Jenkins, J. J., and Jimenez-Pabon, E. (1964): *Aphasia in Adults: Diagnosis, Prognosis and Treatment*. Harper and Row, New York.
37. Shewan, C. M., and Kertesz, A. (1981): Language therapy and recovery from aphasia. Presented at the Academy of Aphasia, London, Ontario. October 13, 1981.
38. Smith, A. (1972): Diagnosis, intelligence and rehabilitation of chronic aphasics. Final report, Department of Physical Medicine & Rehabilitation, University of Michigan.
39. Subirana, A. (1969): Handedness and cerebral dominance. In: *Handbook of Clinical Neurology, Vol. 4*, edited by P. J. Vinken and G. W. Bruyn. Elsevier, New York.
40. Vignolo, L. A. (1964): Evolution of aphasia and language rehabilitation: A retrospective exploratory study. *Cortex*, 1:344–367.
41. Wepman, J. M. (1951): *Recovery from Aphasia*. Ronald Press, New York.
42. Wernicke, C. (1886): Die neueren Arbeiten uber Aphasie. *Fortschr. Med.*, 4:371–377.
43. Wertz, R. T., Collins, M. J., Weiss, D., Kurtzke, J. F., Friden, T., Brookshire, R. H., Pierce, J., Holtzapple, P., Hubbard, D. J., Porch, B. E., West, J. A., Davis, L., Matovitch, V., Morley, G. K., and Resurrecion, E. (1981): Veterans Administration cooperative study on aphasia: A comparison of individual and group treatment. *J. Speech Hear. Res.*, 24:580–594.
44. Yarnell, P., Monroe, P., and Sobel, L. (1976): Aphasia outcome in stroke: A clinical neuroradiological correlation. *Stroke*, 7:516–522.

Advances in Neurology, Vol. 42: Progress in Aphasiology, edited by F. C. Rose.
Raven Press, New York © 1984.

Dysprosody as Part of the Aphasic Language Disorder

Dorothea Weniger

Department of Neurology, University of Zurich, 8091 Zurich, Switzerland

More than a century ago, Hughlings Jackson (16) drew attention to the difference between what he called the intellectual and emotional modes of expression, the former being associated with voluntary use of language, the latter with the more automatic uses. As he argued, the relevance of this distinction becomes apparent in patients whose brain damage has rendered them almost speechless. These patients may utter words like "yes" and "no," but these words often serve no propositional function. As they are usually produced with variations of pitch, they have a certain interjectional value and manifest some state of feeling. Depending on the emotional force of the situation, patients with such extremely reduced speech production occasionally bring forth a word or phrase that, however general in its range of meaning, fits the situational context. The characteristic feature of such automatic speech production is that these utterances, which are spoken with little effort, cannot be repeated. Jackson (16) concluded from this differential availability of words that "the right hemisphere is the one for the most automatic use of words, and the left the one in which automatic use of words merges into voluntary use of words" (p. 130). Basically, this dichotomy regarding hemispheric specialization of language processing has remained undisputed, but it has been subjected to more differentiated interpretations.

The automatic use of words is connected with the assumption that the right hemisphere is also more involved in the processing of the prosodic features of language. What experimental evidence is there to support such a functional asymmetry? Is it observed to the same degree in both speech perception and speech production? Furthermore, both pitch and stress take on linguistic as well as pragmatic functions. For example, we have rules telling us which syllable to stress in some given word or sentence in normal speech; but, depending on the situational context in which a given sentence is uttered, the speaker will ignore these rules and place primary stress on the constituent that marks the focus of information. One might expect such differences in functional status to be reflected in variations of lateralization.

We consider first the findings of some receptive studies. One is often struck by the ability of aphasic patients to follow a conversation rather well, although they do poorly in comprehension tasks. Contrary to conversational discourse, comprehension tasks contain hardly any redundant cues. Gestures, facial expressions, intonation contours, as well as environmental circumstances provide information that aids the comprehension of the spoken utterance. As has been pointed out repeatedly (15,20,23,25,29), right brain-damaged subjects display more difficulties in the perception of affectively intoned speech than aphasic subjects. To determine to what extent aphasics are guided by the emotional tone of a sentence in their comprehension of it, we designed an experiment with two sets of tasks (10); aphasics, right brain-damaged patients, and normal controls served as subjects.

One set (A) consisted of emotionally intonated sentences, which were constructed in such a way that each could be spoken with two different tones of voice. Depending on the tone, the sentential meaning satisfied different referential expectations. The sentence "the cage was left open," spoken with a tone of sadness, refers to some cage which, when left open, leads to some kind of deplorable loss. If the sentence is intonated with a fearful tone of voice, referential expectations of a cage in which some object to be guarded with caution are aroused. Subjects had to identify the meaning conveyed by the emotionally intonated sentence by pointing to the appropriate picture in a multiple choice set of four pictures. Two pictures in the set depicted the sentential meaning of the stimulus sentence, but only one fitted the referential expectations aroused by the tone of voice used. The two other pictures functioned as mere distractors. Four tones of voice were used: fear, anger, happiness, and sadness.

The sentential meanings of the sentences in set A implied no particular emotional attitude; the sentences in set B, however, had sentential meanings that were connected to particular emotional attitudes. The sentence "he won the first prize in the contest" is readily associated with a happy event. Such sentences were intonated with a neutral tone of voice. The same emotions were used as with the sentences in set A, and the task was to identify the emotional attitude conveyed by the sentential meaning by pointing to the corresponding facial expression in a multiple choice set of three facial expressions.

Aphasic subjects were hypothesized to have more difficulties with the sentences of set B, because the correct solution largely depended on comprehending the sentential meaning. Unless the syntactic functions and the meanings of the linguistic units are available, the emotional attitude cannot be inferred. With the sentences of set A, the correct solution could be found by attending to the tone of voice. On the other hand, the group of right brain-damaged subjects was hypothesized to show just the reverse pattern of behavior: whenever the task involves linguistic processing routines (as with the sentences of set B), no difference in performance between normal controls and right brain-damaged subjects ought to be observed. When it is a matter of identifying the emotional tone of an utterance, however, right brain-damaged subjects are expected to do less well than normal controls and aphasic patients. With respect to the sentences of set B, our hypotheses were confirmed; no difference was found between normal controls and right brain-damaged subjects. Although Broca's aphasics performed just like these two experimental groups, the two more severely impaired groups of aphasic patients (global and Wernicke's aphasics) did significantly poorer. With the sentences of set A, clear differences of performance were found between normal controls and right brain-damaged subjects.

The aphasic subjects also differed from the normal controls with respect to the total number of correct responses. When an error analysis was performed, Broca's aphasics did not exhibit a significantly different level of performance than normal controls, as did right brain-damaged subjects. In addition, Broca's aphasics benefited from prosodic information far more than did Wernicke's aphasics, whose speech production is characterized by more or less intact intonation. The difficulties of right brain-damaged subjects in processing emotional material appear to be dependent on the modality in which the material is presented. These subjects showed no impairment when the emotional attitude to be identified was conveyed by the sentential meaning of an utterance, but they were impaired in their identification of the emotional attitudes when these were transmitted prosodically.

As a number of dichotic listening studies (2,4,13,30) have demonstrated, the analysis of the intonational component of an utterance appears to be conducted in the right hemisphere. Contrary to the clear right ear advantages for verbal material, the left ear advantages for tonal material tend to be inconsistent and small when obtained. Blumstein and Cooper (2) report a significant left ear advantage for sets of three consonant–vowel (CV) syllables intonated as declaratives, questions, imperatives, and conditionals when these sets are presented dichotically and must be matched to filtered binaural foils. The left ear advantage is nonsignificant when dichotically presented sentence contours must be judged by their sentence types. Thus it seems that the processing of intonation contours is more a matter of the perceptual task: whenever linguistic decisions must be made, less right hemispheric participation is manifested than when the linguistic medium functions only as carrier of tonal information.

The question is whether there is reason to assume that the two hemispheres are engaged independently and concurrently in the processing of the intonational and phonetic component of verbal stimuli in speech perception. Goodglass and Calderon (12) examined such a hypothesis by having subjects identify dichotically presented pairs of digit triplets, which were either sung or superimposed on a sequence of piano notes. Although their results suggest that "each hemisphere can selectively process that component of a complex stimulus for which it is specifically equipped" (p. 405), their data do not exclude the possibility that tonal information presented to the right ear is analyzed in the left hemisphere together with the phonetic medium. Support for a model of parallel processing could be gained from dichotic listening experiments in which patients with unilateral right and left hemisphere lesions are required to identify both the tonal and the verbal component of the speech signal. A dissociation in the pattern of ear advantages displayed by two such experimental groups would be strong evidence in favor of the model.

A study in which the interaction between side of lesion and class of stimulus (digits versus tonal sequences) was investigated (21) showed left brain-injured subjects to report more tonal sequences correctly from the left ear than the right ear, just like the normal controls. With right brain-damaged subjects, a bilateral decrement of performance for tonal sequences was obtained, but the normal superiority of the left ear/right hemisphere for tones was maintained. On the other hand, both normal controls and right brain-injured subjects correctly identified more digits presented to the right ear/left hemisphere. Patients with a left hemisphere lesion showed severe impairment of the left and right ear for digits; but, in accordance with the normal superiority of the right ear for digits, report from the right ear was slightly better.

Common to both groups of brain-injured subjects in this study is a bilateral decrement of performance with material for which the damaged hemisphere is dominant. These findings raise the question of whether material arriving in the auditory cortex of the hemisphere, which is functionally not dominant for it, is returned across the commissural fibers to the dominant hemisphere. Transfer across the callosal pathways is enhanced when only a verbal or a tonal dichotic stimulus is presented.

In an attempt to find evidence for a dissociation in the pattern of ear advantages in patients with unilateral left and right hemisphere lesions (in support of a model of parallel processing), we carried out the following experiment (14). Six different sets of three CV syllables (BA, DA, GA, LA, MA, NA) were intonated with a tone of surprise, happiness, sadness, and soothing comfort; they were also spoken as questions and imperatives. These sequences were constructed in such a way that either the initial, middle, or final CV syllable of two sequences were identical. This arrangement was constructed to decrease the likelihood that subjects could identify sequences correctly by recognition of only one syllable. The intonation contours had to be matched to a visual analog as well as identified in a multiple choice set of six line drawings, each of which depicted an everyday situation characteristic for the emotional attitude signaled by one of the contours. The rationale for having a task condition with pictorial representations was that matching an acoustic signal to a visual analog could be a qualitatively different task than recognizing the intonation of natural speech. Subjects were asked to listen to the dichotically presented syllable sequences and then point to two syllable sequences in a multiple choice set comprising all six sequences. At the same time, they were required to identify the two intonation contours. In half the tasks, the pictorial representations were used; in the other half, the multiple choice sets of visual analogs were used. Since few numerical differences were found between scores in these two task conditions, they were combined for all analyses.

The analysis of the data was based on the assumption that the intact left hemisphere of right brain-damaged patients is able to identify the phonetic component of the intonated syllable sequences presented to the ipsilateral right ear like normals but deficient in the processing of the intonational component; the intact right hemisphere of aphasic patients is able to identify the intonational component of the intonated syllable sequences presented to the ipsilateral left ear but deficient in the processing of the phonetic component. When the left ear performance of left brain-damaged patients and the right ear performance of right brain-damaged patients were compared with the respective performance of normal controls, no significant differences were found between brain-damaged patients and controls in the identification of the phonetic component by the intact left hemisphere and the identification of the intonational component by the intact right hemisphere. If only the intact hemisphere and that part of the task for which the intact hemisphere is functionally dominant is considered, brain-damaged patients perform as well as normals. If performance of the intact hemisphere on that part of the task for which it is functionally nondominant is considered, however, brain-damaged patients do less well than normals. The numerical differences in performance were significant only for the left brain-damaged subjects' identification of syllable sequences presented to the ipsilateral left ear/intact right hemisphere.

With respect to the processing of the intonational component of the stimuli presented to the ear contralateral to the lesion, both groups of brain-damaged subjects performed significantly worse than normals with their respective ears. Right brain-damaged subjects were significantly less impaired than the aphasic subjects when identifying the phonetic component of the stimuli presented to the ear contralateral to their lesion. This marked "lesion effect" suggests that within the dichotic paradigm used, the input to an intact hemisphere is not, or only deficiently, transferred to the intact hemisphere for processing. As expected, the level of performance displayed by the intact right hemisphere of aphasic patients corresponded to the respective performance of the normal controls. A rather high percentage of intonation contours was also identified by the intact left hemisphere of right brain-injured subjects.

Analogous results were not obtained with respect to the identification of syllable sequences. The processing of intonation contours obviously is not lateralized in the same way as the processing of their phonetic medium. These findings raise doubts as to whether the affective component of language is a dominant function of the right hemisphere, as has been postulated in more recent publications (17,18,26). The results of dichotic listening studies with aphasic subjects do not point to a "functional-anatomic organization of affective language in the right hemisphere which mirrors that of propositional language in the left hemisphere" (17, p. 562).

In a study in which the effects of right and left intracarotid amytal injections were compared, Borchgrevink (3) found the right hemisphere to control pitch and tonality in singing but not in speech production. He also refers to a study in which patients with right temporal lesions were able to discriminate between linguistic forms having a similar sound (e.g., "sil" and "syl" in Norwegian) but failed when required to discriminate between the isolated vowels (sounds) /i/ and /y/ of these same forms. Such results might explain why both hemispheres were observed to be involved in the processing of intonation.

Pitch is another prosodic phenomenon of spoken language, but it differs from intonation in that it has a more "linguistic" status. In tone languages, pitch serves to contrast the meaning of words that otherwise are identical in their segmental sounds. A significant right ear advantage was obtained in a dichotic listening experiment in which native Thai speakers were asked to mark on an answer sheet the "tone-word" (same sequences of segmental sounds spoken with varying pitches) or "consonant-word" (sequence of segmental sounds differing in initial consonant but spoken with the same pitch) heard in the right and left ear (24).

Blumstein and Goodglass (1) investigated the ability of aphasic patients to use stress cues in discriminating between pairs of phonemically identical but semantically different lexical items (e.g., "sóre héad" meaning "head that hurts" and "sóre head" meaning "grumpy"). The two items of a contrast pair were given in randomized order. The task was to point to the picture that represented the meaning of the item heard. Although the aphasic subjects made more overall errors than the normal controls, the pattern of errors was the same in all experimental groups, suggesting that the perception of stress cues is preserved in aphasia.

The above study was replicated with German stimuli (6,27). There are not many words in German that can be stressed contrastively, as there are in English. By pairing compound nouns and verbs with noun phrases and prepositional phrases (e.g., *Eíngriff* meaning "operation" and *ein Ǵriff* meaning "a handle"; *áufbäumen* meaning "to rear" and *auf B́äumen* meaning "on trees"), stress contrasts may be constructed. Since the items of such contrast pairs were presented consecutively, subjects had to identify the meaning of the stimulus item in a multiple choice set of eight pictures. The meaning of each stimulus item was represented by two visually dissimilar pictures (stress errors); two additional pictures were semantically related to each of the two stimulus items constituting the contrast pair (semantic confusion errors). More stress errors were made than semantic confusion errors. Owing to the differential syntactic complexity of the stimuli, aphasic subjects differed in their performance from normals but not in all stimuli conditions from right brain-damaged subjects.

With respect to the vocabulary of a language, a distinction is generally made between a relatively small set of high frequency words (articles, prepositions, conjunctions), which provide the structural information necessary for assigning syntactic functions to the lexical items of an utterance, and a large open set of content words (nouns, verbs, adjectives), which carry the major semantic information load. Words of the former set are referred to as closed class vocabulary items; words of the latter set are open class vocabulary items. Broca's aphasics are known to be impaired particularly in their processing of closed class words. Since major sentential stress tends to fall on open rather than closed class words, the limited ability of Broca's aphasics to access closed class words could be the result of inappropriate expectations concerning word class usage. Normal listeners have been found to react faster to both open and closed class items when they are stressed than when they are unstressed (5).

The question arises of whether Broca's aphasics could benefit from sentential stress cues in distinguishing between these two classes of vocabulary items. Swinney et al. (22) sought to answer this question in a word monitoring task. Broca's aphasics and normal control subjects pressed a button as soon as they heard a specified target word. The target material consisted of open and closed class words;

two sentences, differing only in sentential stress, were constructed for each word. For example, with the open class target word "drink," the two sentences were: "famous people often drínk quite a lot"; and "famous people often drink quíte a lot." With the closed target word "that," the two sentences were: "the car I want is something like thát one over there"; and "the car I want is something like that one over thére." While both groups of subjects responded more rapidly to stressed than to unstressed items, Broca's aphasics also exhibited a word class effect. Reaction times were consistently faster for open than closed class words. Sentential stress does not appear to be used in distinguishing word classes but probably serves as a major cue in locating communicatively important information. Support for this assumption could be gained from word monitoring experiments in which Wernicke's aphasics display the same pattern of performance as Broca's aphasics.

As the reviewed experimental findings demonstrate, the ability of aphasics to process prosodic information in the receptive mode depends on the degree to which the particular prosodic phenomenon is used in the service of a linguistic decision (28). It is interesting to note that when studies are not restricted to Broca's aphasics but also include Wernicke's and global aphasics, the performance of these groups reflects the overall degree of language impairment and not the agility of speech production associated with the different aphasic syndromes. A hierarchy in level of performance is seen from Broca's aphasics to Wernicke's and global aphasics.

Few studies have investigated the prosodic features of speech production in aphasia, in part because a systematic evaluation of the acoustic properties of the aphasic speech wave is not easily achieved. The use of computerized techniques is connected with time-consuming programming and high demands on the recording quality of the data.

Goodglass et al. (11) have examined a factor that can be explored in a paper and pencil manner, namely, the stress saliency of the opening word in an utterance. Characteristic for the speech production of Broca's aphasics is the increased threshold for initiating and maintaining the flow of speech. A stressed word in the initial position may be expected to have a facilitating effect. To assess this hypothesis, Broca's and fluent aphasics were given a repetition test consisting of sentences that began with either a stressed or unstressed function word. Unstressed opening words were omitted more frequently by Broca's than fluent aphasics. The analysis of the repetition ability of an agrammatic Broca's aphasic revealed a 56% decrease in omission rate for function words in medial position as compared to initial position. In these studies, the task was one of repetition; therefore, it remains open to discussion whether the frequent lack of function words in the utterances of Broca's aphasics is only a matter of overcoming an elevated threshold in speech initiation.

The findings of Goodglass et al. (11) are consistent with the results of a more recent computer-aided analysis of the speech prosody in Broca's aphasia. As Danly and Shapiro (7) report, Broca's aphasics exhibit a different timing pattern in reading tasks than do normal controls. In normal speech, the mean duration of words in sentence final position is longer than of words in sentence initial position. Contrary to the normal lengthening of words in the final position, there is an increased mean duration of words in the nonfinal position in Broca's aphasia. Since increased duration is the acoustic correlate of stress, Broca's aphasics may be said to give additional stress to words already stressed. Whether such segmental lengthening is the manifestation of deficits in syntactic planning or the result of difficulties in maintaining the flow of speech cannot be determined unequivocally. However, other prosodic deviations support the assumption that prosodic impairments are attributable to disorders in syntactic organization.

The fundamental frequency (F_0) values tend to decrease throughout the course of an utterance. This gradual tapering off from the initial to the final word of the utterance is referred to as F_0 declination. When reading syntactically simple sentences with only two F_0 peaks, Broca's aphasics were able to produce normal F_0 declination slopes; as soon as the sentences are more complex and contain at least three F_0 peaks, however, little declination was observed. A closer examination of individual performance revealed a correlation between F_0 declination slope and degree of language impairment as measured by an agrammatism index; steeper declination slopes were produced by the less agrammatic subjects.

Depending on the length of a sentence, a new declination line is initiated after a major syntactic boundary. This prosodic phenomenon is known as F_0 resetting. Broca's aphasics made more frequent use of F_0 resetting; they broke sentences into smaller units than normals. Furthermore, they did not distinguish between grammatic structures by variations in the amount of resetting, as do normals.

Longer sentences are noticed to begin with a higher first peak in normal speech. In order for the first peak to be high enough the entire sentence must be preplanned at some low level of processing. No such differences between long and short sentences were manifested in sentences read by Broca's aphasics.

As soon as the utterance has a more complex syntactic structure, properties of F_0 are impaired in Broca's aphasia; to a limited extent, this is also true of Wernicke's aphasics in reading tasks (8). In general, Wernicke's aphasics are able to produce the skeletal forms of sentences, which dictate intonation patterns. These skeletal structures may be filled by neologisms and semantic and phonemic paraphasias, but the intonational specifications are preserved (9).

The lengthening of nonfinal words observed in Broca's aphasia could also be explained in terms of a reduction of laryngeal muscle control rather than as the manifestation of deficient syntactic programming. If pulmonary air necessary for producing variations in F_0 were lacking because of the longer phonation times needed, a correlation between sentence length and range of intonation would be expected. The fact that Ryalls (19) did not find such a correlation suggests that the physiologic aspects of intonation and the properties of F_0 signaling syntactic organization must be separated.

In summary, tasks that require the recognition and identification of intonation contours, pitch, and stress demonstrate quantitative differences in performance between aphasic subgroups. These differences reflect the severity of the language disorder. Measurement of various properties of F_0 in speech production reveals qualitative differences between Broca's and Wernicke's aphasia. These differences appear to be associated with language disturbances characteristic of the particular aphasic syndrome.

REFERENCES

1. Blumstein, S., and Goodglass, H. (1972): The perception of stress as a semantic cue in aphasia. *J. Speech Hear. Res.*, 15:800–806.
2. Blumstein, S., and Cooper, W. E. (1974): Hemispheric processing of intonation contours. *Cortex*, 10:154–168.
3. Borchgrevink, H. B. (1981): Prosody and musical rhythm are controlled by the speech hemisphere. In: *Music, Mind, and the Brain*, edited by M. Clynes, pp. 151–157. Plenum, New York.
4. Carmon, A., and Nachshon, I. (1971): Effect of unilateral brain damage on perception of temporal order. *Cortex*, 7:410–418.
5. Cutler, A., and Foss, D. I. (1977): On the role of sentence stress in sentence processing. *Lang. Speech*, 20:1–10.
6. Dagge, M. (1982): *Der Einfluss des Wortakzentes beim Erkennen der lexikalischen Bedeutung von Wörtern*. MD dissertation, RWTH Aachen.
7. Danly, M., and Shapiro, B. (1982): Speech prosody in Broca's aphasia. *Brain Lang.*, 16:171–190.
8. Danly, M., Cooper, W. E., and Shapiro, B. (1983): Fundmental frequency, language processing, and linguistic structure in Wernicke's aphasia. *Brain Lang.*, 19:1–24.
9. Duchan, J. F., Stengel, M. L., and Oliva, J. (1980): A dynamic phonological model derived from the intonational analysis of a jargon aphasic patient. *Brain Lang.*, 9:289–297.
10. Gensior, M. (1982): *Der Einfluss der satzsemantischen Bedeutung auf die Identifikation von Satzintonationen*. MD dissertation, RWTH Aachen.
11. Goodglass, H., Fodor, I., and Schulhoff, C. (1967): Prosodic factors in grammar—evidence from aphasia. *J. Speech Hear. Res.*, 10:5–20.
12. Goodglass, H., and Calderon, M. (1977): Parallel processing of verbal and musical stimuli in right and left hemispheres. *Neuropsychologia*, 15:397–407.
13. Haggard, M. P., and Parkinson, A. M. (1971): Stimulus and task factors as determinants of ear advantages. *Q. J. Exp. Psychol.*, 23:168–177.
14. Hartje, W., Willmes, K., and Weniger, D. (1984): Is there parallel and independent hemisphere processing of intonational and phonetic components of dichotic speech stimuli? *Brain Lang. (in press)*.
15. Heilman, K. M., Scholes, R., and Watson, R. (1975): Auditory affective agnosia. *J. Neurol. Neurosurg. and Psychiatry*, 38:69–72.
16. Jackson, H. (1931): *Selected Writings of John Hughlings Jackson, Vol. 2*, edited by J. Taylor, pp. 129–145. Hodder and Stoughton, London.
17. Ross, E. D. (1981): The aprosodias. Functional-anatomic organization of the affective components of language in the right hemisphere. *Arch. Neurol.*, 38:561–569.
18. Ross, E. D., Harney, J. H., de Lacoste-Utamsing, Ch., and Purdy, Ph. D. (1981): How the brain integrates affective and propositional language into a unified behavioral function. *Arch. Neurol.*, 38:745–748.
19. Ryalls, J. H. (1982): Intonation in Broca's aphasia. *Neuropsychologia*, 20:355–360.
20. Schlanger, B., Schlanger, Ph., and Gerstman, L. (1976): The perception of emotionally toned sentences by right hemisphere-damaged and aphasic subjects. *Brain Lang.*, 3:396–403.
21. Schulhoff, C., and Goodglass, H. (1969): Dichotic listening side of injury and cerebral dominance. *Neuropsychologia*, 7:149–160.
22. Swinney, D. A., Zurif, E., and Cutler, A. (1980): Effects of sentential stress and word class upon comprehension in Broca's aphasia. *Brain Lang.*, 10:132–144.
23. Tucker, D., Watson, R. T., and Heilman, K. M. (1977): Discrimination and evocation of affectively intoned speech in patients with right parietal disease. *Neurology*, 27:947–950.
24. Van Lancker, D., and Fromkin, V. (1973): Hemispheric specialization for pitch and "tone": Evidence from Thai. *J. Phonetics*, 1:101–109.
25. Wechsler, A. (1973): The effect of organic brain disease on recall of emotionally charged versus neutral narrative texts. *Neurology*, 23:130–135.
26. Weintraub, S., Mesulam, M., and Kramer, L. (1981): Disturbances in prosody. A right hemisphere contribution to language. *Arch. Neurol.*, 38:742–744.

27. Weniger, D. (1978): The recognition of stress patterns as a lexical and syntactic cue. Presented at the 16th Annual Meeting of the Academy of Aphasia, Chicago.
28. Weniger, D. (1979): The influence of prosodic features in language comprehension in aphasic patients. In: *Hearing Mechanisms and Speech*, edited by O. Creutzfeld, H. Scheich, and Chr. Schreiner, pp. 406–413. Springer-Verlag, Berlin, Heidelberg, New York.
29. Yamadori, A., Osumi, Y., Masuhara, S., and Okuto, M. (1977): Preservation of singing in Broca's aphasia. *J. Neurol. Neurosurg. Psychiatry*, 40:221–224.
30. Zurif, E., and Mendelsohn, M. (1972): Hemispheric specialization for the perception of speech sounds: The influence of intonation and structure. *Perception Psychophysics*, 11:329–332.

Advances in Neurology, Vol. 42: Progress in Aphasiology, edited by F. C. Rose.
Raven Press, New York © 1984.

Aphasia with Exclusively Consonant–Vowel Recurring Utterances: Tan-Tan Revisited

Ria de Bleser and Klaus Poeck

Department of Neurology, RWTH Aachen, D-5100 Aachen, West Germany

In a small subgroup (roughly 2%) of aphasic patients, language production is restricted to fluent concatenations of one consonant-vowel (CV) syllable. Examples for German-speaking aphasic patients are *di-di-di-di*... or *mä-mä-mä*.... This is the language production described by Paul Broca (4) in his well-known patient Leborgne, whose recurring utterance (6) was the nasalized French CV syllable *tan* (tã).

Patients with this stereotyped form of recurring utterances are commonly thought to belong to the subgroup of Broca's aphasia (1), an impression based on Broca's original comment that Leborgne understood everything said to him. Furthermore, most of these patients maintain turn-taking conventions relatively well, and they seem to produce their strings of CV syllables "with meaningful modulation or intonation" (5). In summary, the clinical perception is that these patients have good comprehension and are able to convey communicative intentions by means of suprasegmental features.

Formal testing, however, shows that these patients have no language systematic features left, either in comprehension of spoken and written speech or in oral and written production. When the test results are analyzed, CV patients are qualitatively and quantitatively distinguished from Broca's aphasics (Table 1). Except for the fluent output (2), their extremely poor performance places them at the bottom of the category of global aphasics (see Table 1). Consequently, we have suggested (7) that global aphasia be subdivided into standard nonfluent (who make up about one-third of our aphasic population) and nonstandard fluent global aphasia. The discrepancy between the extremely low test scores and the clinical impression that communicative ability is preserved by means of prosody led us to examine the alleged variability of pitch in the production in nine patients with CV-recurring utterances and its perception in one patient.

PATIENTS AND METHODS

We formally tested 12 patients with global aphasia restricted to CV production. Of these, nine patients were selected for the present study; three were excluded because of concomitant dysarthria, which would have confounded the analysis of

TABLE 1. *Aachen Aphasia Test (AAT) results of CV patients, standard globals, and Broca's aphasics*

Sample population	Statistic	ALLOC classification[a]		Spontaneous speech ratings (0–5)[b]						Percentile ranks on AAT subtests[c]				
		Global	Broca	Comm	Art/Pros	Aut	Sem	Phon	Syn	TT	Rep	Writ	Name	Comp
CV patients	Median	100	0	0	3	0	0	0	0	13	3	8	9	15
(*N* = 8)	Range	100	0	0	2–5	0	0	0	0	6–29	2–15	8–27	8–22	1–24
Standard globals	Median	100	0	0	2	1	1	1	0	13	9	8	10.5	15
(*N* = 32)	Range	79–100	0	0–2	0–5	0–4	0–3	0–4	0–2	0–37	2–27	8–44	9–41	1–41
Broca's	Median	0	97	3	2	4	3	2	2	52	46	45	58	65
(*N* = 15)	Range	0–17	74–100	1–3	2–3	0–5	1–4	2–5	1–4	53–95	13–72	20–78	18–83	30–91

[a]ALLOC, Nonparametric discriminant analysis program for *a posteriori* allocation of patients to one of the standard aphasic syndromes on the basis of AAT test results.

[b]Rating scales are abbreviated as follows: Comm, verbal communication; Art/Pros, articulation and prosody (both aspects are rated on one scale because, as a rule, dysarthria causes dysprosody); Aut, automatic speech elements; Sem, semantics; Phon, phonology; Syn, syntax.

[c]AAT subtests are abbreviated as follows: TT, token test; Rep, repetition; Writ, written language (reading and writing); Name, confrontation naming; Comp, auditory and reading comprehension.

TABLE 2. *Sample characteristics*

Patient no.	CV syllable	Sex	Age at onset (years)	Interval onset-AAT (months)	Interval onset-CT (months)
1	do:	M	51	2	2
2	do:	F	49	2	2
3	vaɪ	F	63	3	1
4	da	M	71	(AAT not available)	(CT not available)
5	dɪ	M	61	2	22
6	ma	M	67	4	2
7	ga	M	49	19	19
8	ta	M	69	10	10
9	mæ:	M	74	1	16

TABLE 3. *Major pitch types in CV recurring utterances*[a]

	Length 1		Length 2			Length 3			Length 4	Length 5
Patient	/	–	‾ _	_ ‾	– –	_ ‾ _	_ ‾ ‾	‾ – _	– – – –	︶︶︶︶︶
1[b]			40	29						
2			38	31	31	29	29			
3[b]	36	44						42		
4	22	78						33		
5[b]					100				53	
6										40

[a]Percent of tokens in major pitch types.
Only those pitch types with more than 20% of tokens were included.
[b]Stereotyped pitch.

prosody. The etiology was vascular in all cases. All patients had lesions limited to the left hemisphere, as assessed by computerized tomography (CT) scan, and were right handed. The examination was performed at least 4 weeks after onset, when the aphasia was stable. Sample characteristics are given in Table 2.

Two raters transcribed the pitch characteristics of the spontaneous speech produced by each patient in a semistandardized interview. Units of analysis were the CV syllables between two clear pauses; the rationale for this procedure is discussed elsewhere (3). If the impression of communicative adequacy were correct, the patients would have to show variability of pitch sufficient to convey different intentions. If, on the other hand, the prosodic features were as stereotypic as the sounds carrying them, the view that communicative ability is preserved in these patients could not be upheld.

The number of CV syllables strung together between pauses was quite stereotypic for each patient. The most frequently produced length types were analyzed observing the following pitch features: rising, falling, high, mid, and low level, rise-fall, and fall-rise. The perceptual analysis was done in six patients. The output of

TABLE 4. *Classification German–non-German*

Stimulus sentences	Language
1. Der Junge sieht das Fräulein.	German
2. Ottokonokowa onnao mimasu.	Japanese
3. Le garçon voit la jeune fille.	French
4. Liest der Vater ein Buch?	German
5. Boy, see that young girl!	English
6. Chichiwa uchini imasu.	Japanese
7. Näht das Mädchen die Puppe?	German
8. Der Vater liest ein Buch.	German
9. The girl sews the doll.	English
10. Junge, sieh das Fräulein!	German
11. La fille coud la poupée?	French
12. Naait het meisje de pop?	Dutch
13. Ottokonokowa onnao mimasu.	Japanese
14. Dodo dodo dodo.	CV–Rec.utt.
15. Chichiwa uchini imasu.	Japanese
16. Dodo dodododo?	CV–Rec.utt.
17. Vater, lies ein Buch!	German
18. Dodododododo?	CV–Rec.utt.

TABLE 5. *Classification German–non-German: Reactions by pointing to one of two cards and by nonverbal expressions*

	Pointing		Nonverbal expressions		
Stimulus number	G	NG	Definitely yes	Doubt	Definitely no
German stimuli (*N* = 6)					
1	X		X		
4	X		X		
7		X	X		
8	X		X		
10	X			X	
17	X		X		
Non-German stimuli (*N* = 12)					
2	X				X
3	X			X	
5	X			X	
6	X			X	
9		X		X	
11		X		X	
12	X			X	
13	X			X	
14	X			X	
15		X		X	
16	X			X	
18		X		X	

TABLE 6. *Judgment of seven rising (question) versus ten falling (declarative) pitch contour by pointing to one of two cards*

Pitch contour[a]	Pointing reaction[b]		Facial expression		
	⊡	[?]	Certain	Uncertain	Indecisive
1. 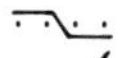	⊕		+		
2. 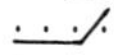		⊕	+		
3. 	-	-			+
	⊕		+		
4. 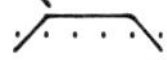		+	+		
5. 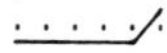	+			+	
6. 	⊕		+		
7. 		⊕	+		
8. 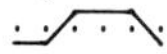	⊕			+	
9. 		+	+		
10. 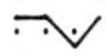	+		+		
11.	⊕			+	
12. 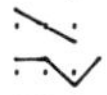		⊕	+		
13. 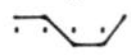	-	-			+
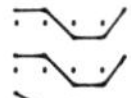	+		+		
14. 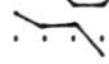		+	+		
15. 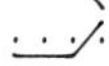	-	-			+
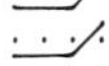	+		+		
16. 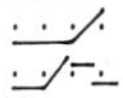	⊕		+		
17. 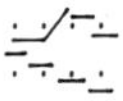		+	+		

[a]Syllable structure was constructed by concatenations of /əm/ in stimuli 1 to 10, by /dɪ/ in stimuli 11 to 17. Stimuli were repeated when there was no pointing reaction, and the facial expression was indecisive.
[b]Correct reactions are encircled.

the three remaining patients was clearly stereotypic with respect to pitch movements. A detailed analysis was not possible by ear, however, because of the extremely long length of recurring utterances; it would have had to be performed by means of a computer. We established a type token ratio for pitch. Using a chi-square statistic, we determined if the different pitch characteristics used were uniformly distributed in each patient.

RESULTS

Table 3 shows the major pitch types in the preferred length of utterance for each of the six patients analyzed. It is evident from Table 3 that level pitch in its high, mid, or low variety is the most frequently used. Pitch is monotonous only in patient 5, with a concatenation of midlevel in 100% of utterances of length 2 and in 53% of utterances of length 4. The minor degree of monotony of the other patients could contribute to the impression of prosodic variability, which is interpreted by the partner as a means of conveying speech intentions. Prosodic variability, however, was present only in half the patients, as shown in Table 3. Since we had excluded three patients from the analysis for lack of variability, we concluded that two-thirds of our patients are stereotypic with respect to pitch, although they are not monotonous.

On the other hand, the impression of communicative adequacy could arise from the preserved receptive ability of the patients to identify the partner's prosodic features. This receptive communicative ability does not necessarily coincide with comprehension as assessed by formal aphasia testing, which examines semantic and syntactic elements. We studied one patient with two tasks. The first examined the ability to identify the native, as opposed to a foreign, language and recurring utterances (Table 4); the second examined whether the patient could distinguish falling from rising intonation contours, i.e., declarative from interrogative sentences. In each task, the patient's answer was requested by having him point to one of two cards. The reactions were videotaped and the accompanying facial and gestural reactions transcribed in order to assess the spontaneous response in addition to task requirements.

The results are shown in Tables 5 and 6. In the first task, the patient's facial and gestural expressions indicated that he could, in fact, distinguish between German and non-German stimulus sentences, even though his pointing reactions were incorrect. In contrast, in the second task, exploring his receptive processing of declarative or interrogative prosodic contours, his pointing reactions were random, while his facial expression showed that he considered his answer to be correct.

DISCUSSION

These findings indicate that our CV patients did not display sufficient prosodic variability to convey communicative intentions. The findings in one patient did not suggest that he could perceive such prosodic variability as would have helped him to identify the communicative intention of the partner. The maintained turn-taking conventions do not express meaningful communicative exchange; rather, what is taking place is some kind of pseudodialogue.

Pseudodialogue linked to fluency of speech production is remarkable in a setting of global aphasia. This fluency cannot be attributed to the activity of the right hemisphere, nor can it be related to intrahemispheric locus of lesion, because variability of lesion size and site is identical in standard nonfluent and nonstandard fluent global aphasics (7). In terms of linguistic processing, the fluency of CV patients is indicative of automatic operations. In this respect, they resemble patients with Wernicke's aphasia more than those with standard global aphasia. They are clearly distinguished from Wernicke's aphasics, however, with respect to language systematic means.

The automatic-controlled processing dimension underlies ("feeds") the fluency–nonfluency dimension; both cut across the aphasic syndromes. It is not justified to equate these dimensions with anterior or posterior localization of brain lesion. Rather, they should be discussed only in functional terms.

REFERENCES

1. Albert, M. L., Goodglass, H., Helm, N. A., Rubens, A. B., and Alexander, M. P. (1981): *Disorders of Human Communication, Vol. 2: Clinical Aspects of Dysplasia.* Springer-Verlag, New York.
2. Benson, D. F. (1967): Fluency in aphasia: Correlation with radioactive scan localization. *Cortex,* 3:373–394.
3. de Bleser, R., and Poeck, K. (1984): Analysis of prosody in the spontaneous speech of patients with CV-recurring utterances. Paper presented at the Academy of Aphasia Meeting, Minneapolis, Minn., October, 1983.
4. Broca, P. (1861): Remarques sur le siège de la faculté du langage articulé suivies d'une observation d'aphémie (perte de la parole). *Bull. Soc. Anat.,* 6:330–357.
5. Hécaen, H., and Albert, M. L. (1978): *Human Neuropsychology.* Wiley, New York.
6. Jackson, J. H. (1879–80): On affections of speech from disease of the brain. *Brain,* 11:203–222.
7. Poeck, K., de Bleser, R., and Graf von Keyserlingk, D. (1984): Neurolinguistic status and localization of lesion in aphasic patients with exclusively consonant-vowel (CV-) recurring utterances. *Brain,* 107:199–217.

Advances in Neurology, Vol. 42: Progress in Aphasiology, edited by F. C. Rose.
Raven Press, New York © 1984.

Praxis in Aphasia

Andrew Kertesz

Department of Clinical Neurological Sciences, University of Western Ontario, St. Joseph's Hospital, London, Ontario, Canada N6A 4V2

Apraxia, as defined by Liepmann (11), clinically means impairment of practiced movement not attributable to comprehension deficit or paralysis. Liepmann further differentiated between limb-kinetic, ideomotor, and ideational apraxia, distinctions that became controversial. The most common variety of apraxia encountered in clinical practice is seen in association with aphasia. The nature of this association is an important issue in behavioral neurology and neuropsychology. First, it should be stated that dissociations are often observed, i.e., there are many aphasics who are not apractic. Similarly, apraxia has been described without significant language impairment, and these patients usually have callosal lesions (16). It is important to examine the association as well as the dissociations in order to understand the mechanisms of practiced movements and language.

Liepmann (11) recognized the association of apraxia with aphasia. In fact, he considered some aspects of aphasia, such as the articulatory disturbance, as apractic. He had a series of 42 left and 41 right hemiplegic patients, five aphasics without hemiplegia, and one patient who had apraxia but no aphasia or paralysis (10). His method of testing patients included mostly traditional gestures of threatening, waving, saluting, raising a hand to swear, and throwing a kiss, in addition to transitive movements, such as knocking, pulling a bell, counting out money, catching flies, and imitating an organ grinder. He also used a category of complex movements. Approximately half of his right hemiplegic patients showed definite impairment of movements with their left hand, and some of the others were slow and imprecise. Fourteen of these apractic patients showed severe speech disturbances; of the 21 nonapractic patients, only four had aphasia. There was also an example of a negative dissociation, a man with severe motor and some sensory aphasia who had no apraxia. The author also discussed the opposite dissociation of six nonaphasic right hemiplegics with apraxia. Liepmann refuted the argument that aphasics do not comprehend and therefore cannot perform these movements. He demonstrated a preserved understanding in other ways. For example, he showed that the beginning of the movement was correct or that approximation indicated good comprehension; finally, he used imitation, which precludes the necessity of verbal commands. Liepmann also noted the high frequency of motor aphasia in cases of apraxia and mentioned specifically three sensory aphasics who had no trouble copying movements; these were considered representative of ideational apraxia. He distinguished ideational apraxia on the basis of these movement confusions in contrast to the amorphic movements which were more characteristic of ideomotor apraxia (11).

Alajouanine and Lhermitte (1), who also emphasized the dissociations, showed cases of anarthria, motor aphasia persisting without buccofacial apraxia. They also demonstrated that buccofacial apraxia is not rare in temporal aphasia where there is no anarthria. In effect, they concluded that there was no direct relationship between apraxia and aphasia. Goodglass and Kaplan (4) did not find very good correlation between the language scores and the apraxia but excluded the severely affected patients, which probably contributed to the lowering of correlation.

The relationship of oral or buccofacial apraxia to speech impairment has been an important issue since the time of Liepmann. Nathan (14) called this speech disturbance apraxic dysarthria because of its association with facial apraxia. DeRenzi et al. (3) found that the severity of oral apraxia correlated with the presence of severe phonemic-articulatory disorder and also pointed out that oral apraxia appeared to be independent from limb apraxia in several instances. They confirmed Alajouanine's initial impression that a large number of jargon aphasics had oral apraxia and also presented four cases with severe phonemic-articulatory disorders without oral apraxia.

We have investigated the relationship of apraxia and aphasia functionally and anatomically (6,8). The praxis test has 20 items of the four categories of intransitive movements, such as waving goodbye, transitive movements, such as using a hammer, buccofacial movements, such as blowing out a light, and complex movements, such as folding a paper and placing it in an envelope. The patients were asked to carry out each movement verbally. If there was no response or if only an approximate response was given, the patient was then shown the movement by the examiner and encouraged to imitate in order. To avoid the comprehension problem, we scored the performance on imitation as well as on verbal command equally on a scale of four, with perfect performance receiving three and no performance zero. For eight items, objects were supplied, and the inability to perform with the objects signified ideational apraxia. The initial study (8) used 230 patients. They had the Western Aphasia Battery (WAB) (5) and the praxis test. Twenty-one normal controls and 72 nonaphasic right brain-damaged individuals and 32 nonaphasic left hemisphere-damaged patients were also seen. The patients were grouped into eight categories, and the sum of the language score (aphasia quotient, AQ) was used as a measure of the severity of aphasia.

The findings in this study showed that there is a hierarchical impairment of gesture in aphasia related to severity, type of aphasia, and the category of gesture. Clearly, global aphasics were the most apractic; this was followed by the isolation syndrome and Broca's aphasia. Wernicke's aphasics had less apraxia as a rule, even though their comprehension was worse than that of Broca's aphasics. Transcortical and conduction aphasics had similarly preserved apraxia scores, even though the language components were affected differently among them. Anomic aphasics had mildly impaired praxis but not quite as good as the right hemisphere group; they were different from controls mostly in the complex, bimanual movements. One of the more interesting findings was that the left hemisphere nonaphasic group did slightly better than the right hemisphere control group, which is opposed to the idea of the left hemisphere being diffusely dominant for the performance of skilled movements.

The most difficult category was complex movements. This was followed by transitive movements, then buccofacial movements, and finally intransitive gestures, which were also the most overlearned and had the most symbolic content.

Of all the language scores, comprehension correlated best with gestural impairment in addition to a high correlation with drawing. Facial praxis scores correlated best with measures of verbal output, such as fluency and repetition. This study also showed a high correlation (0.73) between total praxis and severity of aphasia, which is a different conclusion from that of Goodglass and Kaplan (4).

No significant difference was seen between Broca's and Wernicke's aphasics or transcortical motor and transcortical sensory aphasics who were matched for severity. This contradicts the concept of the posterior left hemisphere specificity for complex sequential patterns contrasted with single acts (9). The relatively mild apraxia found with conduction aphasia is somewhat against the prediction that supramarginal gyrus lesions, that usually cause conduction aphasia, will also produce more gestural disturbance.

A recent extension of this study included lesion localization on the computerized tomography (CT) scan. One hundred fifty-two patients were examined in the acute stage and 143 patients 1 year later. The acute stage was defined as less than 45 days and the chronic stage as beyond 330 days. We used the non-brain-damaged controls to establish the cutoff scores for apraxia in this particular study. We then divided the patients according to the severity of apraxia and aphasia, according to a third of the cutoff scores for each category. A contingency table of patients according to the severity of aphasia and apraxia is shown for the acute patients, indicating that apraxia was not observed in nonaphasic patients, and severe apraxia was present only in severe aphasics (Table 1). There were six cases of severe aphasia without apraxia and four cases of moderate apraxia showing only mild aphasia. In one of these cases, a small lesion involved the superior temporal gyrus, producing a severe state of Wernicke's aphasia; the sparing of occipital-parietal to frontal connections explains the good performance on imitation of praxis. In another patient, a small central, cortical-subcortical lesion caused a hemiparesis and severe nonfluent aphasia that was associated with only minor buccofacial errors on the praxis test. The lesion spared the premotor region and also the parietofrontal connections. In four other cases, rather large left hemispheric lesions were present with severe aphasia and sparing of apraxia. Two of these patients showed initial apraxia, which recovered quickly. Two other patients had atypical skull asymmetries, which may relate to bilateral cerebral representation for language and praxis, allowing for greater recovery.

TABLE 1. *Relationship of the severity of aphasia and apraxia in acute and chronic groups*

Aphasia (AQ)	Apraxia (total apraxia score) No Apraxia (>51)	Mild (>33–50<)	Moderate (>17–33<)	Severe (<17)
Acute patients				
Not aphasic (>93.8)	9	—	—	—
Mild (>62–93.7)	44	6	3	—
Moderate (>31–61<)	12	17	4	—
Severe (<30)	4	7	15	31
Chronic patients				
Not aphasic (>93.8)	17	—	—	—
Mild (>62–93.7<)	60	10	1	—
Moderate (>31–61<)	7	11	4	—
Severe (<30)	2	9	13	9

Modified from Kertesz et al. (6).

ANATOMIC CORRELATIONS IN APRAXIA

Few studies document the anatomic aspects of apraxia. Many authors have doubted that apraxia is associated with a lesion in any particular area (2,13). In our study (7), the CT scans were traced on templates by a radiologist independently from the test scores. The lesion size was objectively measured by digitizer program, and a percentage of hemispheric volume was calculated. Lesions were then grouped into small, if they were less than one-tenth of the volume, and large, if they were more than one-third the left hemispheric volume; moderate lesions were between the two. This study indicated that there is significant correlation between lesion size and gestural impairment ($r = 0.39$ in the acute and $r = 0.5$ in the chronic groups, both significant at $p > 0.001$).

The most interesting cases were those where relatively small lesions produced moderate to severe ideomotor apraxia. Seven patients had subcortical infarcts, mostly in the frontal lobe and the anterior half of the periventricular white matter; these are overlapped on Fig. 1. These patients were severe motor aphasics with a right hemiplegia; they performed with their left hand only. There were two other cases with small lesions with more posterior localization. One was in the posterior cerebral artery distribution, and the other had Wernicke's aphasia with a parietal infarct and a supramarginal and angular gyrus lesion, which is similar to the classic localization described by Liepmann and Maas (12).

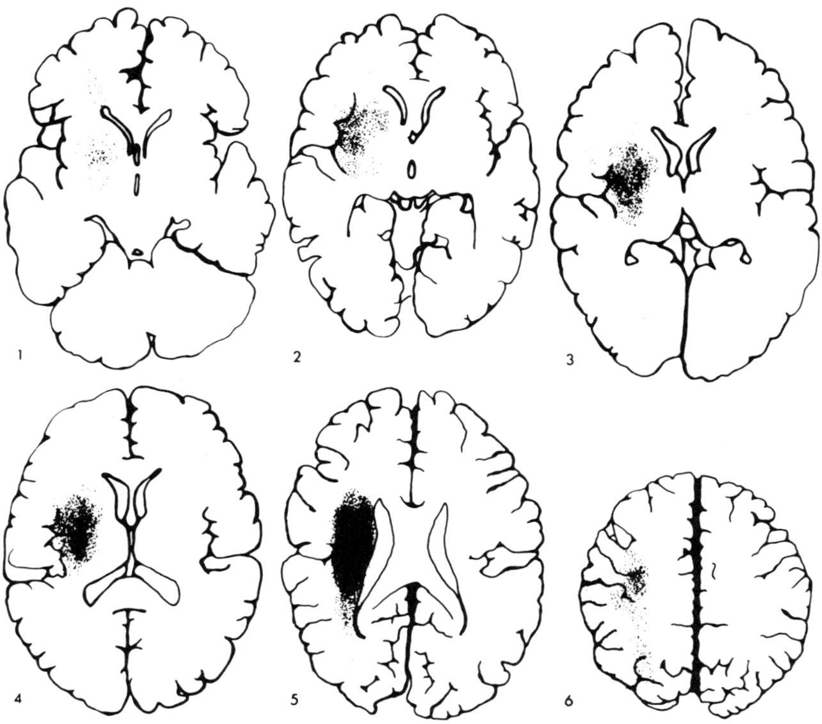

FIG. 1. The small lesions, $N = 7$ (less than 10% of hemispheric volume) that produce apraxia overlapped. 1 to 6, bottom to top. (Modified from Kertesz and Ferro, ref. 7, with permission.)

Patients with large left hemispheric lesions without apraxia were also encountered in substantial numbers. Eighteen percent of acute and 30% of the chronic patients in this study were not apractic. There was a relatively high incidence of uncommon patterns of skull asymmetries (50%), suggesting that this may be related to better recovery in apraxia.

The interaction of lesion size and location is crucial to the understanding of the impaired mechanisms of gesture. It is evident from this study that lesion size alone does not account for all the variability in apraxia scores, and that location of the lesions is also important. The crucial areas that cause a persisting and severe ideomotor apraxia seem to be the anterior half of the periventricular white matter and frontal lobe, which is an area that can disconnect parietofrontal and occipitofrontal connections, as well as temporofrontal connections converging on the prefrontal motor regions. This disconnection prevents the visuokinesthetic information from evoking frontal motor patterns. Previous theories placed much emphasis on the parietal location of lesions producing apraxia, but we had relatively few cases supporting this localization. The specific role of the parietal lobe in forming visuokinesthetic patterns remains to be investigated.

In summary, the association of gesture and language is complex and seems to have an anatomic as well as a functional component. The topographic component may be peculiar to vascular lesions because damage to language and praxis areas are both included in middle cerebral artery territory lesions. The left hemisphere is clearly dominant for praxis mechanisms as well as for language. The amount of dissociation between gestural and language impairment suggests that there is a certain degree of independence of one from the other. In recent studies of sign language, impairment in lesions of the left hemisphere suggests an analogy to aphasic deficits. A recent study observed a separation of the linguistic components of sign language and nonlinguistic gesturing in brain-damaged signers (15). Because of this dissociation of praxis from language disturbance, the possibility of using sign language for aphasics as an alternative communication has a certain practical value. Sign systems that are less abstract and relatively simple, such as the Amerind sign language, seem to be more suitable than the complex linguistic systems taught for the congenitally deaf.

REFERENCES

1. Alajouanine, T., and Lhermitte, F. (1960): Les troubles des activities expressives du langage dans l'aphasie leurs relations avec les apraxias. *Rev. Neurol.*, 102:604–629.
2. Basso, A., Luzzatti, C., and Spinnler, H. (1980): Is ideomotor apraxia the outcome of damage to well-defined regions of the left hemisphere? *J. Neurol. Neurosurg. Psychiatry*, 43:118–126.
3. DeRenzi, E., Pieczuro, A., and Vignolo, L. A. (1966): Oral apraxia and aphasia. *Cortex*, 2:50:73.
4. Goodglass, H., and Kaplan, E. (1963): Disturbance of gesture and pantomime in aphasia. *Brain*, 86:703–720.
5. Kertesz, A. (1982): *The Western Aphasia Battery*. Grune & Stratton, New York.
6. Kertesz, A., Ferro, J., and Shewan, C. M. (1984): Apraxia and aphasia. *Neurology*, 34:40–47.
7. Kertesz, A., and Ferro, J. (1984): Lesion size and location in ideomotor apraxia. *Brain (in press)*.
8. Kertesz, A., and Hooper, P. (1982): Praxis and language. The extent and variety of apraxia in aphasia. *Neuropsychologia*, 20:275–286.
9. Kimura, D., and Archibald, Y. (1974): Motor function of the left hemisphere. *Brain*, 97:337–350.
10. Liepmann, H. (1905): Die linke Hemisphare und das Handeln. *Munch Med. Wochenschr.*, 2:2375–2378.
11. Liepmann, H. (1913): Motor aphasia and apraxia. *Monatsschr. Psych. Neuro.*, 34.
12. Liepmann, H., and Maas, O. (1907): Ein Fall von linksseitiger Agraphie und Apraxie bei rechtsseitiger Lahmung f. *J. Psychol. Neurol.*, 10:214–227.
13. Monakow, C. von (1914): *Die Lokalisation im Grosshirn und der Abbau der Funktionen durch corticale Herde*. Bergmann, Wiesbaden.
14. Nathan, P. W. (1947): Facial apraxia and apraxic dysarthria. *Brain*, 70:449–478.
15. Poizner, H., Bellugi, U., and Iragui, V. (1984): Apraxia and aphasia in a visual-gestural language. *Am. J. Physiol. (in press)*.
16. Watson, R., and Heilman, K. (1983): Callosal Apraxia. *Brain*, 106:391–403.

Advances in Neurology, Vol. 42: Progress in Aphasiology, edited by F. C. Rose.
Raven Press, New York © 1984.

The Language of Dementia

Robert J. Joynt

Department of Neurology, University of Rochester, School of Medicine and Dentistry, Rochester, New York 14642

The first descriptions of Pick's disease in 1892 (13) and Alzheimer's disease in 1907 (2) emphasized the language disturbance as part of the clinical findings. Pick's paper, entitled "On the relation between aphasia and senile atrophy of the brain," contained an extensive section on the language abnormality encountered in a 71-year-old patient: "The patient showed a profound speech difficulty of an apathetic character; speech comprehension is significantly, though not totally, destroyed; simple questions about his general circumstances are understood; other questions he does not understand at all." In concluding, Pick states:

> In observing the speech disorder we lay greatest emphasis on the fact that we are not dealing with a disorder which can be exclusively, or even primarily, attributed to the simple amnestic effects of the senile process, but rather, it more closely parallels those which are the result of focal lesions; it resembles those disorders which Wernicke-Lichtheim described as transcortical sensory aphasia insofar as we could determine that the patient's primary symptoms were a loss of understanding of speech and writing, paraphasia and partially retained ability to repeat speech.

Part of the basis for Pick's report was to emphasize the presence of a focal sign, aphasia, as part of a general process, cerebral atrophy, and to refute the contention of Wernicke that general paralysis of the insane is the only mental disorder that has focal manifestions.

Alzheimer (2) reported the findings of intellectual deterioration in a 51-year-old woman who, in addition to paranoid and aggressive behavior, had a marked language problem, a prominent feature described as follows:

> When shown objects she could name them relatively correctly. However, even her perceptions were extremely disturbed. Immediately after naming the objects she would forget them. She drifted from one line to the next while reading—either enunciating the individual letters or speaking in a meaningless tone. While writing, she repeated single syllables, omitted others, and quickly became confused. She used perplexing phrases when speaking or made paraphasic errors ("milk pourer" instead of "cup"). She would hesitate during speech. She did not understand some questions put to her. She appeared to have forgotten the use of several objects.

Alzheimer went on to describe the structural lesions noted in the brain.

Since these original clinical descriptions of the most well-known presenile dementias, language disorders have always been emphasized, usually under the broad designation of aphasia. Indeed, it is only in recent years that efforts have been made to characterize more accurately the language disorders in dementia; one of the major problems has been the use of the term *aphasia*, which has classically been a focal sign.

Critchley (6), in 1964, asked a critical question: what are we to call the type of speech disorder seen in a patient with brain atrophy but without gross focal lesions? He reviewed and rejected for various reasons the following suggestions: latent aphasia, generalized aphasic difficulty, nonaphasic speech impairment, and pseudoaphasia. In his summary, he recommended the term *dyslogia* but pointed out that Kleist had already employed this term in another context.

The confusion in terminology is symptomatic of the other problems we encounter in the field of dementia and language, particularly highlighted in the past 10 years by the burgeoning interest in the field of dementia. The problems in what I have termed the "language of dementia" center around three points: (a) our changing concept of the underlying defect in dementia, (b) the lack of knowledge about speech in the elderly and what is happening to the normal aging brain, and (c) the inadequate descriptions of the language disturbances in dementia, which is partly related to the variability of the dementing process. It is recognized that dementia is a symptom and may be the end result of a number of illnesses; in general, this discussion centers around Alzheimer's disease, which is by far the most common of the presenile and senile dementias.

The first problem, the structural basis of the disease, poses problems for the classic aphasiologist. Most of the disturbances affecting language have been studied in patients with focal lesions—traumatic, neoplastic, or vascular in origin. In dementia, we are faced with partial or incomplete syndromes defying categorization, which is based on regional and not system involvement. Indeed, when we finally became comfortable with the notion that Alzheimer's disease involved the large cortical neurons, it became obvious that this simple concept has to be abandoned. Neurochemical analysis in recent years has shown a remarkable deficiency in choline acetyltransferase (7), when it was thought that Alzheimer's disease represented a central cholinergic deficit, just as it was first thought that Parkinson's disease was a striatal dopamine deficiency syndrome. In both cases, the explanation has not turned out to be that simple. Other enzymes, neurotransmitters, and neuropeptides have been found to be deficient in Alzheimer's disease. Selective studies of different brain areas have revealed an inordinate loss of nerve cells in the locus ceruleus and basal nucleus of Meynert in brains from patients with Alzheimer's disease. These areas project to the cortex, and Rossor (14) has recently suggested that they constitute a core of nerve cells running through the central neuraxis and projecting to the cerebral cortex without relaying in the thalamus. The destruction of this system (the isodendritic core) in old age may then account for some of the age-related degenerative disorders, such as Alzheimer's disease and Parkinson's disease. Thus the structural basis for language disturbance seen in dementia has no anatomic similarity with other diseases typically used for our present classification and knowledge of the aphasias.

The second problem is our lack of knowledge about the normal changes in speech seen with the aging brain and the basis for this change. Few studies have looked at language in the elderly. Without these normative data, it is dangerous to make statements about language in elderly dements. Martin Albert (1), a student of this area, has emphasized three principal changes noted in his and his colleagues' studies: first, speech discrimination and comprehension fall off; second, discourse becomes more fluent at the syntactic level but less so at the prosodic level; and third, use of the lexicon or store of words is decreased in active usage but not in passive use as word recognition. What is the basis for these changes? Various quantitative studies have shown a decrease in the number of nerve cells with aging, particularly in the superior temporal gyrus (4). Dementia was attributed to an accelerated loss of nerve cells so that, in aging and in dementia, the loss of function was ascribed to loss of nerve cells.

Another intriguing possibility for these changes in aging and dementia is the finding by Buell and Coleman (5) that, while the number of nerve cells decreases with age, there is good evidence of dendritic proliferation in the remaining cells. This suggests that aging may not be a simple decline in function proceeding *pari passu* with cell loss but may be a reorganization with increasing dendritic growth accounting for a different neural network. The result may be a change rather than a decline in neural function. The authors also found that this capacity for dendritic proliferation was absent in Alzheimer's disease. Thus the language changes seen with aging and with dementia do not represent a simple decline in the number of nerve cells but may represent a different neural organization in aging and an incapacity to form these new pathways in dementia. This evidence of plasticity in the aging nervous system suggests new approaches to therapy if the factors enhancing plasticity could be determined.

The third problem is the lack of uniformity of the descriptions of the language disturbances in dementia, which is likely to be related to the variability of the disease. Attempts have been made to single out specific language abnormalities in dementia. Recently, the prevalence of intrusion errors on retrieval of words from semantic memory has been noted in Alzheimer's disease (10); in other words, a word used, which may have been an appropriate answer, often is inappropriately used again and again in later conversation. This phenomenon has also been noted in subjects treated with anticholinergic medication. The word intrusions were found in 90% of patients with Alzheimer's disease but in only 35% of those patients with other forms of dementia. Also, the frequency of intrusions in testing was found to correlate with a low level of choline acetyltransferase and increase of senile plaques in the brain post-mortem. Therefore, one of the language abnormalities noted in Alzheimer's disease appears to correlate with the new neuroanatomy now being revealed with this disorder.

Critchley (6) pointed out some characteristic abnormalities seen in dementia; for example, the demented patient does not hesitate to name an object even though the anomic errors may be severe. The anomia of the aphasic patient is usually characterized by hesitancy and a searching for the correct word. Other language abnormalities seen in dementia were similar to those of the patient with an early sensory or receptive aphasia. Critchley also noted the decrease or absence of appropriate gestures by the demented patient. Benson (3) points out that the aphasia seen with dementia is almost always confined to anomia. Albert (1) suggests that dements with language problems most closely resemble patients with Wernicke's aphasia.

The language disturbance seen in Alzheimer's or Pick's disease has been used for differential diagnosis, but the overlap of specific speech abnormalities is too great for differentiation of the two disorders. Most authors agree that the lack of language disorders in the face of profound dementia is a hallmark of so-called subcortical dementias, as with that accompanying Huntington's disease (8).

The presence or absence of a severe language disturbance accompanying dementia has been used as an indicator of early mortality and of familial occurrence. The presence of an expressive language defect in a group of hospitalized patients with dementia was found to be an excellent predictor of mortality within 1 year of hospitalization (11). In a genetic study, it was found that a dementia syndrome with prominent aphasic or agraphic features suggests a familial disorder (9), and the authors suggested that familial Alzheimer's disease is an entity characterized by a dementia syndrome with prominent aphasia and agraphia.

It is obvious from the above discussion that there is a great variability in the language disorder seen in dementia, from almost none to the most prominent feature of the dementia. Indeed, it appears that an aphasia-like syndrome may be the only manifestation of dementia for many years. At times, the aphasia may be so severe that testing for signs of dementia must be precluded. Mesulam (12) has recently reported the occurrence of a slowly progressive aphasia in six right-handed patients, five of whom started with an anomic aphasia. The patients did develop additional impairments of reading, writing, and comprehension. Four of the six did not develop other signs in the 5- to 11-year follow-up. Computerized axial tomography showed selective degeneration in the left perisylvian area. These cases again emphasize the extreme variability of language disorders in dementia and raise the question of whether or not they are part of a dementing process or a localized, yet progressive, atrophy without dementia.

In conclusion, three problems in the language of dementia have been raised: (a) our present categorization of language disturbances based on focal lesions does not fit the neuroanatomic lesions in dementia; (b) the lack of adequate knowledge about the changes in language with normal aging and the effect of plasticity in the aging nervous system on these changes; and (c) the great variability in the language disorders seen in dementia, which suggests variations in the disease process. The study of language disorders has provided information about focal brain damage, but this has not been the case with the language disorders in dementia; it represents a new challenge for the aphasiologist.

REFERENCES

1. Albert, M. L. (1980): Language in normal and dementing elderly. In: *Language and Communication in the Elderly*, edited by L. K. Obler and L. M. Albert. Lexington Books, Lexington, Massachusetts.
2. Alzheimer, A. (1907): Uber eine eigenartige Erkrankung der Hirnrinde. *Allge. Ztschr. Psych. Psychgerichtlich Med.*, 64:146–148.
3. Benson, D. F. (1979): *Aphasia, Alexia, and Agraphia*. Churchill Livingstone, New York.
4. Brody, H. (1976): An examination of cerebral cortex and brain-stem aging. In: *Neurobiology of Aging*, edited by R. Terry and S. Gershon. Raven Press, New York.
5. Buell, S., and Coleman, P. (1979): Dendritic growth in the aged human brain and failure of growth in senile dementia. *Science*, 206:854–856.
6. Critchley, M. (1964): The neurology of psychotic speech. *Br. J. Psychiatry*, 110:353–364.
7. Davies, P., and Maloney, A. J. (1976): Selective loss of central cholinergic neurones in Alzheimer's disease. *Lancet*, II:1403.
8. Fisher, J., Kennedy, J., Caine, E., and Shoulson, I. (1983): Dementia in Huntington's disease: A cross-sectional analysis of intellectual decline. In: *The Dementias*, edited by R. Mayeux and W. G. Roseau. Raven Press, New York.
9. Folstein, M., and Breitner, J. (1981): Language disorder predicts familial Alzheimer's disease. *Johns Hopkins Med. J.*, 149:145–147.
10. Fuld, P., Katzman, R., Davies, P., and Terry, R. (1982): Intrusions as a sign of Alzheimer dementia: Chemical and pathological verification. *Ann. Neurol.*, 11:155–159.
11. Kaszniak, A., Fox, J., Gandell, D., Garron, D., Huckman, S., and Ramsey, R. (1978): Predictors of mortality in presenile and senile dementia. *Ann. Neurol.*, 3:246–252.
12. Mesulam, M-M. (1981): Slowly progressive aphasia without generalized dementia. *Ann. Neurol.*, 11:592–598.
13. Pick, A. (1892): Uber die Beziehungen der senilen Hirnatrophie zur Aphasie. *Prag. Med. Wochenschr.*, 17:165–167.
14. Rossor, M. N. (1981): Parkinson's disease and Alzheimer's disease as disorders of the isodendritic core. *Br. Med. J.*, 283:1588–1590.

Advances in Neurology, Vol. 42: Progress in Aphasiology, edited by F. C. Rose.
Raven Press, New York © 1984.

Computed Tomography Localization of Standard Aphasic Syndromes

Klaus Poeck, Ria de Bleser, and Diedrich Graf von Keyserlingk

Department of Neurology, RWTH Aachen, D-5100 Aachen, West Germany

The obvious usefulness of computed tomography (CT) scanning for the diagnosis of brain diseases led to the expectation that this method would also lend itself to the clinical localization of brain lesions underlying neuropsychologic syndromes. This approach included two hypotheses: (a) that CT technology was refined enough to permit exact assessment of a brain lesion; and (b) that a given neuropsychologic syndrome is related to only one specific localization of lesion. In this chapter, we show that both these assumptions are only partially confirmed. Consequently, the problems of CT localization in neuropsychology have technical and conceptual aspects.

STANDARDIZATION OF CT LESIONS AND DATA PROCESSING

Obviously, the original CT images are not well suited for research purposes, because they do not permit interindividual comparisons. Interindividual differences exist with respect to the anatomic characteristics of brain shape, size, and macroscopic structure, as well as in the technical aspects of scanning, such as inclination and starting level. Furthermore, it is not possible to subject the original CT data to computerized data processing.

The first problem was met by developing methods of standardization. There are two approaches: the template method (3,7,10) and the lateral diagram (1,16,20). In the template method, the CT lesion is transferred onto schematic horizontal drawings corresponding closely to the CT slices. Orientation is obtained by specific anatomic landmarks, such as the ventricular system, basal ganglia, or sylvian fissure. Thus lesions are brought on the same scale, and their site and size can be assessed across individuals at the expense of individual features. Interindividual comparability is attained at the expense of intraindividual information (Fig. 1).

Lateral diagrams are obtained by transferring the individual CT lesion into a schematic lateral view of the left hemisphere, which approximates most closely the patient's brain (15). The advantage of this approach is that the patient's individual anatomy is considered in the anteroposterior dimension; the drawback is that the lesion can be localized only roughly with respect to intracerebral landmarks.

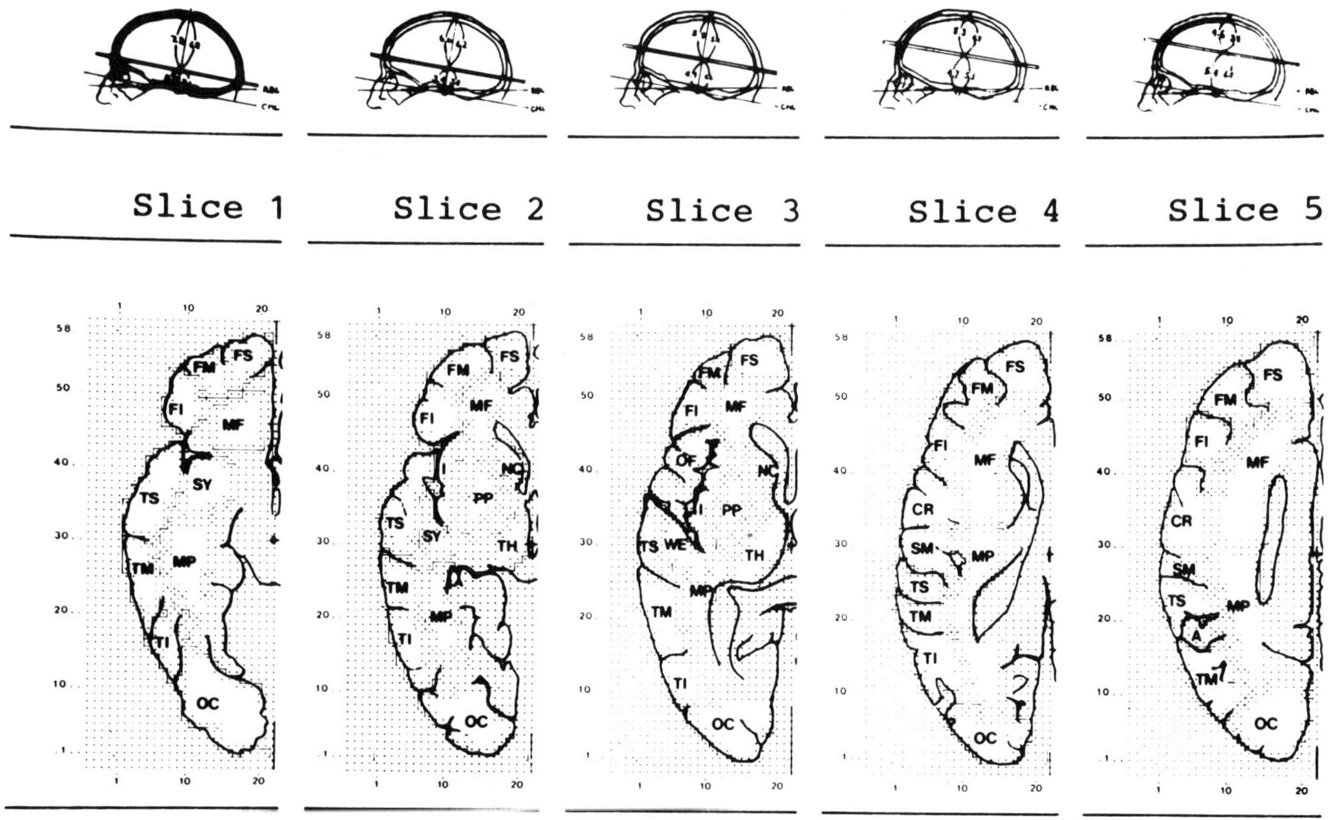
Slice 1
Slice 2
Slice 3
Slice 4
Slice 5
FS
FM
FI
MF
SY
TS
TM
MP
TI
OC
NC
PP
TH
OF
WE
CR
SM
A

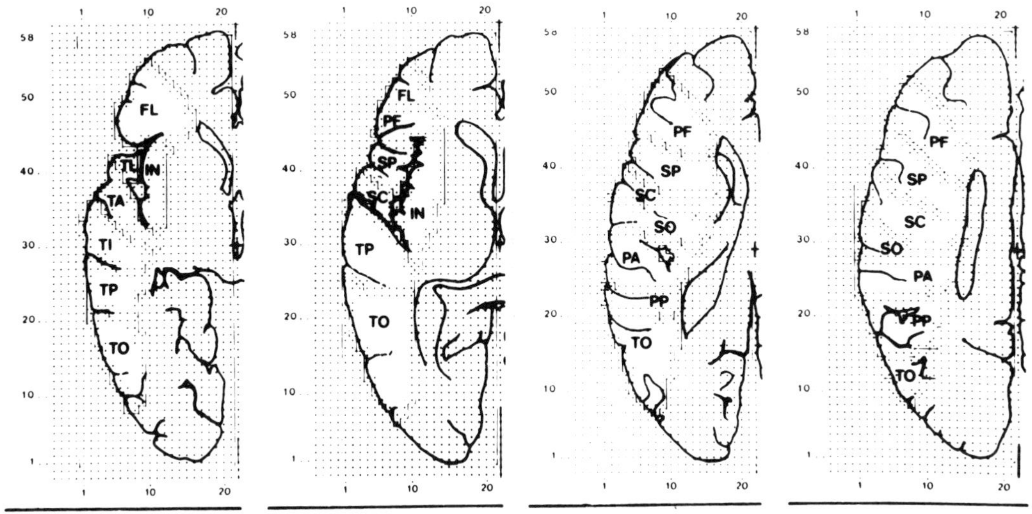

FIG. 1. Standardized templates after Matsui and Hirano, with anatomic landmarks. Lateral views of skull on top indicate level of slice. CML, canthomeatal line; RBL, Reid's baseline. **Top:** (standardized morphologic areas): FS, superior frontal gyrus; FM, medial frontal gyrus; FI, inferior frontal gyrus; OF, frontal operculum; I, insula; MF, frontal white matter; NC, caudate nucleus; PP, putamen and globus pallidus; TH, thalamus; CR, central region; SM, supramarginal gyrus; TS, superior temporal gyrus; WE; Wernicke's area; SI, sylvian fissure; A, angular gyrus; TM, medial temporal gyrus; TI, inferior temporal gyrus; OC, occipital lobe; MP, posterior white matter. **Bottom:** (standardized territories of branches of middle cerebral artery): FL, R. frontobasalis lateralis; PF, R. prefrontalis; SP, R. sulci precentralis (prerolandii); SC, R. sulci centralis (rolandii); SO, R. sulci postcentralis (postrolandii); PA, R. parietalis anterior; PP, R. parietalis posterior with R. gyri angularis; TO, R. temporo-occipitalis; TP, R. temporalis posterior; TI, R. temporalis intermedius; IN, Rr. insulares; TA, R. temporalis anterior; TL, R. temporopolaris.

Moreover, interindividual comparison is constrained by similarity of brain size (Fig. 2).

In the majority of studies cited so far, the standardized lesions have not been transformed into binary matrices which can be processed by computer. This is important if one must work on large amounts of data, as was done by Blunk et al. (3). These authors transferred the lesions manually onto standardized templates in the form of grids, which could then be converted into 1/0 matrices, an entry of "1" indicating a grid point covered by a lesion; "0", the absence of a lesion. Standardized anatomic areas could then be defined as specific sets of grid points for each slice.

This procedure was simplified by Hündgen et al. (8) and Schmachtenberg et al. (21) who used a joy stick to transfer the lesion immediately from the CT onto a grid schema on the automatic evaluation unit. This information is stored as 1/0 entries on a matrix. Also, reduction of lesion information is possible for specific questions. This reduction is achieved by considering only a certain percentage of "1" entries as indicating the presence of a lesion. This is done to avoid the fuzziness of the outer boundaries of a lesion due to incomplete interrater agreement. We decided to judge an area as lesioned if at least 30% of its grid points have an entry of "1". On the basis of matrices with full or reduced information, one can do frequency counts of lesions either for specific anatomic areas or for certain aphasic syndromes (Fig. 3).

The method of standardization described here was used to examine the relationship between standard aphasic syndromes and lesion localization in patients with aphasia caused by ischemic stroke. The first study was based on a total of 70 patients (20 Broca's, 20 Wernicke's, and 30 global aphasics). We did not examine patients with amnesic aphasia because the aphasiologic status of this syndrome is unclear. Also, the syndrome is often observed during the recovery of patients with one of the other standard syndromes.

Absolute frequency counts of lesioned areas per aphasic syndrome using the 30% criterion gave the results illustrated in Fig. 4. The lesioned areas for Wernicke's

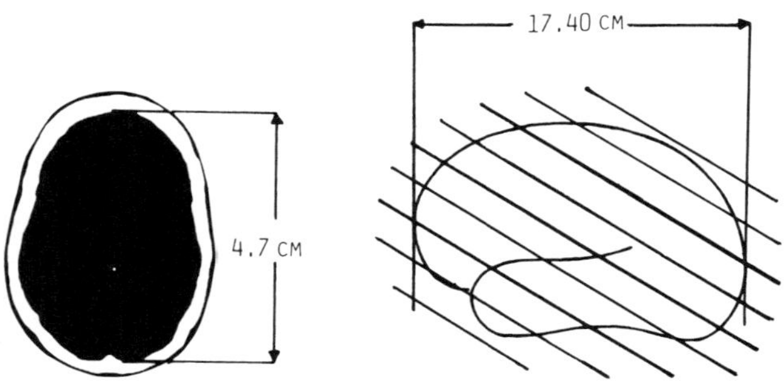

FIG. 2. Lateral diagram, after Luzzatti et al. (15). The maximal anteroposterior diameter of the patient's brain is measured on CT and multiplied by a factor of 3.7. The standardized lateral diagram approximating the patient's brain size most closely is chosen for mapping the lesion. The parallel lines are tracings for the CT scanning sections.

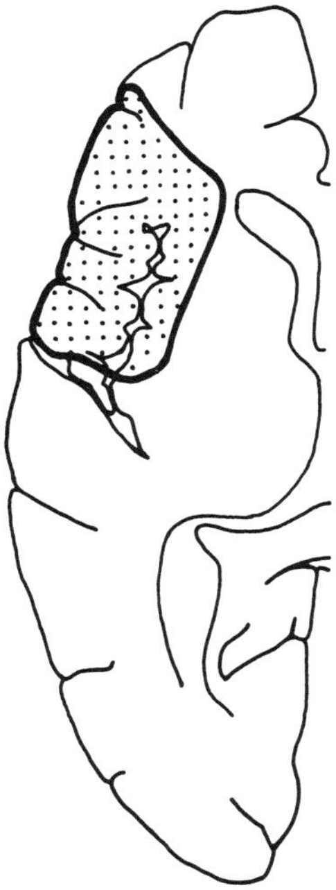

FIG. 3. Standardized lesion in slice 3 of an aphasic patient and corresponding binary matrix, using the 30% criterion. For abbreviations of anatomic regions, see Fig. 1.

and Broca's aphasia were a mirror image of each other but with considerable overlap between the two groups. Overlap occurred mainly in the frontal operculum and insula and in the posterior perisylvian region, including Wernicke's area. In other words, there were patients with Broca's aphasia whose lesion was predominantly in or extended to Wernicke's area, and vice versa.

Since we presupposed at this stage that there should be one typical lesion underlying distinct aphasic syndromes, the overlapping lesions had to be considered "atypical." Consequently, we subtracted the lesions of one syndrome from those of the other and considered the remaining lesioned areas "the typical" lesion for the group (Fig. 5). Lesions of Broca's aphasics rarely involved the foot of the third frontal convolution but characteristically included the rostral insula in slice 3. They reached a peak in the frontal white matter in slice 4, that is, above Broca's area. Wernicke's aphasics had a relatively circumscribed cortical lesion in the superior temporal gyrus, predominantly in Wernicke's area (Fig. 6). Whereas lesion size did not differ significantly for the groups of Broca's and Wernicke's aphasics, patients with global aphasia had significantly larger lesions which, as expected, included the lesions found for Broca's and Wernicke's aphasia. These findings were confirmed in a replication study, which included another sample of 82 patients, 20 with Broca's, 20 with Wernicke's, and two with global aphasia (8,21) (Fig. 7).

An alternative position to the assumption of a direct correlation between an aphasic syndrome and one particular lesion site would accept that lesions of different localization may give rise to the same aphasic syndrome. This view would imply that overlapping lesions should not be eliminated by data processing, but rather

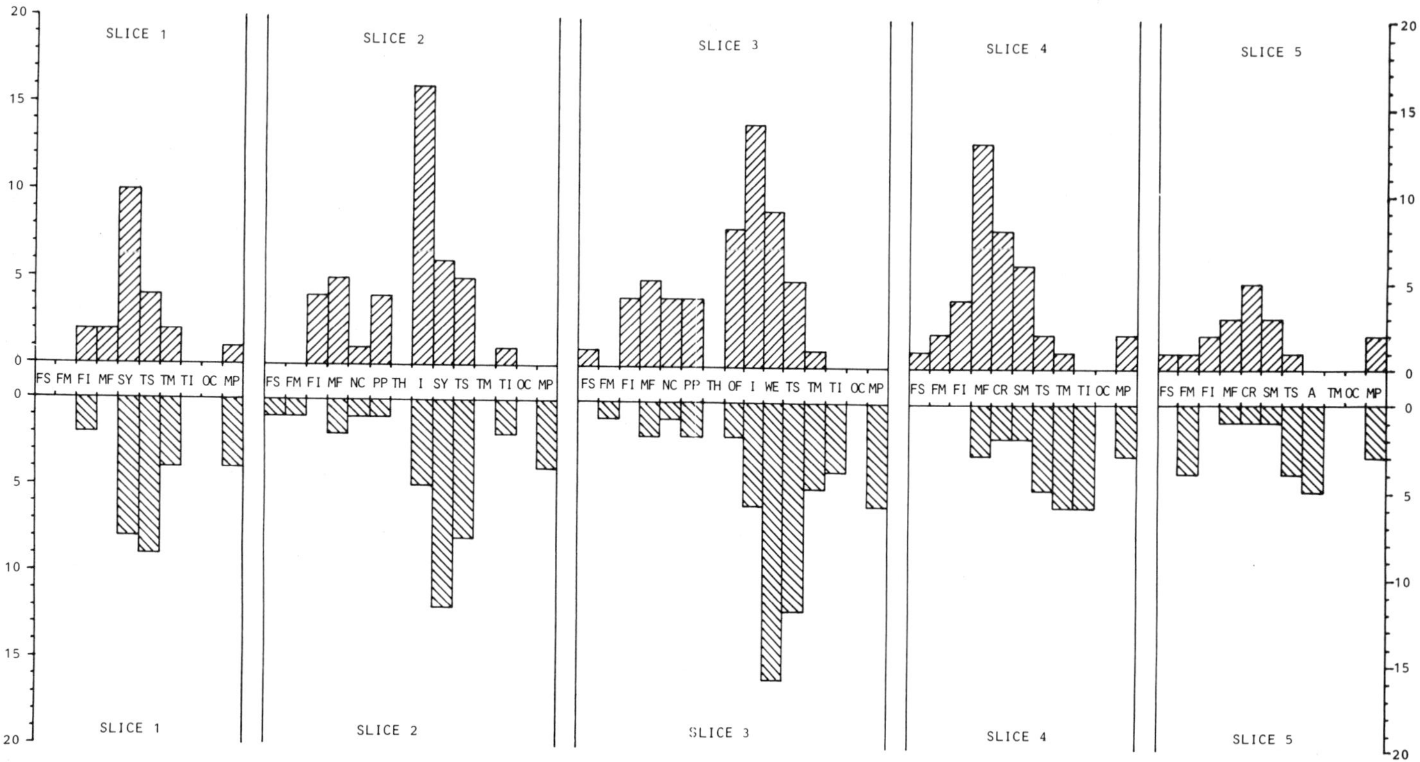

FIG. 4. Lesioned areas for the syndrome of Broca's *(upper)* and Wernicke's *(lower)* aphasia, using the 30% criterion. For abbreviations of anatomic regions, see Fig. 1.

that the individual cases should be studied for possible differences within a group and for similarities across groups.

We have done this first for 32 patients with global aphasia with and without recurring utterances (19). Less than half these patients had the expected large perisylvian lesion, indicating infarction of the entire territory of the middle cerebral artery (Fig. 8). Even those patients with the most severe form of global aphasia who only produced one and the same CV recurring utterance and who have no language systematic elements left, in either production or comprehension, had very different lesion sites and sizes; in other words, they did not have a characteristic "strategically placed lesion," and their lesions were by no means the largest.

A cluster analysis was done on selected patients with Broca's aphasia, Wernicke's aphasia with and without jargon, mixed transcortical and transcortical sensory aphasia, and very severe and moderate global aphasia (6). No cluster of lesions included patients with only one aphasic syndrome. The majority of patients with jargon Wernicke's aphasia were found in the large postrolandic lesion cluster, and the majority of patients with very severe standard global aphasia could be found in the cluster of large perisylvian lesions. Even in those clinical groups the exceptions were remarkable. The remaining five syndromes were distributed over various lesion clusters (Table 1). Lesions restricted to the basal ganglia could give rise to any aphasic syndrome (Table 2).

TABLE 1. *Five-cluster solution for standardized lesions over five slices*

	Lesion clusters				
Patient subgroup	Pre- and postrolandic	Unclassifiable	Small prerolandic	Large postrolandic	Small postrolandic
Global severe (*n* = 7)	6	1			
Mixed transcortical (*n* = 7)		6	1		
Global moderate (*n* = 7)	2	1	2	1	1
Broca (*n* = 7)		2	2	1	2
Wernicke with jargon (*n* = 6)	1			5	
Transcortical sensory (*n* = 6)		4	1	1	
Wernicke without jargon (*n* = 6)		1		2	3
Patients/cluster	9	15	6	10	6

THREE-DIMENSIONAL RECONSTRUCTION OF CT LESIONS

The procedures of CT localization of lesions in aphasic patients described so far presuppose that all brains are alike in size, shape, and internal structure. The similarity of the brains is either tacitly assumed in the evaluation of original CT scans or overtly produced in the idealization of standardization procedures. There is considerable individual variability, however, both in macroscopic anatomy (11) and in the extension of cytoarchitectonic areas (22). These differences are so

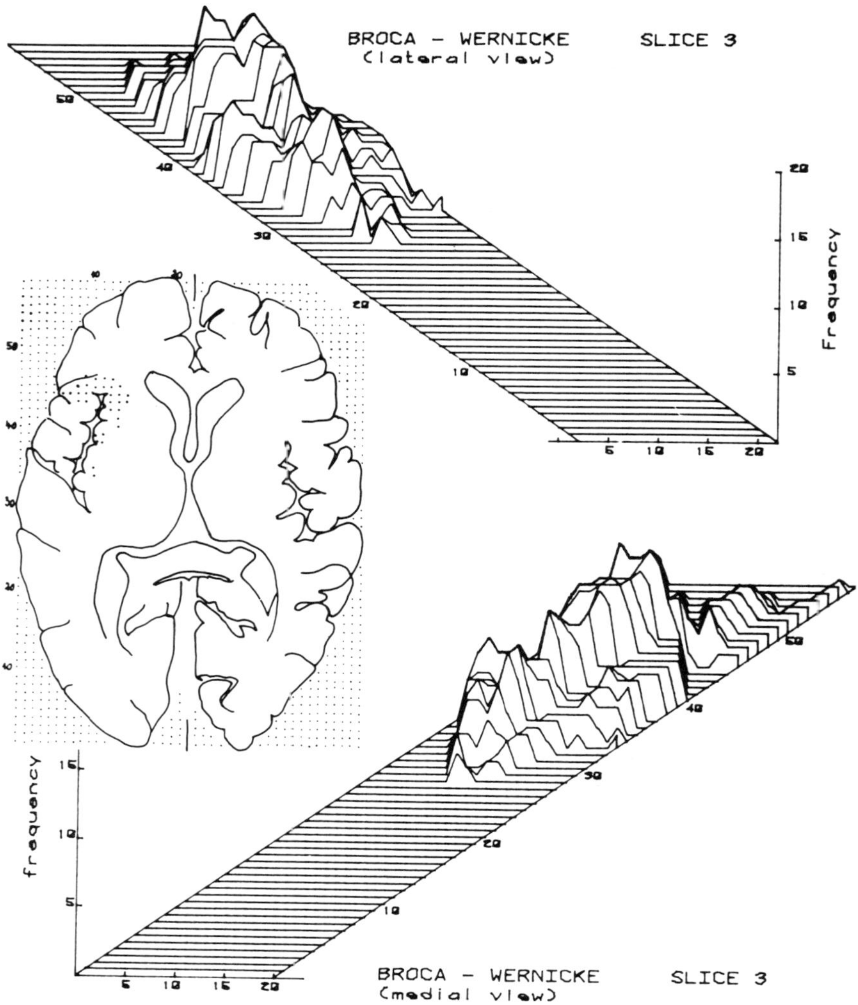

FIG. 5. Broca's aphasia. Subtraction of the absolute lesion points in Wernicke's aphasics from that of Broca's aphasics. The lesion points remaining after subtraction are displayed in the three-dimensional graphics. *Upper*, lateral view; *lower*, medial view. Points of highest frequency were transferred on a two-dimensional slice, thus showing the "typical lesion." **A:** Slice 3 shown here.

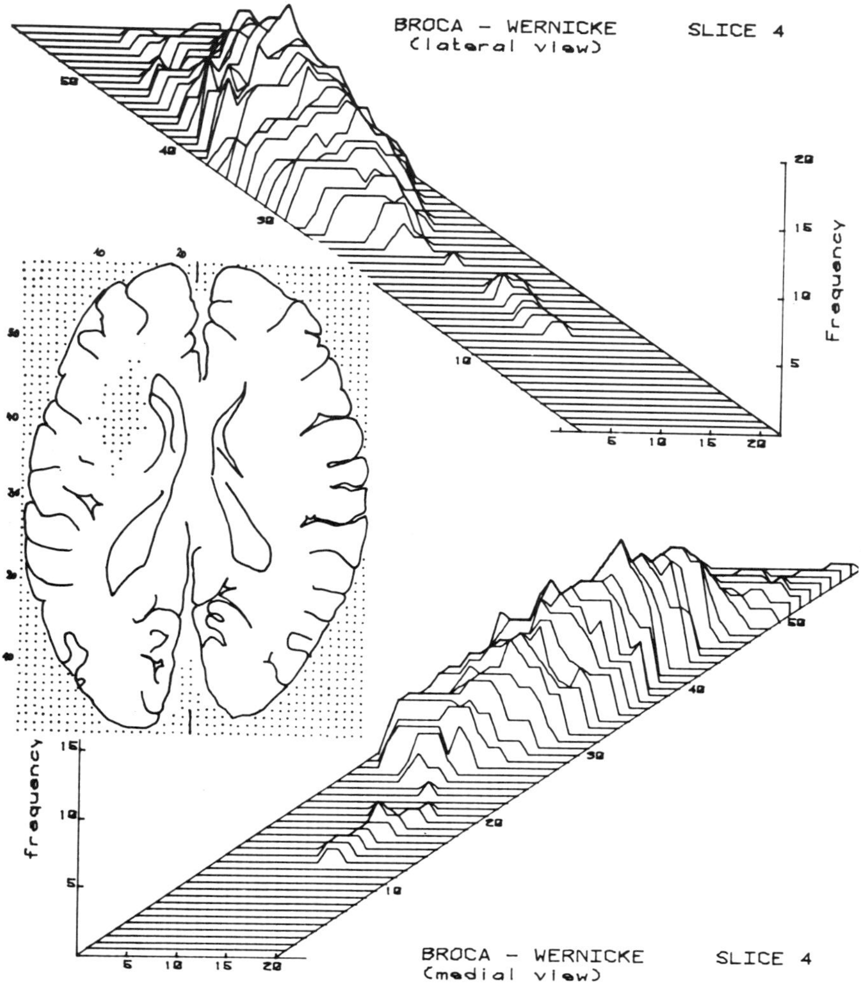

FIG. 5. *(continued)* Broca's aphasia. **B:** Slice 4 shown here.

important that apparently identical CT lesions may actually involve different neighboring structures and the reverse. Methodical limitations of this sort do not play a role with respect to problems like the occurrence of Broca's aphasia with a lesion in Wernicke's area, and vice versa. They should not be ignored, however, if one tries to link, e.g., specific aphasic disturbances to the anterior or posterior putamen (17). Differential localization in neighboring areas cannot be achieved with either of the currently used methods (lateral diagram or template method), because each of these two-dimensional representations covers only one kind of variability, i.e., shape and size or internal structure. In order to assess the lesion in both its "true"

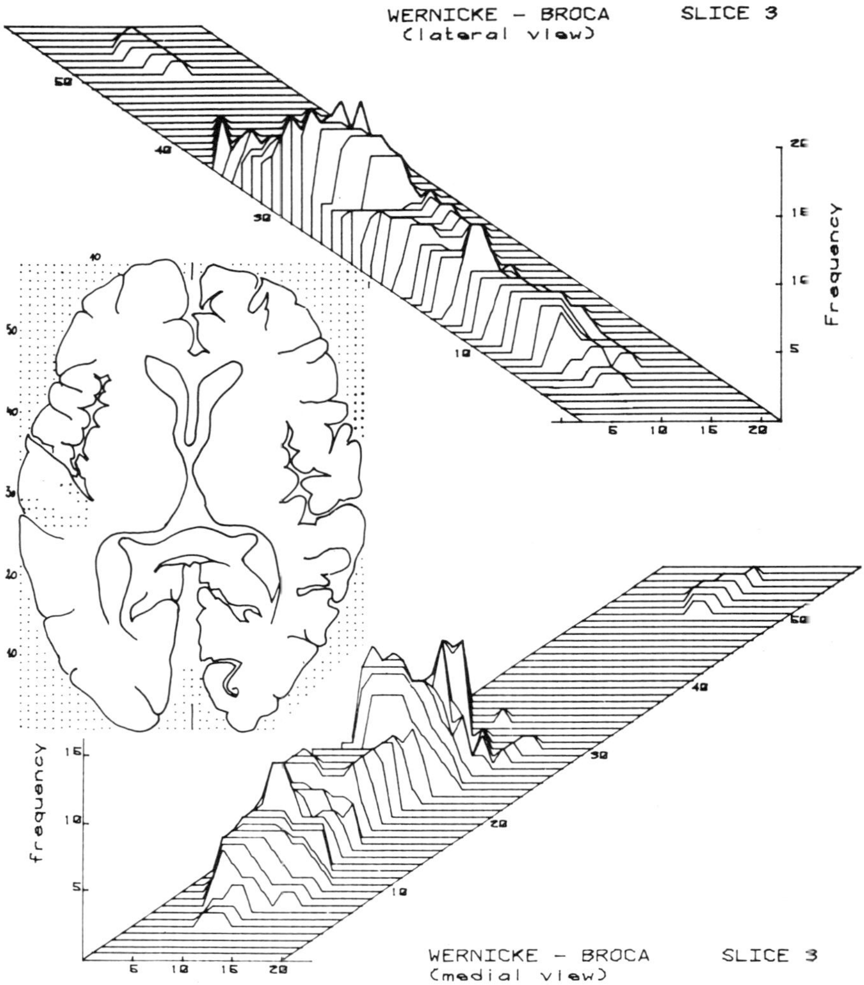

FIG. 6. Wernicke's aphasia, slice 3. Same mode of representation as in Fig. 5, this time Wernicke minus Broca.

size and site and its relation to adjacent structures, a three-dimensional reconstruction of the CT lesion is needed. This method goes beyond merely depicting schematically the CT lesion on a succession of horizontal templates. Rather, it utilizes completely the spatial information contained in series of CT sections. It allows the examination of an object from different points of view by graphic rotation, enlargement, and perspective transformation (Fig. 9).

By means of a computerized data storing and plotting system, brain contours and sulci, as taken from the actual CT series, and the lesion in relation to them can be reproduced as stereopictures. Depending on the problem under study, selective information can be retrieved and used for graphic display. The method

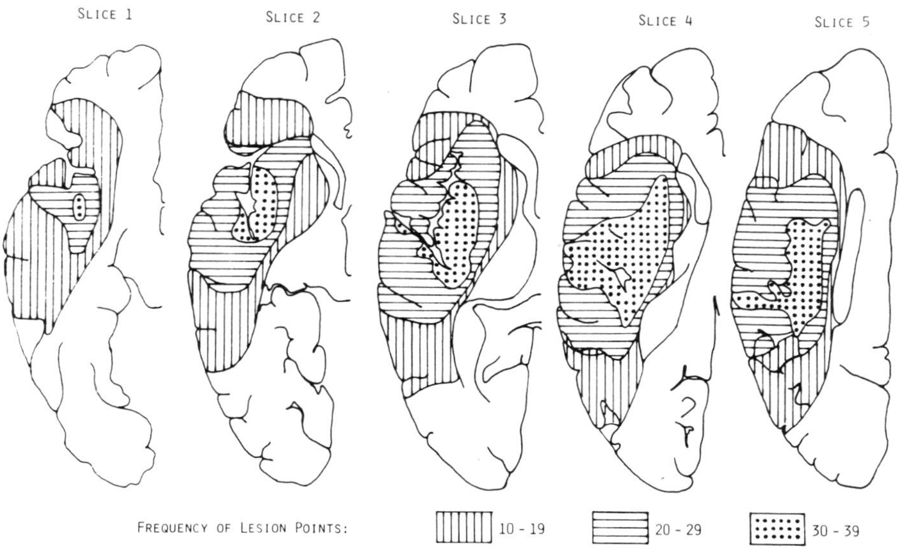

FIG. 7. Absolute frequency of lesion points in 42 patients with global aphasia. Note relatively small extension of regions with highest frequency of lesion points (30 to 39 of the 42 patients). No lesion point is common to all patients.

allows one to produce a maximum amount of individual anatomic information with a minimal amount of noise. Moreover, additional anatomic information, like standardized pial arteries or stylized fiber tracts, can be superimposed onto the reconstructed three-dimensional brain model. The superimposition of different kinds of stored information is not accomplished schematically or automatically; rather, one kind of structure is gradually transposed into the coordinate system of another until the best possible fit is reached (12) (Fig. 10).

LIMITATIONS OF CT LOCALIZATION OF APHASIA

Earlier, we emphasized two sets of problems, one related to CT techniques, the other to the concept of localization in neuropsychology. Even though CT has provided valuable knowledge on the clinical localization of brain lesions, which was impossible to obtain *in vivo* before, one should not ignore its inherent limitations.

A crude but widespread error is to choose too short an interval between onset and CT scan in vascular patients. For practical reasons, it is often impossible to scan the patient 6 weeks post onset, when the lesion is stable. At a technical level are poor control of variables, such as recording artifacts, partial volume effects, and differences in angularization. Small lesions may remain undetected even though they are stable and technical requirements are met. Multiple small lesions of this sort may lead to severe functional impairment. Patients with Alzheimer's disease who have severe semantic/cognitive disorders may have a normal CT scan. This

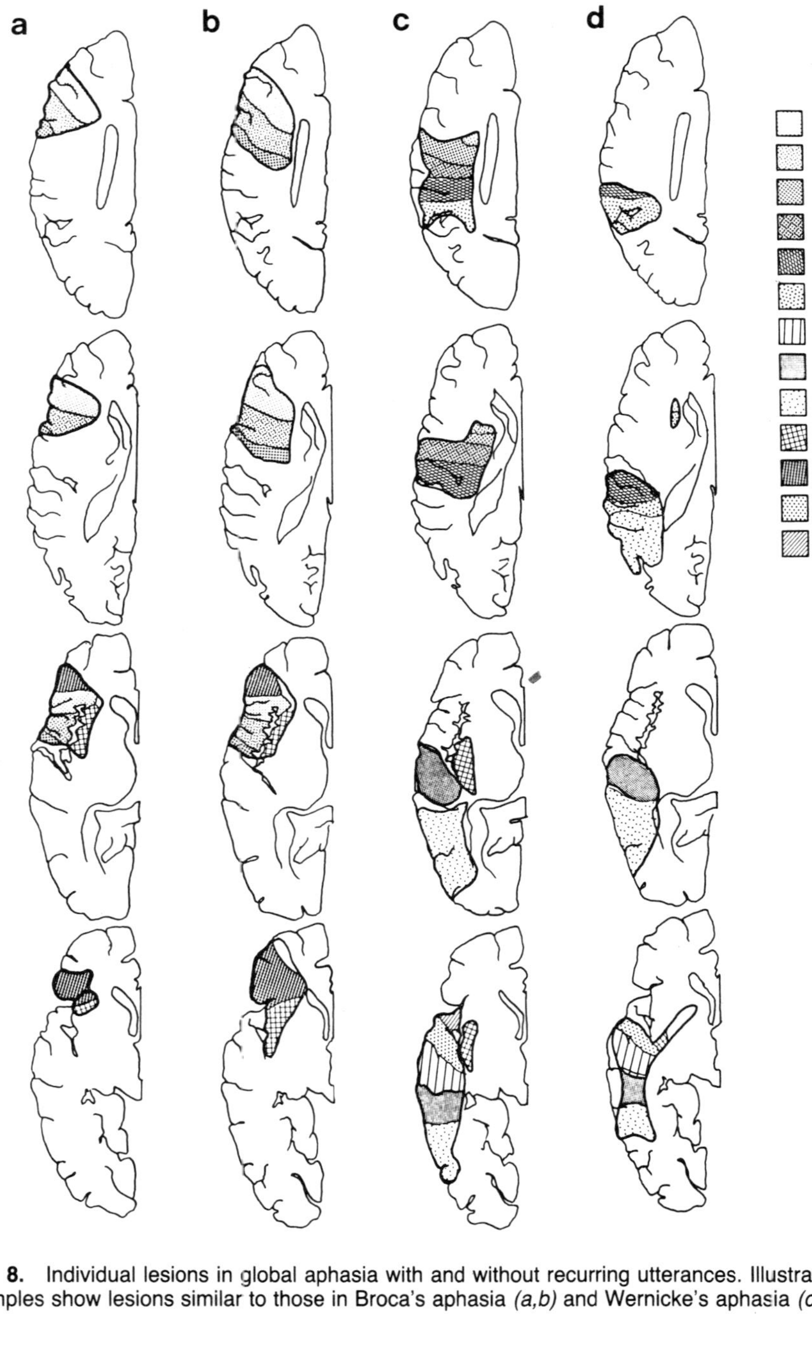

FIG. 8. Individual lesions in global aphasia with and without recurring utterances. Illustrative examples show lesions similar to those in Broca's aphasia *(a,b)* and Wernicke's aphasia *(c,d)*.

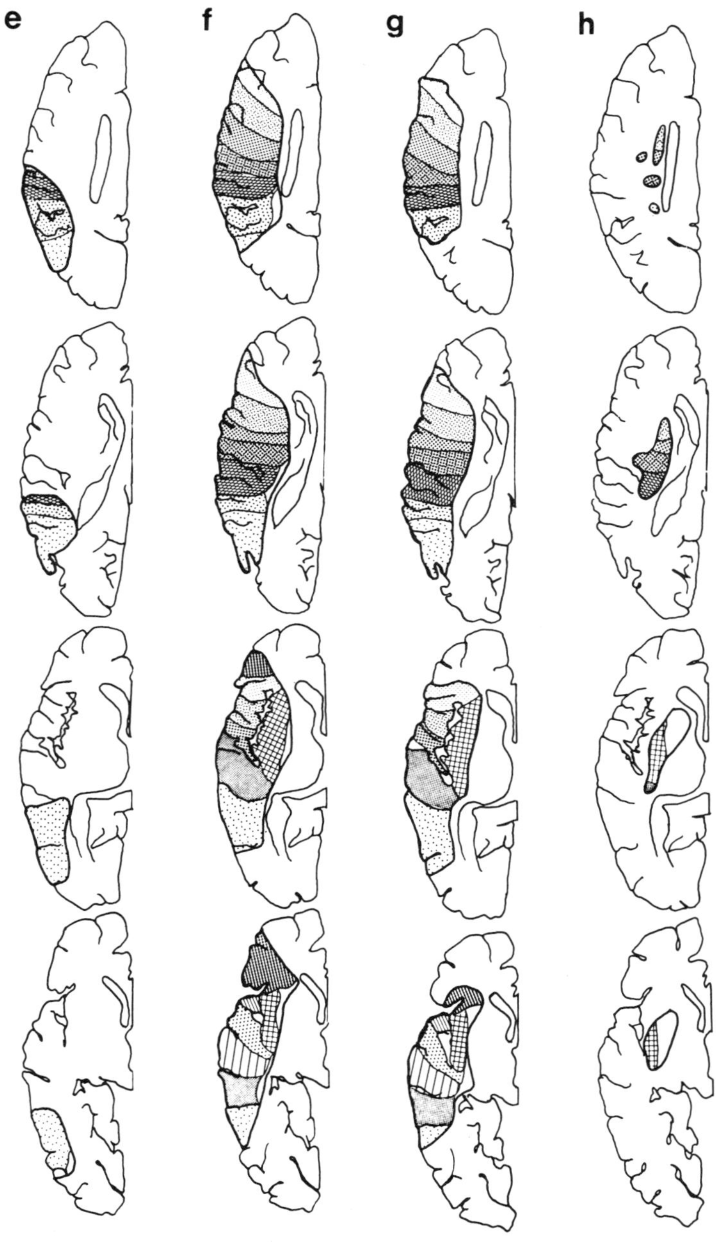

FIG. 8. *(continued)* Individual lesions in global aphasia. Illustrative examples show lesions similar to transcortical sensory aphasia *(e)*, "typical" infarction of middle cerebral artery *(f,g)*, and isolated basal ganglia lesion *(h)*.

TABLE 2. *Basal ganglia lesions and aphasic patients*[a]

	Anterior putamen	Posterior putamen	Global putamen
Global severe		1	
Mixed transcortical	2	1	
Global moderate			1
Transcortical sensory	2		
Wernicke without jargon	1		
Patients/subgroup	5	2	1

[a]Basal ganglia lesions were contained in the unclassifiable lesion cluster (see Table 1) together with small prerolandic lesions and small temporal lobe lesions in which the superior temporal gyrus was not involved.

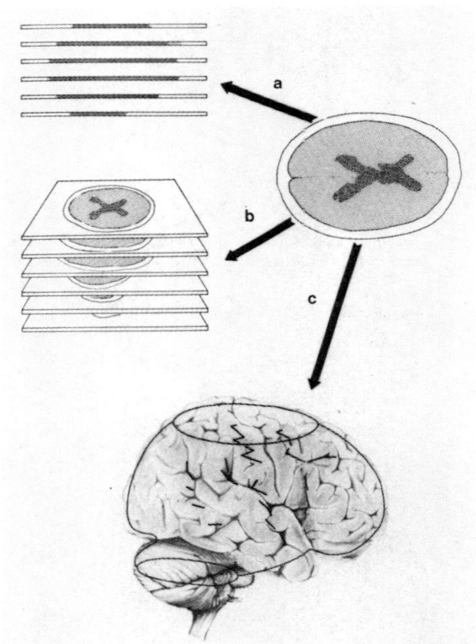

FIG. 9. Comparison of three modes of schematic representation of CT images. *a*, Lateral diagram (see Fig. 2); *b*, template representation (see Fig. 1); *c*, three-dimensional reconstruction.

probably is due to qualitative deficiency of brain tissue, which does not alter its density. Heterogenous etiology makes comparison across studies difficult.

Although these technical drawbacks are trivial, the most severe limitation of CT is that it is not suited for the detection of functional lesions. It is unrealistic to assume that only the visibly destroyed tissue is related to the patient's behavioral disturbance. On the other hand, functional methods, such as rCBF or PET scan, have a resolution that is insufficient for answering scientific questions on locali-

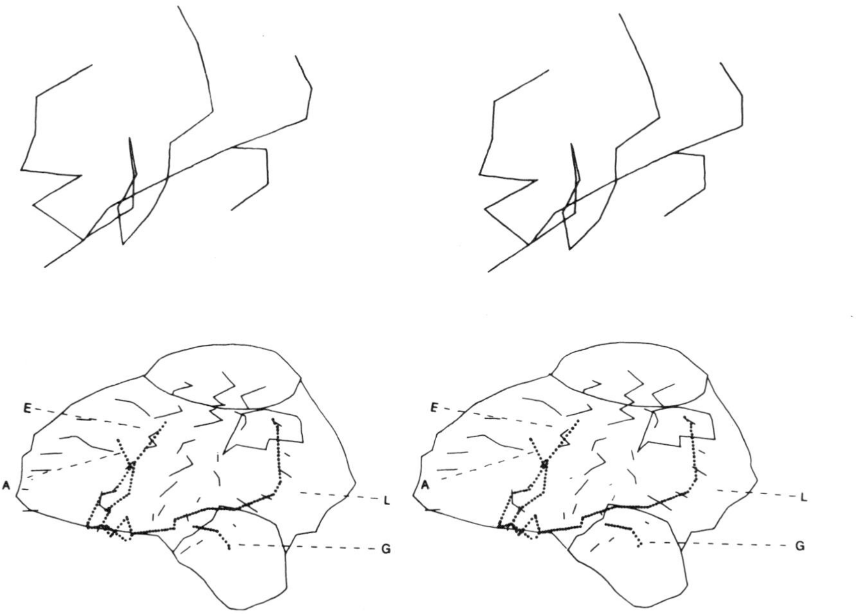

FIG. 10. Top: Stereoimages of four reconstructed branches of middle cerebral artery. **Bottom:** Stereoimages of reconstructed brain, based on CT series of one patient. Letters indicate four superimposed pial arteries.

zation, and they cannot be used on a large scale for clinical localization. With the present state of technology, it is desirable that the structural and functional methods would complement each other. This could be done only on single cases, however, and is feasible only in a few institutions. Even there, test–retest examinations will be possible only to a limited extent.

Until now, there has been no sufficient information on lesion localization in neuropsychologic syndromes by means of nuclear magnetic resonance (NMR). The standardization and reconstruction methods discussed here for CT scan will be applicable also to other brain imaging techniques, however, and the problems of data assessment, reduction, and processing will be the same.

Conceptually, studies on correlations between CT lesions and neuropsychologic syndromes, particularly aphasia, are still based on the traditional psychoanatomic theory focused on centers and their connecting pathways. This neoclassic approach aims at confirming or rejecting localizationist views that had been developed—and were controversial—a century ago. There is a tendency even today to underemphasize negative cases and to either eliminate them by statistical procedures or to minimize them by ad hoc arguments. Individual consideration of single patients in groups shows that there is by no means a one-to-one relationship between specific aphasic syndromes and particular regions within the language area.

Elsewhere, we have maintained that the standard aphasic syndromes are artifacts of cerebral vascularization and not linguistically meaningful entities; in other words,

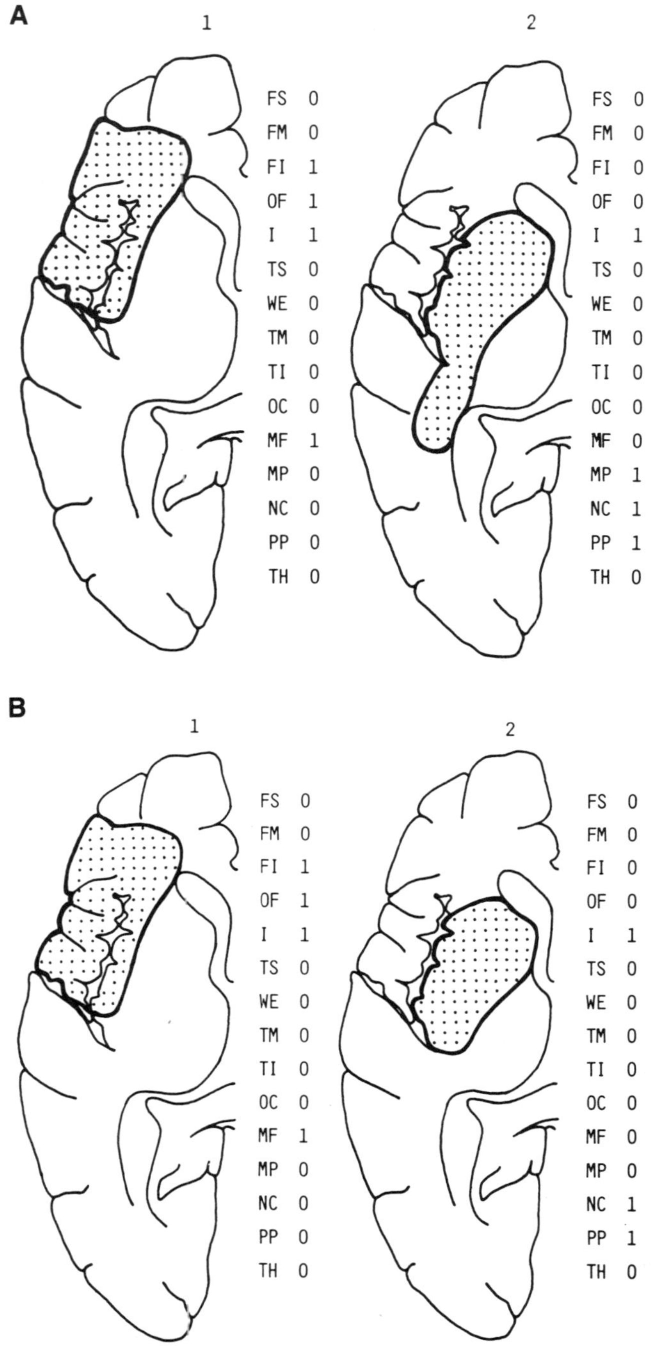

FIG. 11. Illustrative examples of lesioned areas in slice 3. **A:** Two patients with moderate global aphasia. **B:** two patients with mixed transcortical aphasia. A1 and B1 are identical; A2 differs from B2 only by a slightly larger white matter lesion. For abbreviations, see Fig. 1, legend.

the constituent symptoms do not entail each other (18). The logical consequence is either the specification of the constituent symptoms or the selection of patients who have predominantly one dissociated disorder and to take up the localization problem again.

Illustrative examples for the latter approach are the hypotheses that either the syntactic parser (2) or phonology (9) is localized in Broca's area. We are not optimistic that this "modular" psychoanatomic approach will provide insight that is satisfactory to the demands of both linguistics and anatomy. For example, it was impossible to find a typical CT localization for patients with only one preserved modality, such as repetition. When patients with mixed transcortical aphasia were compared with those with moderate global aphasia, who were similar in all linguistic disturbances but could not repeat, there was no consistent difference of lesion localization and consequently no reason to assume an anatomic correlate for repetition (6) (Fig. 11).

In order to verify the lesions postulated for specific syndromes or symptoms, we have chosen an alternative approach (5). The lesions reported for six cases of conduction aphasia (4) were transferred onto our standardized grids (Fig. 12), and patients with this lesion were then examined for their aphasic disturbance, as assessed by Aachen Aphasia Test (AAT). Of the 122 patients whose standardized lesions had been stored at the time of this study, only three patients had a lesion identical to those in Damasio's conduction patients. Two patients were without aphasia, and one had Broca's aphasia.

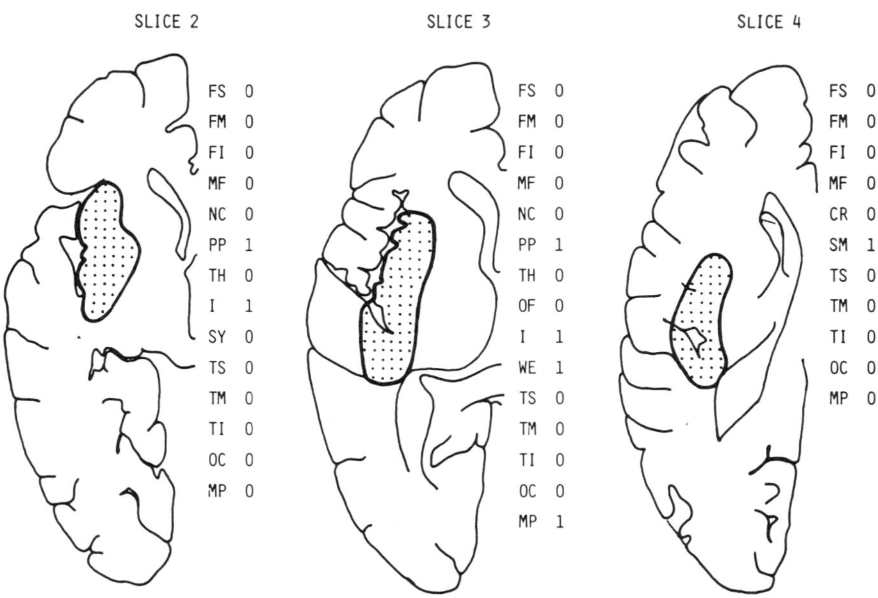

FIG. 12. Transference of the lesion in case no. 5 of Damasio and Damasio (4) onto our standardized slices 2, 3, and 4.

CONCLUSIONS

The deficit theory of localization has not been strengthened by the *in vivo* localization of lesions in CT scans. On the contrary, one has recognized more negative cases than expected by the classic doctrine on the differential localization of aphasic syndromes within the left hemisphere. Even its modernistic version in modularity theory too often relies on conventional concepts.

If one considers that the language area is association cortex, one has every reason to assume that its neuronal organization is characterized by the same intricate wiring known, for instance, in the multimodal convergence of the parietal cortex (13,14), not to mention the efferent aspect, which is extremely difficult to examine. Consequently, one must conceive of partial linguistic functions as related to neuronal networks, which are intricately intermingled in the language area. It follows that localization of function should be envisioned at the level of neuronal networks, the interruption of which in different places leads to similar symptoms. This view excludes the assumption that psychoanatomic localization is present at the gross anatomic level, and that it is meaningful to search for one lesion in relation to one symptom.

With these considerations, we do not mean to propose a null hypothesis with respect to the clinical localization of aphasic syndromes; nor do we intend to imply that research on the relationship between brain lesions and functional disturbance is unproductive in principle. Rather, this research should be continued with the best means available. Regardless of the method of brain imaging that provides the raw data, stylized reconstruction simulating the three-dimensional imagibility of neuroanatomy is a promising approach for localization studies in neuropsychology. On the basis of clinicoanatomic investigation of selected patients, questions should be generated that can then serve as hypotheses to be empirically verified or rejected in larger samples. The new techniques should not be implemented to reexamine problems that were raised a century ago but rather to support the development of new concepts.

REFERENCES

1. Alexander, M., and Lo Verme, S. (1980): Aphasia after left hemispheric intracerebral hemorrhage. *Neurology*, 30:1193–1202.
2. Berndt, R. S., and Caramazza, A. (1980): A redefinition of the syndrome of Broca's aphasia: Implications for a neuropsychological model of language. *Appl. Psycholinguistics*, 1:225–278.
3. Blunk, R., de Bleser, R., Willmes, K., and Zeumer, H. (1981): A refined method to relate morphological and functional aspects of aphasia. *Eur. Neurol.*, 20:69–79.
4. Damasio, H., and Damasio, A. (1980): The anatomical basis of conduction aphasia. *Brain*, 103:337–350.
5. De Bleser, R., Hojo, K., and Willmes, K. (1982): The morphological correlates of aphasia with preserved repetition or comprehension ability. Presented at the 5th INS European Conference.
6. De Bleser, R. (1984): Localization of aphasia. Science or fiction. In: *Proceedings of the First European Workshop on Cognitive Neuropsychology*, edited by F. Denes. Erlbaum *(in press)*.
7. Hayward, R. W., Naeser, M. A., and Zatz, L. M. (1977): Cranial CT in aphasia. Correlation of anatomical lesions with functional deficits. *Radiology*, 123:653–660.
8. Hündgen, R., Zeumer, H., and Schmachtenberg, A. (1981): An improved computer assisted

method designed to relate morphological data acquired by CT to clinical aspects of brain lesions. Presented at the 10th Congress of the European Society of Neuroradiology, Milan.
9. Kean, M. L. (1977): The linguistic interpretation of aphasic syndromes. In: *Explorations in the Biology of Language*, edited by E. Walker. Harvester Press, Hassocks, Sussex, England.
10. Kertesz, A., Harlock, W., and Coates, R. (1979): CT localization, lesion size, and prognosis in aphasia and nonverbal impairment. *Brain Lang.*, 8:34–50.
11. Keyserlingk, Graf von D., and Lange, S. (1979): Lagevariation von Hirnstrukturen im Bezugssystem der Computertomographie. *Anat. Anz.*, 146:245–255.
12. Keyserlingk, Graf von D., de Bleser, R., and Poeck, K. (1983): Stereographic reconstruction of human brain CT series. *Acta Anat.*, 115:336–344.
13. Kornhuber, H. H. (1983): Functional interpretation of the multimodal convergence in the central nervous system of vertebrates. In: *Fortschritte der Zoologie, Vol. 28*, edited by Horn, pp. 99–111. Fischer, Stuttgart.
14. Kornhuber, H. H., and DaFonseca, J. S. (1964): Optovestibular integration in the cat's cortex: A study of sensory convergence on cortical neurons. In: *The Oculomotor System*, edited by M. B. Bender, pp. 239–279. Hoeber, New York.
15. Luzzatti, C., Scotti, G., and Gattoni, A. (1979): Further suggestions for cerebral CT-localization. *Cortex*, 15:483–490.
16. Mazzocchi, F., and Vignolo, L. A. (1979): Localization of lesions in aphasia: Clinical CT-scan correlations in stroke patients. *Cortex*, 15:627–654.
17. Naeser, M., Alexander, M., Helm, N., Levine, H., Laughlin, S., and Geschwind, N. (1982): Aphasia with predominantly subcortical lesion sites. Description of three capsular/putaminal aphasia syndromes. *Arch. Neurol.*, 39:2–14.
18. Poeck, K. (1984): What do we mean by "aphasic syndromes"? A neurologist's view. *Brain Lang.*, 20:79–89.
19. Poeck, K., de Bleser, R., and Keyserlingk, Graf von D. (1984): Neurolinguistic status and localization of lesion in aphasic patients with exclusively consonant-vowel (CV)-recurring utterances. *Brain*, 107:199–217.
20. Rothi, L. J., McFarling, D., and Heilman, K. M. (1982): Conduction aphasia, syntactic alexia, and the anatomy of syntactic comprehension. *Arch. Neurol.*, 39:272–275.
21. Schmachtenberg, A., Hündgen, R., and Zeumer, H. (1983): Ein EDV-adaptiertes Rastermodell des Gehirns zur topographischen Analyse von Läsionen im cranialen Computertomogramm. *Fortschr. Rontgenstr.*, 135:499–502.
22. Whitaker, H. A., and Selnes, O. A. (1978): Anatomic variations in the cortex: Individual differences and the problem of the localization of language functions. In: *Origins and Evolution of Language and Speech, Vol. 280*, edited by S. Harnad, H. Steklis, and J. Lancaster, pp. 844–854. Annals of the New York Academy of Sciences, New York.

Advances in Neurology, Vol. 42: Progress in Aphasiology, edited by F. C. Rose.
Raven Press, New York © 1984.

Aphasias Associated with Computed Tomography Scan Lesions Outside Broca's and Wernicke's Areas

L. A. Vignolo

Department of Neurology, University of Milan, 20122 Milan, Italy

This chapter discusses the main types of aphasia associated with lesions outside Broca's and Wernicke's areas and the connecting structures, i.e., with lesions sparing the left perisylvian region. The marginal language areas, including the occipital lobe, and some subcortical structures, such as the thalamus and basal ganglia are considered next. The language disorders associated with such lesions are less frequent and less well defined than those associated with strictly perisylvian areas. As a consequence, consensus regarding the role of the damaged structures in language is far from universal. We have collected cases from our previous work and mention the work of others in order to illustrate these rarer forms of aphasia and their computed tomography (CT) scan counterparts. Some syndromes that should belong to this chapter, such as those of alexia with agraphia and the language disorders following excision of the left temporal pole, are not considered because of lack of suitable CT scan figures.

MATERIALS AND METHODS

The cliniconeuroradiologic correlations described were carried out in adult patients who harbored cerebrovascular lesions. Aphasia and agraphia were evaluated by a detailed standard examination of language. The site and extent of the lesion was assessed by CT apparatus, a correlation explained by Mazzocchi and Vignolo (18).

RESULTS

Aphasias Associated with Lesions of Marginal Language Areas

This group comprises the transcortical aphasias of traditional classification, amnestic or anomic aphasia (discussed with the transcortical sensory), and "pure" agraphia.

Transcortical motor aphasia may be defined by the following characteristics: reduced, nonfluent speech without articulation disorders, preserved naming and repetition, and good comprehension. The syndrome is caused by damage (sometimes bilateral) of the marginal frontal language areas, located above and in front of Broca's region and also including the mesial premotor area (1,17,26). Broca's area may remain intact or be only slightly damaged in this syndrome, in which case the clinical picture may be contaminated by slight articulation defects (11).

The only case of transcortical motor aphasia in the first large series that we have examined (18) had a typical clinical picture. As expected, the CT showed bilateral damage to the centrum semiovale, undermining the anterior marginal areas of language, as shown in Fig. 1A. This syndrome also may follow unilateral left subcortical damage, such as a lesion near the anterior horn of the left lateral ventricle (7) or in the anterior capsuloputaminal region, interrupting the thalamic-frontal connections (28). Crossing into the postrolandic region, we find two syndromes: amnestic and transcortical sensory aphasias.

Amnestic or anomic aphasia (fluent speech with frequent word-finding difficulties and good repetition and comprehension) results from lesions in the posterior marginal areas surrounding Wernicke's zone from behind and below. Anomic aphasia usually is associated with damage that is either abrupt but small and well circumscribed or slowly diffusing to the cortical areas in question. Instead, when damage to the same zone is massive and extensive, transcortical sensory aphasia results, a form defined clinically by fluent speech with predominantly lexical-semantic paraphasias and strikingly good repetition, in contrast to poor comprehension with semantic confusion. Von Monakow (21) called this form "associative" sensory aphasia, but we suggest that both syndromes can be considered "associative" or "semantic," each being regarded as different degrees of the same basic defect, namely, the inability to associate the entire word with its meaning. When damage is slight, the defect is seen only in the most difficult performance, i.e., spoken language (hence anomic aphasia); when the damage is severe, the defect is apparent in both expression and comprehension (hence transcortical sensory aphasia).

Amnestic aphasia, as defined above, is not frequent. We found only one clear-cut case (in a series of 90 aphasias). In this patient, a small zone of the posterior part of T2 was damaged, somewhat marginally located with respect to Wernicke's area, as could be predicted (Fig. 1C). With respect to the transcortical sensory aphasia, the lesions underlying two recent cases (Fig. 1B) were in agreement with

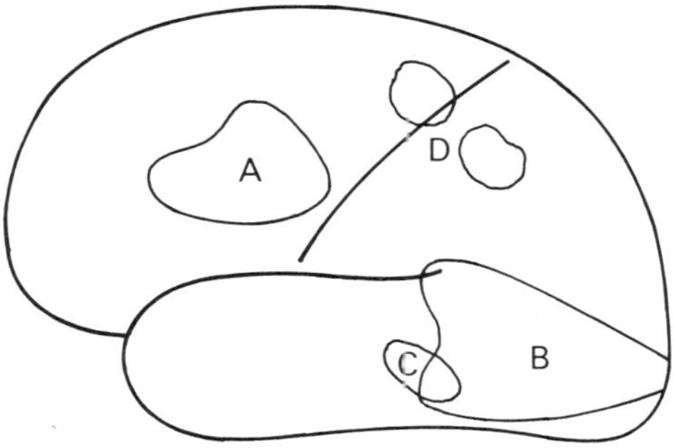

FIG. 1. Diagram of left hemispheric surface. The maps indicate the CT scan lesions, lying largely outside the perisylvian areas, that have been found to be associated with different types of aphasia. *A*, transcortical motor; *B*, transcortical sensory; *C*, amnesic; *D*, pure agraphia.

expectations; they destroyed a large part of the posterior marginal region, encroaching only a little upon Wernicke's area. Analogous location has been found in other CT scan studies (7,15). When good repetition is associated with both comprehension defects and severe expressive inertia, this should be called a mixed (sensory and motor) transcortical aphasia, a condition that may also be referred to as a syndrome of isolation of the speech area, since the lesions partially surround the older, perisylvian speech region, damaging both the parietooccipital and frontal marginal language areas.

Good repetition, which is the hallmark of all the transcortical aphasias, usually points to integrity of the perisylvian language areas of the left hemisphere. A convincing case of isolation of the speech areas, with autopsy, was reported by Geschwind et al. (12). Both CT scan and autopsy evidence of lesions in this syndrome indicate that the damaged posterior marginal areas may include the medial aspect of the left parietal lobe (25). Less severe clinical pictures, with features resembling the transcortical aphasias (selectively preserved repetition, in particular) may be due to subcortical vascular lesions confined to the thalamus and, in a few cases, centered on the putamen (see below).

A lesion in either the left parasagittal or the medial parietal areas seems to be crucial in determining a rare syndrome, the so-called pure agraphia. In a case with this disorder, we found two small lesions, one in the upper half of the central region, the other in the posterior and superior parietal lobule (Fig. 1D). The latter site had already been pointed out by Russell and Espir (27) and was confirmed by our own work (2). If one considers how many sensory and motor skills are needed to acquire writing, it is worth recalling that this area, and especially the depth of the intraparietal sulcus, is a locus of multisensorimotor convergence (14). This may not be the most crucial, but only a particularly important, lesion site. The possibility that slight damage in other language zones, such as the left perisylvian region, may bring about isolated writing disturbances of long standing has recently been suggested by a CT scan case report (24).

Alexia Without Agraphia and the Occipital Lobe

We now discuss deeper lesions, beginning in the occipital lobe with the syndrome of alexia without agraphia. In one case (18), this syndrome was associated with the destruction of a large portion of the left occipital lobe. Similar lesions have been found in a subsequent study in five additional cases showing analogous reading disorders (Fig. 2). The anatomic finding of decisive importance seems to consist of the destruction of the posterior callosal pathways coursing leftward from the intact right occipital lobe. Such interruption, according to traditional interpretation, would not permit the written letters, visually perceived in the intact right occipital lobe, to reach the left angular gyrus where they can be deciphered. Regardless of the interpretation, in our cases, these callosal fibers were consistently interrupted by the anterior extension of large occipital lesions, which encroached upon incoming callosal radiations. A separate infarction of the splenium (9) is not needed where the left occipital lesion reaches the callosal radiations anteriorly.

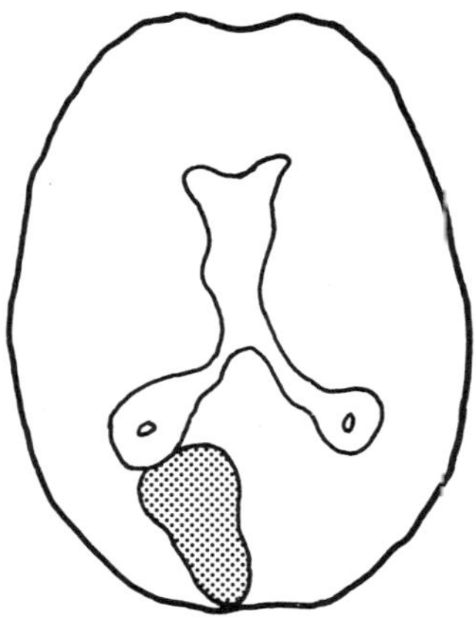

FIG. 2. Template of CT scan section showing a lesion *(dotted)* of the left occipital lobe associated with alexia without agraphia.

The most frequent cause of this syndrome is a large occipital infarct in the territory of the left posterior cerebral artery [see also the CT scan cases of Orgogozo et al. (22) and Damasio (7)]. However, the occurrence of a parietal hematoma undercutting the left angular gyrus (and thereby preventing access from both occipital lobes to it) has been shown to produce a different type of pure alexia without agraphia: "subangular alexia" (10,13,23). Alexia without agraphia has been reported in association with a left occipital tumor in only four cases; in one, the symptoms were due to compression and disappeared after surgery (29).

Thalamic Aphasia

Proceeding frontally into the depth of the left hemisphere, we encounter the thalamus, destruction of which may produce language disorders. Aphasia caused by a lesion of the left thalamus had occasionally been described in the older literature (for a review, see ref. 16), and an increasing number of CT scan cases are being reported (for updated references, see ref. 19). During a period of almost 2 years, Cappa and Vignolo (6) performed a systematic study of all intracerebral hemorrhages observed in a consecutive series of CT scans. They found 10.6% of thalamic hemorrhages, a figure that agrees with those observed by pioneer authors, notably Miller Fisher (20), in the epoch preceding the use of the CT scan. Aphasia was present in seven of eight cases of left thalamic bleeding (see example in Fig. 3) and in none of six cases of right thalamic hemorrhage.

All these cases were examined during the acute period, i.e., within 3 weeks after stroke. Whenever a detailed language examination was performed, aphasia appeared to be characterized by semantic paraphasias and word-finding defects in spontaneous speech and partially defective comprehension, in sharp contrast to undamaged repetition. This emphasizes the intactness of the phonemic level of language. This dissociation is similar to that of the transcortical aphasias and is present in other case reports of left thalamic hemorrhages and infarcts studied by means of the CT scan (19). The integrity of repetition suggests that the function

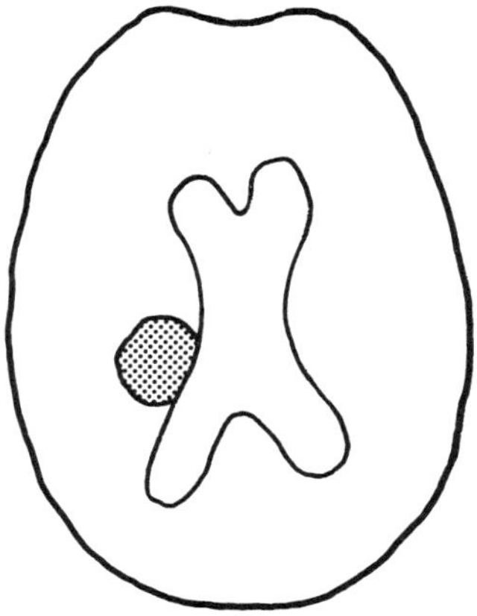

FIG. 3. Template of CT scan section showing a hemorrhagic lesion *(dotted)* of the left thalamus associated with aphasia (exhibiting transcortical sensory features).

of the thalamus is related mainly to that of the so-called marginal language zones, as it concerns principally the use of complete meaningful words rather than phonemes.

Another point of interest is that most thalamic aphasias are transient; they are no longer present when the patient is examined after the acute period. This indicates that the function of the thalamus in language, however relevant, is perhaps not as crucial as believed by some authors (notably Penfield and Roberts).

Aphasia and the Basal Ganglia

The findings concerning lesions of purely subcortical structures other than the thalamus, i.e., basal ganglia and internal capsule, are far less homogeneous. It is possible that small differences of localization entail quite different pictures.

In general, one of the assets of the CT scan is to permit visualization of relatively small and purely deep lesions, i.e., lesions that do not reach the surface of the hemisphere. Some of these lesions, however, are deep but not subcortical, because they involve the cortex buried in sulci. Examples of this are deep lesions damaging the left insular cortex; such lesions, albeit deep, are cortical in nature. They entail nonfluent aphasias, which can be explained by the fact that the anterior insular cortex belongs to the anterior language area, as mentioned by Dejerine in 1914 (9). Other lesions are truly subcortical and are confined to either the left thalamus (as we have seen) or the left basal ganglia and neighboring white matter. We confine ourselves here to truly subcortical lesions.

Few convincing cases of mild, nonfluent aphasias with some dysarthria have been described (8), following small infarcts of the anterior limb of the internal capsule, encroaching upon the caudate nucleus. Aphasic pictures reportedly similar to those caused by thalamic hemorrhages have been observed in association with putaminal hemorrhages. In our experience (5), language disorders following strictly subcortical cerebrovascular lesions confined to the basal ganglia and adjacent structures (excluding the thalamus) are rare (about one of three cases with such lesions on CT scan), generally mild, and presumably transient. Two cases of logorrheic jargonaphasia with intact repetition have been observed following a small caudate hemorrhage (4) and an anatomically verified putaminal infarction (3). A typical transcortical motor aphasia has been described in association with an internal capsuloputaminal infarct, probably disconnecting the dorsomedial thalamic nucleus from the frontal cortex (28).

Recently, we undertook two studies in order to investigate the frequency and characteristics of aphasia following strictly subcortical left hemisphere lesions (5). In study 1, all patients whose CT scan, carried out within a given period, showed subcortical lesions in both hemispheres were evaluated for presence and type of aphasia. Conversely, in study 2, the records of all patients referred to our Aphasia Unit for language evaluation within a given period were examined for presence of subcortical lesions on the CT scan. In study 1, aphasia was found in two of six patients. In study 2, stabilized, strictly subcortical lesions of the left hemisphere were found in six of 250 patients; four of six were aphasic. Closer scrutiny of the type of language disorder in the aphasics from both studies ($N = 6$) suggests the possibility of differentiating two types of defect: an atypical nonfluent aphasia, sometimes associated with anterior capsuloputaminal lesions, as shown, for example, in Fig. 4—left, and a mild fluent aphasia, sometimes associated with posterior capsuloputaminal lesions, as shown in Fig. 4—right.

CONCLUSIONS

In addition to the classic areas of Broca and Wernicke, other regions of the left (dominant) hemisphere play an important role in language processing, so much so that their damage brings about diverse forms of aphasia. Some such regions (for example, the so-called marginal language areas) were well known by the late 19th

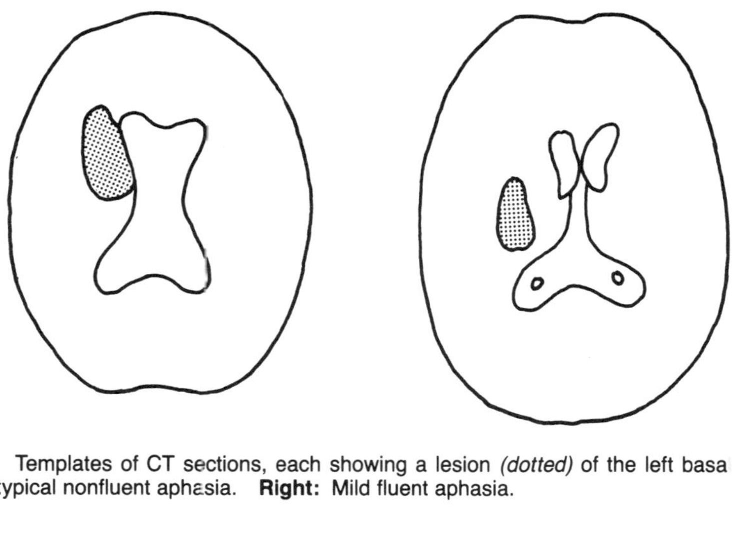

FIG. 4. Templates of CT sections, each showing a lesion *(dotted)* of the left basal ganglia. **Left:** Atypical nonfluent aphasia. **Right:** Mild fluent aphasia.

century neurologists, while others are a comparatively recent acquisition to our knowledge in this field. This is true, in particular, of the subcortical structures, lesions of which may entail language disorders. The discovery of subcortical lesions *in vivo* is specifically attributable to the use of the CT scan and constitutes a real advance in aphasiology; but its consequences still appear too dishomogeneous to permit reliable systematization. The possible meaning of damage to the subcortical structures in the cerebral function of language deserves further study.

REFERENCES

1. Alexander, M. P., and Schmitt, M. A. (1980): The aphasia syndrome of stroke in the left anterior cerebral artery territory. *Arch. Neurol.*, 37:97–100.
2. Basso, A., Taborelli, A., and Vignolo, L. A. (1978): Dissociated disorders of speaking and writing in aphasia. *J. Neurol. Neurosurg. Psychiatry*, 41:556–563.
3. Barat, M., Mazaux, J. M., Bioulac, B., Giroire, J. M., Vital, C., and Arné, L. (1981): Troubles du langage de type aphasique et lesions putamino-caudées. *Rev. Neurol.*, 137:343–356.
4. Cambier, J., Elghozi, D., and Strube, E. (1979): Hémorragie de la tête du noyau caudé gauche. *Rev. Neurol.*, 135:763–774.
5. Cappa, S. E., Cavallotti, G., Guidotti, M., Papagno, C., and Vignolo, L. A. (1983): Subcortical aphasias: Two clinical-CT scan correlation studies. *Cortex*, 19:227–241.
6. Cappa, S. F., and Vignolo, L. A. (1979): "Transcortical" features of aphasia following left thalamic hemorrhage. *Cortex*, 15:121–130.
7. Damasio, H. (1981): Cerebral localization of the aphasias. In: *Acquired Aphasia*, edited by M. T. Sarno. Academic Press, New York.
8. Damasio, A. R., Damasio, H., Rizzo, M., Varney, N., and Gersch, F. (1982): Aphasia with nonhemorrhagic lesions in the basal ganglia and internal capsule. *Arch. Neurol.*, 39:15–20.
9. Dejerine, J. (1914): *Séméiologie des Affections du Système Nerveux*. Masson, Paris.
10. Ducarne, B., Bergego, C., and Gardeur, D. (1984): Alexie "sous angulaire" et signes neuropsychologiques associés: Étude clinique et tomodensitométrique. *Cortex*, 19:115–124.
11. Freeman, M., Alexander, M. P., and Naeser, M. A. (1982): Predictive CT scan anatomy in anterior aphasia. *Neurology (NY)*, 32:A189.
12. Geschwind, N., Quadfasel, F. A., and Segarra, J. (1968): Isolation of the speech area. *Neuropsychologia*, 6:327–340.
13. Greenblatt, S. H. (1976): Subangular alexia without agraphia or hemianopsia. *Brain Lang.*, 3:229–245.
14. Hyvärinen, J., and Poranen, A. (1974): Function of the parietal associative area 7 as revealed from cellular discharge in alert monkeys. *Brain*, 97:673–692.
15. Kertesz, A., Sheppard, A., and MacKenzie, R. (1982): Localization in transcortical sensory aphasia. *Arch. Neurol.*, 39:475–478.
16. Lecours, A. R., and Lhermitte, F. (1979): *L'aphasie*. Flammarion, Paris.
17. Masdeu, J. C., Schoene, W. C., and Funkenstein, H. (1978): Aphasia following infarction of the left supplementary motor area: A clinicopathologic study. *Neurology*, 28:1220–1223.
18. Mazzocchi, F., and Vignolo, L. A. (1979): Localization of lesions in aphasia: Clinical CT scan correlation in stroke patients. *Cortex*, 15:627–654.
19. Mc Farling, D., Rothi, L. J., and Heilman, K. L. (1982): Transcortical aphasia from ischemic infarcts of the thalamus: Report of two cases. *J. Neurol. Neurosurg. Psychiatry*, 45:107–112.
20. Miller Fisher, C. (1959): The pathological and clinical aspects of thalamic hemorrhage. *Trans. Am. Neurol. Assoc.*, 84:56–59.
21. Monakow, C. von (1914): *Die Lokalisation in Grosshirn und der Abbau der Funktionen durch korticale Herde*. Bergmann, Wiesbaden.
22. Orgogozo, J. M., Péré, J. J., and Strube, E. (1979): Alexie sans agraphie, "agnosie" des couleurs et atteinte de l'hémichamp visuel droit: Un syndrome de l'artère cérébrale postérieure. *Sem. Hop. Paris*, 25(31–32):1389–1394.
23. Pirozzolo, F. J., Kerr, K. L., Obrzut, J. E., Morley, G. K., Haxby, J. V., and Lundgren, S. (1981): Neurolinguistic analysis of the language abilities of a patient with a "double disconnection syn-

drome": A case of subangular alexia in the presence of mixed transcortical aphasia. *J. Neurol. Neurosurg. Psychiatry*, 44:152–155.
24. Rosati, G., and De Bastiani, P. (1979): Pure agraphia: A discrete form of aphasia. *J. Neurol. Neurosurg. Psychiatry*, 42:266–269.
25. Ross, E. D. (1980): Left medial parietal lobe and receptive language functions: Mixed transcortical aphasia after left anterior cerebral artery infarction. *Neurology (NY)*, 30:144–151.
26. Rubens, A. (1975): Aphasia with infarction in the territory of the anterior cerebral artery. *Cortex*, 11:239–250.
27. Russell, W. R., and Espir, M. (1961): *Traumatic Aphasia*. Oxford University Press, London.
28. Sterzi, R., and Vallar, G. (1978): Frontal lobe syndrome as a disconnection syndrome: Report of a case. *Acta Neurol.*, 33:419–425.
29. Turgman, J., Goldhammer, Y., and Braham, J. (1979): Alexia, without agraphia, due to brain tumor: A reversible syndrome. *Ann. Neurol.*, 6:265–268.

Advances in Neurology, Vol. 42: Progress in Aphasiology, edited by F. C. Rose.
Raven Press, New York © 1984.

Language Disorders and Their Relationship to Thalamic Lesions

Francois Lhermitte

Clinique de Neurologie et de Neuropsychologie, Unite de Recherches Neuropsychologiques, INSERM, Hôpital de la Salpêtrière, 75013 Paris, France

The history of speech and language disorders of thalamic origin is recent. The initial facts were discovered by neurosurgeons, first by electrical stimulation of the thalamus and then by stereotactic thalamotomies in the left cerebral hemisphere, a period that extended from 1959 to 1975. It was under these conditions that neurologists described the different elements of a coherent syndrome which recalled aphasia. The computed tomography (CT) scan was helpful as it allowed diagnosis while the patient was still alive.

Few cases had been recorded before that time (12,16,21), but neurologists were not surprised: the thalamus is situated in Pierre Marie's famous *quadrilatère*, and the lesions could extend into, or have repercussions on, the internal capsule. Penfield and Roberts (28) and Bell (1) recorded two cases of this at a time when neurosurgical data were becoming well-known.

Cases of language disorders caused by lesions of the left thalamus are rare. About 30 cases have been published in the last 20 years, half since 1970, with sufficient semiologic precision for understanding the nature of language disorders.

For more than 100 years, neurologists have been trying to describe aphasia as provoked by lesions of the cerebral cortex and of the subcortical white matter in the so-called language areas. In recent years, neurologists have become more interested in language disorders provoked by lesions outside these cortical areas but which interfere with the activities of the latter. Here we can list the frontal lobe, the hippocampomamillothalamic system, and the reticular formation. It is in this field that thalamic lesion disorders belong. In this chapter, we present the facts already known and discuss their physiopathology.

ELECTRICAL STIMULATION OF THE THALAMUS

Table 1 summarizes published data. It can be seen that speech disorders are provoked by stimulation of the ventrolateral (VL) nucleus of each hemisphere. These results, also obtained by stimulation of the primary cortical areas of both hemispheres, are logical, the explanation lying in the connections between the VL nucleus and the motor and premotor cortical areas. They are comparable to the speech dis-

TABLE 1. *Stimulation of the thalamus*[a]

	Left hemisphere		Right hemisphere	
Speech disorder	Ventrolateral nucleus	Pulvinar	Ventrolateral nucleus	Pulvinar
Vocalization	0	0	0	0
Tachylalia, spluttering	+ +	0	+ +	0
Palilalia and other speech disorders	+ +	0	0	0
Arrest	+ +	0	+	0
Hesitation	+ (?)	+	+ (?)	0
Naming	+ +	+ +	0	0
Perseveration	+ +	+ +	0	0
Verbal paraphasias	0	+ +	0	0

Adapted from Lecours and Lhermitte (17).

orders seen in Parkinson's disease, with the obvious proviso that stimulation is not taken to mean activation of a normal motor pattern. They confirm that systems that control the speed of vocal utterances make use of both cortical and subcortical levels of motor function. The results also show the existence of left hemispheric dominance for palilalia, a symptom associated with tachylalia in patients suffering from Parkinson's disease but not necessarily in cases with dementia. Furthermore, it has not been proved that palilalia provoked by stimulation of the sensorimotor cortex or the VL nucleus of the left hemisphere is dependent on the same mechanisms responsible for the very complex palilalia observed in neurologic diseases.

The important fact is that language disorders *per se* are provoked only by stimulation of the VL nucleus and pulvinar of the left hemisphere. Stimulation of the right thalamus does not produce language disorders. Moreover, only stimulation of the pulvinar is able to induce verbal paraphasias, probably the same as those obtained by stimulation of the left parietotemporal cortical areas. We agree with Ojemann's (27) conclusion:

> Left thalamus appears to be related to language processes. This is suggested by the ability to evoke the same types of object naming errors from left thalamus as can be evoked from the cortex concerned with language. Indeed, only portions of the left thalamus, including anterior superior pulvinar, and medial central ventrolateral nucleus may be thus related to language.

Ojemann incriminated a limited part of the pulvinar, corresponding to that part of the medial nucleus that sends projections to, and receives projections from, the posterior parietal region, which is just in front of that part of the pulvinar that sends projections to the visual associative area.

The naming is based on pictures, an experimental condition that may play a role. If the naming depended on auditory stimuli, the sensory area of the pulvinar could stretch toward the lateral nucleus of the pulvinar. This is linked to the posterior regions of the temporal lobe, which are also part of the cortical areas of language.

TABLE 2. *Thalamotomies*[a]

	Cryogenic (%)		Unilateral (%)		
Speech disorder	Right	Left	Right	Left	Bilateral (%)
Diminished volume	13×	45×	10	28	66
Dysarthria	32×	80×	21×	29×	83
Dysphasia	0×	29×	0×	33×	25

[a] Data from Bell (1).

A final point is that the different stimulation of the VL nucleus and of the pulvinar provoked disorders known as hesitation, anomia, and perseveration. First, these words describe only different kinds of behavior and have a wide meaning, covering both linguistic perturbations which differ from each other and, obviously, varied physiologic systems. Second, from a neuropsychologic point of view, a language/speech dichotomy is justified on the condition that they are not separated by a barrier; between mind and speech, sets of patterns are activated successively in such a way that linguistic formulation appears, then becomes articulatory movements. Even if we do not know precisely about the sets of patterns, physiology and pathology force us to accept this continuum.

THALAMOTOMY

A great number of thalamotomies were performed in cases of Parkinson's disease and other pathologic states. These operations were directed mostly to the VL nucleus but also to the pulvinar and other structures. Neurosurgeons have not often paid special attention to postoperative language disorders, which have had a reputation for being rare and transitory. This is true only in part. The disorders usually are divided into three categories: (a) lowering of voice volume, (b) speech impairment or abnormality, dysarthria, slurring, and stuttering in the absence of true aphasia and changes in patterns of rate and rhythm, and (c) language disturbances, aphasic difficulties, dysphasia, and true disorders of language.

These disorders are not rare. Three publications have been chosen as examples. Bell's (1) results are summarized in Table 2; voice and speech disorders are frequent and are statistically significant when thalamotomy is effected in the left hemisphere; dysphasia also is frequent. Riklan and several of his collaborators (29,30) have studied patients operated on by Cooper since 1969, basing their studies on the Wechsler scale. In their latest publications, Riklan et al. (29,30) underlined the transitory fall in marks obtained with verbal subtests following destruction of the left VL nucleus (an average drop of 8.7 in nine patients) and of the left pulvinar (an average drop of 10.2 in 16 patients). They concluded that the principal disorder observed was a diminution of verbal fluency. Although they insisted on the predominance of left thalamic lesions, they considered that the disorders after right thalamic lesions are "more in the nature of a continuum than a dichotomy," but this is far from certain.

Darley et al. (8) used a complete protocol for language examination, their results being precise with an outline of the pathologic basis. Nearly 25% of 123 patients had disorders of language, which were found essentially after left thalamotomy; they did not affect basic functioning but rather higher functions in the mind-language field (i.e., comprehension of texts and precision and accuracy of the definition of words). These authors wrote: "impairments were predominantly of higher language function." In the majority of their cases, the VL nucleus was involved by thalamotomy; unfortunately, the number of pulvinar thalamotomies were not mentioned.

For more than 20 years, the cause and nature of this dysarthria and these language disorders have been discussed. To explain the dysarthria, an associated lesion of the internal capsule, induced either by direct destruction or by adjacent edema, has been invoked. This is possible, perhaps frequent, but a lesion of the VL nucleus is not excluded. The anatomic cases of Hassler et al. (13) support such a hypothesis. Their essential points are as follows: (a) Such a dysarthria is different from Alajouanine's phonetic disintegration observed in cases of lesions of the foot of F3 and the inferior part of FA; and (b) it is different from disorders of speech, which occurred with lesions of the inferior part of PA, as we described (19). Thus thalamic lesions never induced a dislocation of a cortical sensorimotor activity in its intracortical components.

Regarding dysphasia, these authors (19) initially stressed its existence only with lesions of the left hemisphere and its analogy with such disorders observed in true aphasia as perseveration, garbled words, similar errors in both written and spoken speech, and disorders of high level psycholinguistic activities. Discussion regarding the technical errors of thalamotomy or neighboring edema is no longer topical. Spiegel and Wycis (31) described only one case of disorder of speech—and not of language—in their series of 90 dorsomedial thalamotomies. The thesis of disturbance of speech mechanisms at the subcortical level is true for lesions of the VL nucleus; this applies also to language mechanisms, partly from lesions of the left VL nucleus but in larger part from the left pulvinar.

SPONTANEOUS PATHOLOGY

As already mentioned, these disorders of language have been described correctly only since 1970. Sixteen cases of vascular accidents have been reported with precise data (2–4,6,9,10,18,24,26). Fourteen of these cases were hemorrhages, and two were infarcts. The rarity of infarcts could be explained by arterial patterns of supply, but thalamic infarcts may not be visible on the CT scan. A postmortem study of thalamic infarcts has provided additional information about the nuclei of the thalamus that do not affect language(5). Language disorders have been mentioned in cases of thalamic tumors, but these cases cannot be used because a precise anatomoclinical correlation is impossible, except for one case of an intrathalamic cyst (3). The two cases we reported (18) clearly illustrate the linguistic and neuropsychologic syndrome of speech and language disorders.

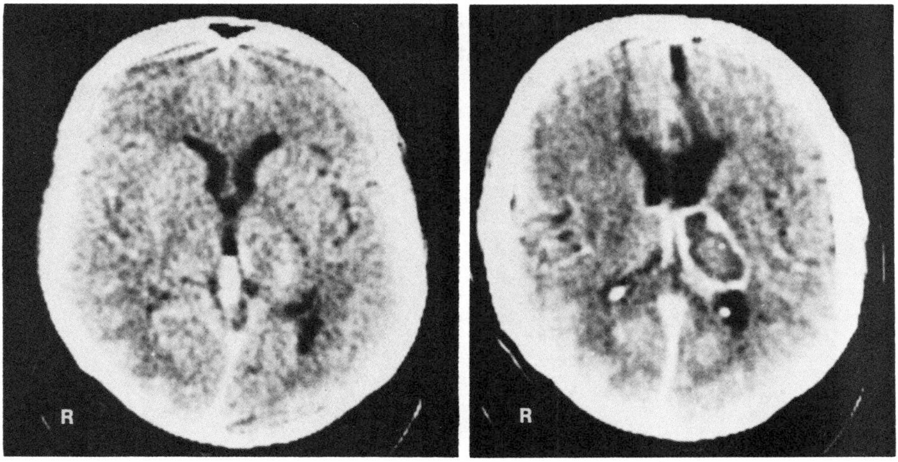

FIG. 1. Case 1. CT scan: Hematoma of the left thalamus. **Left:** Without enhancement. **Right:** With enhancement.

Today, clinical diagnosis is possible:

Case 1: A right-handed, hypertensive male engineer, aged 56 years, developed a right hemiplegia over several hours, followed by speech difficulties. His blood pressure at that time was 230/120. On examination, he had a complete hemiplegia, including a right Babinski sign. Joint position sense was absent, and there was complete astereognosis of the right hand. No tactile or painful stimuli were perceived on the right half of the body or face. Visual fields were normal, and there was no visual extinction. The head and eyes were deviated to the right; eye movements were normal (3,18).

The EEG showed slow activity in the left hemisphere. The CT scan, performed 1 month after the vascular accident, exhibited an area of increased density corresponding to a left thalamic hemorrhage (Fig. 1). Neuropsychologic examination was carried out 1 week after the accident.

Case 2: A right-handed man, 69 years old, presented one evening with somnolence, titubation, and confused speech. Neurologic examination the next day showed a right central facial paralysis, without motor or sensory deficit in the limbs. Upward movement of the eyes was limited and convergence impossible. The patient was inert and did not join in conversation. The CT scan, performed 15 days later, showed an area of decreased density in the left thalamus, finely encircled by contrast medium, and corresponding to the infarct (Fig. 2). Neuropsychologic examination was carried out as soon as possible (3,18).

Language disorders cannot really be expressed by signs such as 0, +, or + +, but it is useful to present them in a profile form (Fig. 3). The voice and speech disorders do not require additional comment. The first fact is the integrity of fundamental activities of language. Word, phrase, and sentence repetition were normal except in long sentences, as in reading aloud and writing under dictation (and even spontaneous writing). This means that cortical and juxtasubcortical systems of receptive areas of oral and written language are normal. In other words, the systems from input to output are normal. Furthermore, anatomic listing of series (words and

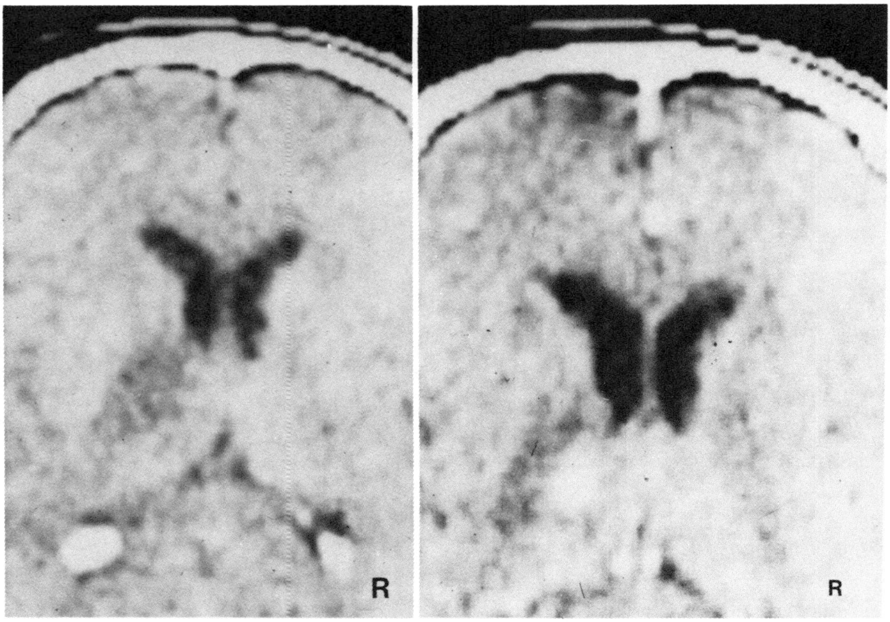

FIG. 2. Case 2. CT scan: Infarct of the left thalamus.

numbers) is normal. Disorders that affect these fundamental circuits in one or several points of their temporospatial development occur in all cases of cortical aphasia.

Neither phonetic nor phonologic disintegration in the form of phonemic paraphasias were present. Moreover, the mental values of language are partly preserved: both oral and written comprehension were normal, as were naming pictures and sounds. The value of the naming test in cases of aphasia is well known.

There are seven characteristics of language disorders (see Fig. 3):

1. The more difficult the mental and psycholinguistic task, the more disturbed is linguistic production. These tasks call for the possibility of precise thought and the evocation of suitable linguistic units on higher levels. This fact becomes clearer if we compare acceptable conversational language (the examiner encourages the patient to speak) with that used for describing the patient's profession, more so with that used for recalling childhood stories or fables, and still more so in the case of word definition. The so-called verbal fluency test is another proof of this; word evocation based on categories, for example, of animals, succeeds better than word evocation based on first letter, which calls for more abstraction and a more difficult strategy. We wonder why this test is called a "fluency" test; the fact of speaking fluently has nothing to do with this test, which is first and foremost a test of speed in prelinguistic mental activities. As another example, making sentences with words provided by the examiner is more easily done than storytelling, since these words

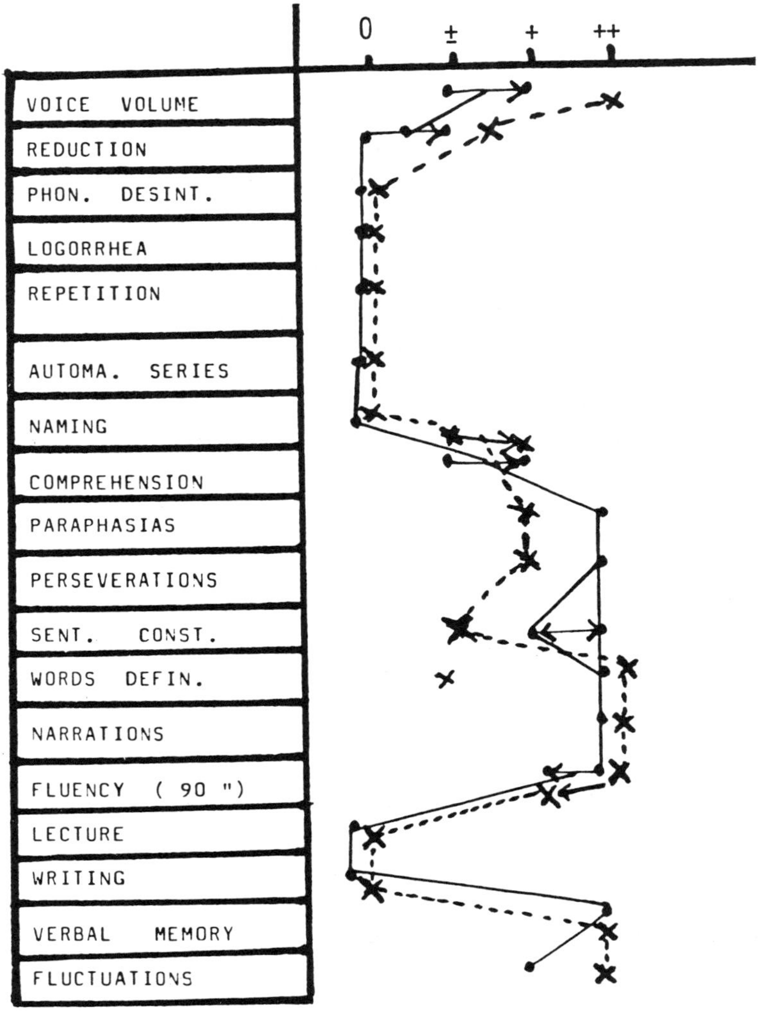

FIG. 3. Clinical profile of case 1 (*circles*) and case 2 (*crosses*).

and their meanings are already known by the patient, which helps him to group them together into sentences.

2. Hesitations and certain silences express the difficulty of evoking a word with only the back-up of thought; this is in contrast to good performance in naming of images which, on recognition, suggest the corresponding words.

3. Perseverations are frequent and become even more so as the examination proceeds. Perseveration is seen in many neurologic disorders; it has no specific character but expresses only a defect in the inhibition of a formerly activated pattern. As in

true aphasia, the perseverations are not only words or bits of phrases but also ideas, which had been expressed before and which reappear formed by new words. As in true aphasia, it is not necessary for the perserved word or idea to have been just said, it can recall another subject evoked 10 sec or more before.

4. The paraphasias are verbal and not phonemic, except for rare neologisms, which are difficult to interpret. Verbal paraphasias are easy to understand, either because they are semantically related to the right word or because they are only perseverations; in certain cases, the origin cannot be traced. Paraphasias seem to be incoherent; but we frequently call others incoherent when we cannot understand them. We can observe the same phenomenon in true aphasia and in language disorders in relation to left frontal lobe lesions.

5. Another disorder connected with aphasia is the dislocation of the logical sequences of a speech. Here the patient cannot control the order of his ideas. The series of "performances" underlying a narration is no longer chronologic; a passage from one story slides into another story. One word can give rise to new words which are linked to it semantically speaking but which no longer carry out the patient's original intention. In true aphasia, these disorders are also met, as in certain cases of complex left frontal lobe lesions.

6. A defect in verbal memory, the last linguistic disorder, was studied in four cases of vascular accidents (3). Short-term verbal memory was diminished; learning word couples from the WAIS test and memorization of texts were both badly performed. This defect was specific for verbal information and not for visual information or in daily life. Finally, it persisted for a long time after the regression of the other language disorders. This fact has no relation to the mamillothalamic tract or to the anterior and dorsomedial nuclei of the thalamus but is linked to the pulvinar and, probably, to the VL nucleus lesion, confirming data observed in stereotactic stimulation. Ojemann (27) elaborated a sophisticated protocol showing that VL nucleus stimulation had an alarm effect concerning information from outside (specific alerting response). Thus the stimulation favored or cramped the verbal amnesic capacity, depending on the moment when the stimulation occurred during the experimental protocol. Fedio and Van Buren (11) showed that pulvinar stimulation had the same effect; in both experiments, only the stimulation of the left thalamus was effective.

7. In 1975, Mohr et al. (26) underlined the surprising fluctuations in the condition of one patient who, for short periods and under the influence of continual stimulation by the examiner, was able to understand and speak almost normally. This was followed by a longer period, where his attention could not be captured and where his language was a mixture of verbal paraphasia, perseveration, dyssyntaxia, and then murmurs that became inaudible. This phase sometimes included sleepiness. In aphasia, language fluctuations are well known. They express a functional exhaustion of the affected cortical and subcortical networks, but the intensity and the length of the phases are not as great as in this case, where there was an exhaustion of an activating system of specialized circuits in the cerebral cortex.

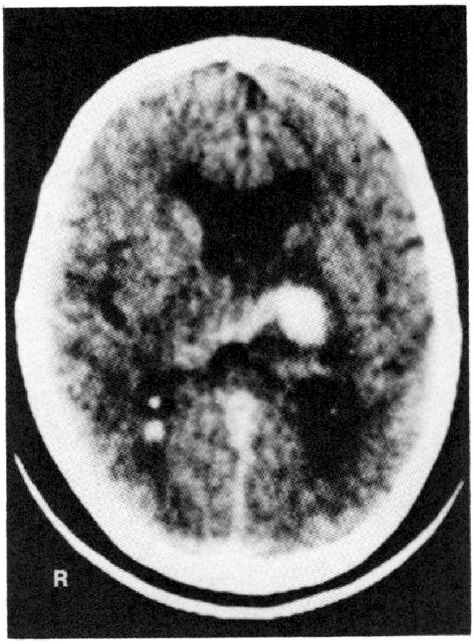

FIG. 4 Hematoma of the anterior and lateral parts of the left thalamus.

From another point of view, constructional apraxia is frequently associated with language disorders and disturbances of logical and intellectual activities in WAIS and PM47 tests, of behavior analogous to those related to frontal lobe lesions. All these disorders are related to the multiple connections of the thalamus. Underlying these disorders is the problem of dementia from thalamic lesions. Global memory defects are also frequent, since they depend on the mamillothalamic tract and the anterior nucleus of the thalamus. These are discussed later in this chapter.

Classic gestural apraxia has never been observed, even though the thalamus projects to all associative regions of the parietal lobe. Perhaps this is because the neurologic examination of symbolic gestures and the utilization of objects are not sufficiently sophisticated.

Anatomic Data

In most cases, hemorrhage involves the whole thalamus and the internal capsule; in some cases, it is possible on CT scan to see that some nuclei are spared where hemorrhage involves only the posterior thalamus and/or the pulvinar and/or the lateral nucleus. Seldom does the hemorrhage involve the anterior part of the thalamus together with its lateral part. However, we have observed such a case:

A right-handed male, 50 years old, presented with blood pressure of 260/160 mm Hg. The CT scan showed a left thalamic hemorrhage extending to the VL nucleus and not to the pulvinar (Fig. 4). There were definite abnormalities of voice: tachylalia, palilalia, dysprosody, and monotony. There was an alternation of subnormal voice and jargon aphasia. The disorders of language were as follows: jargon aphasia with neologisms; disturbances of denomination and psycholinguistic tests; and jargon agraphia. During follow-up, language disturbances improved, but the voice abnormalities did not.

This case is interesting because of the association between voice and language disorders. The voice disorders are nearly the same as those observed in thalamotomies and posterior thalamic hematoma. The language disturbances have several explanations. Activities of the nuclei surrounding the hemorrhagic focus are probably altered during a period of several weeks. It is also possible that in anterior thalamic hematomas extending to the anterior limb of the capsule, some fiber systems are damaged, i.e., projections from the frontal cortex to the pons, from the auditory cortex to the head of the caudate nucleus, from the motor thalamus to the frontal premotor cortex, from the head of the caudate nucleus toward the pallidum, and from the mediodorsal thalamus to the prefrontal cortex (7). Finally, ascending pathways from the midbrain may also interfere with such lesions. At present, it is not possible to identify all these different anatomoclinical entities, except that, when speech disorders are dominant, the lesion involves the left VL nucleus. When language disorders are dominant, the lesion involves other thalamic nuclei, pulvinar caudally and probably cranially. It is not yet possible to distinguish between these two lesions.

NEUROPHYSIOLOGIC APPROACH

For more than 10 years, numerous reports have shown the activating and inhibitory roles of intralaminar reticular formations of the thalamus and of the pulvinar on the cerebral cortex. The model of Heilman, Watson, and Walenstein is too well known to be described here (32) but can be applied to the left hemisphere in the case of language. Apart from the connections with intralaminar formations, the pulvinar receives nonspecific polysensory afferents from specific sensory nuclei in the thalamus. From this meeting point, the afferents pass through the posterior part of the internal capsule and project onto the parietotemporooccipital association areas as far as secondary sensory areas. The pulvinar is thought to receive efferents from these same cortical areas. All the secondary areas are also linked together by associative cortical and subcortical tracts. The efferents from these vast cortical areas project onto the motor cortex of the frontal lobe on the one hand; on the other hand, they project onto the medial side of the frontal lobe, the cingulum. Finally, the fibers of the cingulum project to the hypothalamus and then to the mesencephalic reticular formation. Autoactivation of each hemisphere is thus realized via the corpus callosum and the white anterior commissure, producing activity in both cerebral hemispheres.

Another model has been elaborated for the VL nucleus, which does not have an activating role but is part of the motor system; its precise participation in language activities is not yet known. For this reason, it is easy to postulate an activating role for the pulvinar on the cortex and the variations in activation and inhibition probably result in modulation of cortical functions and neuronal activities that underlie language.

Neurophysiologic models are necessary in neuropsychology, which has no meaning without them. These models are also traps; I prefer not to use such words as "selective attention" and "intention" which have psychologic meaning but cannot be used for neurophysiologic models. In order to express psychologic concepts in terms of a physiologic network, a neuronal activity should be correlated with a psychologic activity. For this reason, the following formulations are unsatisfactory: (a) thalamic structures are in charge of the elaboration of the message in prelinguistic stages; (b) the thalamus is a "strategy" point; and (c) the mutism seen in cases of tegmentothalamic infarct could reflect the disorganization of expression on a "prehistory of language" level. If the pulvinar has an activating, and perhaps an inhibiting, role in the parietotemporal cortex of the left hemisphere, there is no relationship either with the preverbitum or with linguistic units, whether received or produced.

Observation of facts raises another problem: quasiimmediate and transitory language disorders are two discrete entities. When a lesion suddenly appears, it brings on functional upsets not observed in progressive lesions, a well-known phenomenon depending on activities of those structures normally controlled by specific and nonspecific systems. Cortical activities become highly disturbed and, at this stage, symptomatology is most characteristic. If it is true that the thalamus activates cortical areas to create harmonious functioning, regression occurs usually after several weeks. The concept of perturbations of the formulations surrounding the thalamus cannot be defended (in contrast to hemiplegia), nor can the notion of plasticity and equipotentiality of the different nuclei of the thalamus.

The thalamic nuclei are integrated into circuits that have different activities, e.g. if the whole thalamus is hemorrhagic. The activating role of the right hemisphere through the corpus callosum does not agree with physiologic facts: the callosal fibers transfer information patterns from one hemisphere to the other, which does not concern a nonspecific activating function. In different pathologic cases, the right hemisphere, through the medium of the corpus callosum, has been blamed for semantic verbal paraphasias and perseverations (25), an interpretation that is attractive but incorrect if these language disorders are thoroughly analyzed:

1. All neurologic disorders must be interpreted in terms of suppression, perturbation, and disinhibition, although the notion of perturbation has tended to be forgotten. Thalamic hemorrhage can be the immediate cause of abnormal activities. It is not a normal condition for brain activities to receive exogenous electrical stimulation, which provokes abnormal discharges of the neurons stimulated, and not normal patterns. The same applies to an electrical or cryogenic probe.

2. The VL nucleus is involved in speech motor systems, being one unit of the whole; the activity of the pulvinar is different. We must remember the contrast between the integrity of the basic system of the language itself and the alterations of higher psycholinguistic activities. The role of the pulvinar very likely takes place at the level of psycholinguistic systems in the left parietotemporal lobe.

3. Most cases are related to hemorrhagic events; this is not by chance. In the white matter, a hematoma separates the nerve fibers and only minimally destroys them; functional recuperation is often remarkable, but this is in fact the same with hemorrhages in the gray matter. The sequelae manifest themselves as thin cavities in the pulvinar with normal neurons (Fig. 5). It is undoubtedly the most important factor in the regression of language disorders. In contrast, pulvinar infarcts are rare (two of 16 cases). The explanation lies in the fact that arterial vascularization is multiple and variable (e.g., the thalamogeniculate trunk; branches from the posterior choroidal artery, usually anastomosing with the anterior choroidal artery; arteries specific to the pulvinar, of which the topographic layout varies; the frequency of an occlusion of the origin of the posterior cerebral artery or of the basilar trunk). Under these conditions, either the vascularization of the pulvinar can benefit from a collateral supply or, as usually happens, the infarct is associated with other tegmentomesencephalic and thalamic lesions provoking serious disorders (coma) and often death.

4. Somatesthetic and visual neglect and/or inattention provoked by lesions of the right thalamus are also regressive (14,15). This fact must be explained in the same way as the recovery of language after lesions of the left hemisphere. These disorders are not like those produced by cortical lesions, contrary to the claim of others (3). This indicates that the pulvinar does not play as decisive a role in the cortical activities of the left cerebral hemisphere as in the right. It is remarkable that even the most severe symptoms of the Anton-Babinski syndrome are transitory, despite the marked corticosubcortical necrosis. Even in these cases, would the asomatognosia and anosognosia not result to some extent in inhibitory effects far from the lesion?

5. In vascular accidents involving several nonspecific activation areas after a coma lasting several weeks, clinical recovery comes about (even when the activating system has been destroyed), as if other activating areas remaining intact had undergone a functional reorganization, or as if the cortical activities themselves had become reorganized and could autoactivate alone. Twenty years ago (20), we reported the case of a woman whose ascending reticular formation had been destroyed (confirmed by postmortem examination). She had been in coma, followed by akinetic mutism. A small voluntary movement in the forearm enabled us to check on her normal mental activities. Other cases showed the same phenomenon, so that we no longer believe in the existence of genuine coma lasting for years.

6. We cannot agree with the schemes of a tridimensional conception of language proposed by Penfield and Roberts (28) and then by Ojemann (27). Language implies a global activity of the brain. As many dimensions can be found as one wishes, e.g., a fourth counting the left frontal lobe, a fifth with the right hemisphere, a sixth with the neoarchipallium and deep matter in relation to affective behaviors, and so on. The expression *dynamic aphasia* proposed by Luria (22) for language disorders caused by left frontal lobe lesions is accepted; but this is not real aphasia. Luria (23) has spoken about quasiaphasia for disorders from thalamic lesions, but this is not ideal terminology since "quasi" means "almost" or "more or less," and has a vague meaning. Under these conditions, there would be many and varied quasiaphasias.

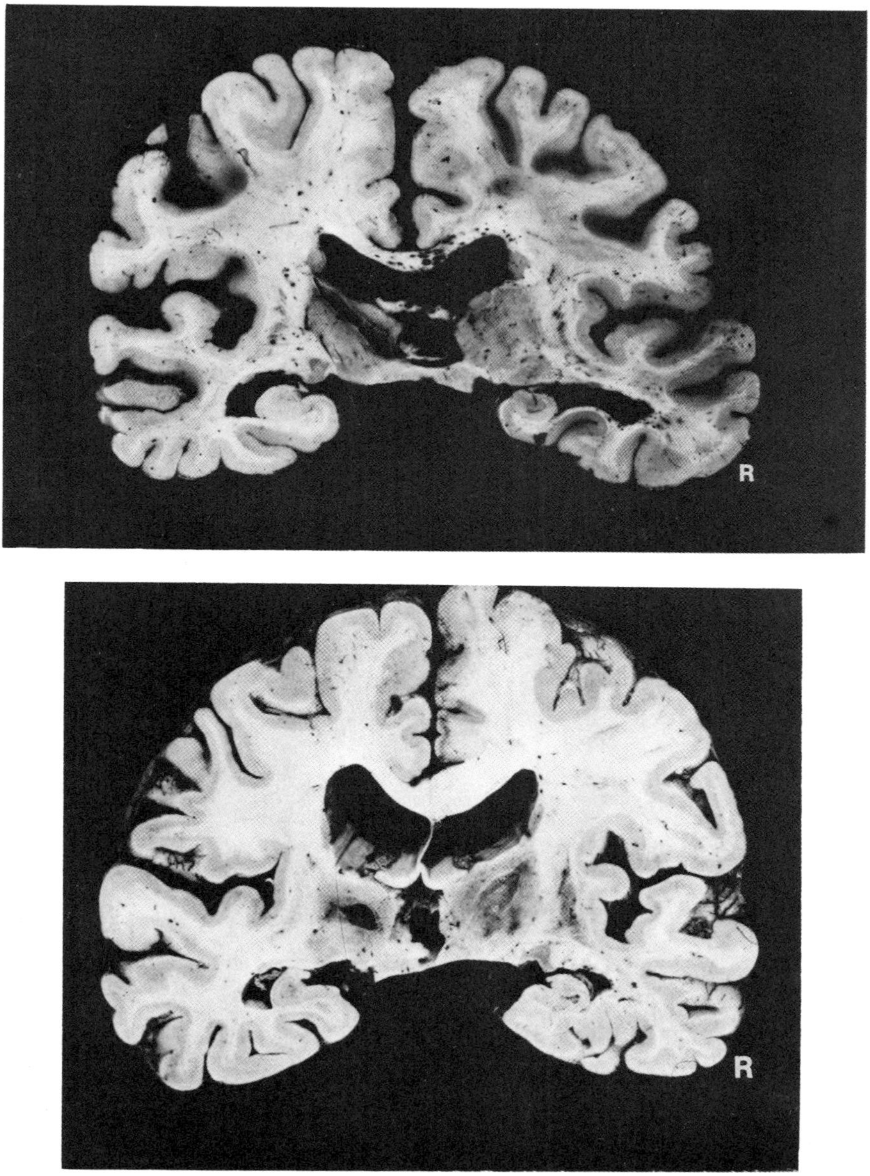

FIG. 5. Two anatomic cases of old hemorrhages of the left pulvinar. (Courtesy of R. Escourolle and F. Gray, Hôpital de la Salpêtrière.)

Without doubt, these speech and language disorders are related to dysfunction of the cortex and the subcortical white matter, but their cause is related to the disorganization of the nonspecific activating and inhibiting activities of thalamic nuclei. We say nuclei because the physiology is complex and implies many different systems; and the physiologic disturbances are not of a single nature. The best expressions are "language disorders related to thalamic lesions" or "dysphasia of thalamic origin." The word *origin* implies the site of the lesion and something about its physiologic role. "Thalamic aphasia" is the favorite expression. The French writer Paul Valery was a purist in everything concerning language. He wrote:

> Excellent not to be able to find the right word—that can prove that we really envisage a mental fact and not the shadow of a dictionary. I have spent all my life making *my* definitions.

ACKNOWLEDGMENT

We thank Dr. O. Lyon-Caen and Dr. M. Serdaru for their invaluable help.

REFERENCES

1. Bell, D. S. (1968): Speech functions of the thalamus inferred from the effects of thalamotomy. *Brain,* 91:619–638.
2. Bugiani, O., Conforto, C., and Sacco, G. (1969): Aphasia in thalamic hemorrhage. *Lancet,* 24:1052.
3. Cambier, J., Elghozi, D., and Graveleau (1982): *Neuropsychologie des lésions du thalamus.* Masson, Paris.
4. Cappa, S. F., and Vignolo, L. A. (1979): "Transcortical" features of aphasia following left thalamic hemorrhage. *Cortex,* 15:121–130.
5. Castaigne, P., Lhermitte, F., Buge, A., Escourolle, R., Hauw, J. J., and Lyon-Caen, O. (1981): Paramedian thalamic and midbrain infarcts: Clinical and neuropathological study. *Ann. Neurol.,* 10:127–148.
6. Ciemins, V. A. (1970): Localized thalamic hemorrhage: A cause of aphasia. *Neurology,* 20:776.
7. Damasio, A. R., Damasio, H., Rizzo, M., Varney, N., and Gersh, F. (1982): Aphasia with nonhemorrhagic lesions in the basal ganglia and internal capsule. *Arch. Neurol.,* 39:15–20.
8. Darley, F. L., Brown, J. R., and Swenson, W. M. (1975): Language changes after neurosurgery for parkinsonism. *Brain Lang.,* 2:65.
9. Elghozi, D., Strube, E., Signoret, J. L., Cambier, J., and Lhermitte, F. (1978): Quasi-aphasie lors de lésions du thalamus. Relation du trouble du langage et de l'activation élective de l'hémisphère gauche dans 4 observations de lésions thalamiques gauches et droites. *Rev. Neurol. (Paris),* 134:557–574.
10. Fazio, C., Sacco, G., and Bugiani, O. (1973): The thalamic hemorrhage: An anatomo-clinical study. *Eur. Neurol.,* 9:30–43.
11. Fedio, P., and Van Buren, J. M. (1975): Memory and perceptual deficits during electrical stimulation in the left and right thalamus and parietal subcortex. *Brain Lang.,* 2:78–100.
12. Fisher, C. M. (1959): The pathologic and clinical aspect of thalamic hemorrhage. *Trans. Am. Neurol. Assoc.,* 84:56.
13. Hassler, R., Mundiger, F., and Riechert, T. (1979): *Stereotaxis in Parkinson Syndrome.* Springer-Verlag, New York.
14. Heilman, K. M. (1979): Thalamic neglect. *Neurology,* 29:690–695.
15. Heilman, K. M., and Watson, R. T. (1977): Unilateral neglect syndrome. In: *Advances in Neurology, Vol 18: Hemi-Inattention and Hemispheric Specialization,* edited by E. A. Walenstein and R. P. Friedland, pp. 93–106. Raven Press, New York.
16. Hillemand, P. (1925): *Contribution à l'Etude des Syndromes de la Région Thalamique.* Thèse, Paris.
17. Lecours, A. R., and Lhermitte, F. (1979): *L'Aphasie.* Flammarion, Paris.
18. Lhermitte, F., Cambier, J., and Elghozi, D. (1981): Thalamic control of lateralized hemispheric function. In: *Studies in Cardiovascular Disease.* Masson Italia, Milan.

19. Lhermitte, F., Desi, M., Signoret, J. L., and Deloche, G. (1980): Aphasie kinesthésique et syndrome pseudo-thalamique. *Rev. Neurol. (Paris)*, 136:675–688.
20. Lhermitte, F., Gautier, J. C., Marteau, R., and Chain, F. (1963): Troubles de la conscience et mutisme akinétique. Etude anatomo-clinique d'un ramollissement paramédian bilatéral du pédoncule cérébral et du thalamus. *Rev. Neurol. (Paris)*, 109:115–131.
21. Lhermitte, J. (1936): Symptomatologie de l'hémorragie du thalamus. *Rev. Neurol. (Paris)*, 65:89–93.
22. Luria, A. R. (1966): *Human Brain and Psychological Processes*. Harper & Row, New York.
23. Luria, A. R. (1977): On quasi-aphasie speech disturbances in lesions of the deep structures of the brain. *Brain Lang.*, 4:432–459.
24. Mazaux, J. M., Orgogozo, J. M., Henry, P., and Loiseau, P. (1979): Troubles de langage au cours des lésions thalamiques. Etude par le test de Goodglass et Kaplan. *Rev. Neurol. (Paris)*, 135:59–64.
25. Michel, F., Schott, B., Boucher, M., and Kopp, N. (1979): Alexie sans agraphie chez un malade ayant un hémosphère gauche déafférenté. *Rev. Neurol. (Paris)*, 135:347–364.
26. Mohr, J. P., Watters, W. C., and Duncan, C. W. (1975): Thalamic hemorrhage and aphasia. *Brain Lang.*, 2:3–17.
27. Ojemann, G. A. (1975): Language and the thalamus: Object naming and recall during and after thalamic stimulation. *Brain Lang.*, 2:101–120.
28. Penfield, W., and Roberts, L. (1963): *Lañgage et Mécanismes Cérébraux*. P.U.F., Paris.
29. Riklan, M., and Cooper, I. S. (1975): Psychometric studies of verbal functions following thalamic lesions in humans. *Brain Lang.*, 2:45.
30. Riklan, M., Weissman, D., and Cooper, I. S. (1974): Psychological functions following pulvinectomy in man. In: *The Pulvinar-LP Complex*, edited by A. Cooper, M. Riklan, and R. Rakio, p. 138. Charles C Thomas, Springfield, Illinois.
31. Spiegel, E. A., and Wycis, H. T. (1962): *Stereoencephalotomy. II. Clinical and Physiological Applications*. Grune & Stratton, New York.
32. Walenstein, E. A., and Friedland, R. P., editors (1977): *Advances in Neurology, Vol. 18: Hemi-Inattention and Hemisphere Specialization*. Raven Press, New York.

Advances in Neurology, Vol. 42: Progress in Aphasiology, edited by F. C. Rose.
Raven Press, New York © 1984.

Intracarotid Amytal Test in the Assessment of Language Dominance

Susan M. Oxbury and John M. Oxbury

Department of Neurology, The Radcliffe Infirmary, Oxford OX2 6HE, England

The idea that non-right-handed individuals may have bilateral cerebral language representation has been inferred from findings that they are as likely as right-handers to develop aphasia from left hemisphere pathology and more likely than right-handers to do so from right hemisphere pathology (6). It has also been inferred from the apparent tendency of non-right-handers to recover better from aphasia caused by focal pathology (7). The extent of any bilateral language representation in right-handers is obscure. Brown and Hécaen (1) suggested that right-handers with aphasia from right hemisphere pathology have bilateral, as opposed to right unilateral, language representation. Rasmussen and Milner (5), however, using the carotid amytal technique, which enables the language capabilities of each hemisphere to be examined independently, did not find any case of bilateral language representation among 140 right-handers who had no evidence of left hemisphere damage sustained early in life, even though six had right hemisphere dominance. Evidence of bilateral language representation was found in 15 to 20% of non-right-handers, regardless of whether or not they had sustained left hemisphere damage early in life; this was found also in three of 42 right-handers with such early damage. Our own data, admittedly derived from a much smaller number of carotid amytal examinations, suggest that bilateral language representation of some degree might be less rare among right-handers; it is these data that we report in this chapter.

The subjects were 23 patients with long-standing epilepsy resistant to drug treatment who had bilateral intracarotid amytal examinations and who subsequently had an *en bloc* anterior temporal lobectomy carried out by Mr. C. Adams in the Department of Neurological Surgery at The Radcliffe Infirmary, Oxford, England. Approximately 50 patients have had this operation during the last 12 years. The 23 considered here are all but one of those who had carotid amytal examinations during the preoperative assessment; the other had been treated previously with a cortical excision from her left frontal lobe and is excluded. We are not considering those patients who had carotid amytal examinations prior to other types of epilepsy surgery or those in whom an operation was not carried out; part of our purpose is to relate the behavioral findings to the underlying cerebral pathology presumably responsible for the epilepsy and perhaps also for differences in cerebral organization. The portion of brain excised *en bloc* usually measured 5½ to 6½ cm in an anteroposterior dimension from the anterior tip of the temporal lobe, weighed 45 to 50 g, and in most cases contained the anterior 1 to 2 cm of the hippocampus. Histologic examination was carried out in the Department of Neuropathology at The Radcliffe Infirmary, predominantly under the auspices of Dr. J. Trevor Hughes.

The median age of the 23 patients at the time of the amytal examinations was 19 years (range, 12–42 years); 14 were male; and 14 subsequently had a right temporal lobectomy. Seventeen were right-handed, the other six being non-right-handers, i.e., left-handed or ambidextrous. Handedness was assessed on the Edinburgh Inventory (4). The primary indications for the amytal examinations were: left-handedness in six patients and a minor degree of left preference in two others, a strong family history of left-handedness in five, concern about the adequacy of memory function in seven, and an unexpectedly large performance versus verbal IQ discrepancy in the "wrong" direction in three.

As a routine, amytal is injected into the internal carotid artery contralateral to the proposed lobectomy at the first examination and into the ipsilateral internal carotid artery on a subsequent day. During the last few years, the injection has been made through a catheter introduced into the internal carotid artery via the transfemoral route, which has proved much less traumatic than the previous technique of direct carotid artery puncture. This has enabled much younger people to be examined without difficulty. The catheterizations have been carried out by Dr. Philip Sheldon and Dr. Andy Molyneux in the Department of Neuroradiology at The Radcliffe Infirmary. No premedication is given, and a small amount of contrast medium is injected during the passage of the catheter from the femoral artery to the carotid cistern to check that it is situated correctly in the internal carotid artery. Occasionally, formal carotid angiography is carried out after the amytal examination, but never before. As a routine, 200 mg sodium amytal dissolved in 4 ml water for injection (i.e., a 5% solution) is injected over a period of 3 to 4 sec; the dose is decreased to 175 mg, still as a 5% solution, for particularly young and small people. The same dose is always administered on the two sides.

On the day prior to the first examination, one of us (S.M.O.) explains the procedure to the patient, who is then asked to name the common objects that will be presented during the amytal examination; the occasional item that cannot be correctly named is excluded from the collection. It is also established that he can recite the days of the week, the months of the year, and numbers 1 to 20 both forward and backward without error. (All the patients have undergone an extensive neuropsychologic examination as part of the assessment prior to the decision to undergo epilepsy surgery.) When the catheter is situated in the internal carotid artery, and before the amytal is injected, the patient is instructed about various items for recall later in the examination; this aspect is not described any further, because memory is not being considered here. The patient is asked to hold his arms out in front of him, wiggle his fingers and toes, and begin counting. He is told that he must continue to hold up his arms, wiggle his fingers and toes, and count until asked to stop. The amytal is injected shortly after these activities have commenced. The contralateral arm falls with a flaccid paralysis within 2 to 3 sec, and the toes on the contralateral foot stop moving. The ipsilateral limbs continue as before the injection unless, as occasionally happens, the patient has a seizure, in which case the examination is repeated at a later date. Movement usually begins to return to the paralyzed limbs within 2 to 3 min, but motor function is not fully restored for 5 to 6 min.

When the amytal injection is ipsilateral to the language dominant hemisphere, there is usually a period of complete speech arrest lasting 2 to 3 min. During this period, the patient is conscious, continuing to hold up the ipsilateral arm with the fingers wiggling and with the toes on the contralateral foot still moving, but he usually does not obey verbal commands. The examiners make vigorous attempts to get him to speak, either counting, naming common objects, or repeating a word. When speech returns, common objects are presented for naming, and the patient is required to recite "series" (days of week, months of year, counting) both forward and backward, repeat simple sentences (e.g., "we shall have tea at four o'clock"), read single words, and spell; he is also presented with items of the Token Test. Items for memory testing are interspersed with the language tests, and other neuropsychologic functions can also be tested. Limb power and hand facility are tested periodically to determine the extent of recovery from paralysis. Testing of visual fields and sensation also can be carried out. Injection to the nondominant side produces a contralateral limb paralysis of the same type. Occasionally, there is a brief period of speech arrest, and speech often becomes moderately dysarthric or dysprosodic. An audio recording has always been made of the entire examination, and the more recent examinations have also been video recorded, which has greatly facilitated the subsequent analysis. As yet, we have not experienced any complication of the procedure. The patients recover within 15 to 20 min of the amytal injection and usually report that it was not unpleasant.

Eight of the 23 patients made aphasic errors after left-sided injections, in all cases including naming and/or series errors, but no aphasic errors (naming, series, repetition, reading, spelling, Token Test) after right-sided injection. One patient did the opposite; that is, he made aphasic naming and series errors after right injection but no aphasic error after left injection. Fourteen patients made naming and series errors after both left and right injections. The eight patients who made aphasic errors only after left-sided injection can clearly be classed as left hemisphere dominant. All but one had a period of more than 30 sec speech arrest following left injection. The one exception was left-handed with left temporal lobe pathology sustained in early childhood; she had prolonged convulsions when 2 years old. Histologic examination of her excised left temporal lobe showed severe neuronal loss from all zones of the hippocampus, i.e., a severe Ammon's horn sclerosis. Although she had no speech arrest, she made as many aphasic errors as the others. The median duration of speech arrest after left-sided injection was 150 sec (see Table 1). Only one of these eight had any speech arrest at all after right injection and it was short, lasting only 18 sec. The one patient who made aphasic errors only after right injection had a period of 270 sec of speech arrest after the right injection, with only 18 sec after left injection. He was clearly right hemisphere dominant for language. He was left-handed. His

TABLE 1. *Performance during carotid amytal examination in three groups defined according to whether they made errors after amytal injection into one or both carotid arteries*

Performance	Injection	Aphasic errors with injection on		
		Left only	Both	Right only
Speech arrest (sec.)	R:L	0:150	5:113	270:18
Naming errors	R:L	0:2.5	1:5	1:0
Series errors	R:L	0:2	2:2	4:0
Total errors	R:L	0:5	3:7	5:0

All figures are median.

epilepsy had begun when he was 8 years old, and pathologic basis was not established because the excised portion of his left temporal lobe showed only nonspecific histologic changes. The hippocampus was not included in the excision because of worries about the adequacy of his memory function.

The 14 patients who made aphasic errors with both left and right injections are the main subjects of interest. Their performance, and also that of the nine patients who had clearly lateralized dominance, is summarized in Table 1. Their significantly higher incidence of errors after right injection was on both naming ($p < 0.01$) and series ($p < 0.001$). They also made significantly more naming errors after left injection ($p < 0.05$), although there was no difference for series errors (see Table 1). The duration of speech arrest did not differ for these two groups, regardless of the side of injection. Various other characteristics of the groups are shown in Table 2, and the histologic findings on neuropathologic examination of the excised temporal lobes are shown in Table 3. It is important to note that the first symptom did not

TABLE 2. *Characteristics of groups defined according to whether they made errors after amytal injection into one or both internal carotid arteries*

Parameter	Aphasic errors with injection on		
	Left only	Both	Right only
Number of patients	8	14	1
Age at first symptom (median years)	3	10	8
Age at amytal (median years)	21	21.5	15
Sex M:F	5:3	8:6	1:0
Handedness R:L	7:1	10:4	0:1
Operation side R:L	5:3	9:5	0:1

TABLE 3. *Histologic findings in groups defined according to whether they made errors after amytal injection into one or both carotid arteries*

Histology[a]	Aphasic errors on injection: Left only	Both	Right only
MTS/AHS	5	7	
Alien	2	2	
Nonspecific		5	
Indefinite[b]	1		1

[a] AHS, Ammon's horn sclerosis (see text); MTS, mesial temporal sclerosis (hippocampal neuron loss but not severe in all zones); Alien, cryptic glioma (2 patients), papilloma (1 patient), cortical malformation (1 patient).
[b] Hippocampus not excised.

occur at a younger age in the group who made aphasic errors after both right and left injections, and there is no reason to believe that they had cerebral pathology from a younger age.

The relative extent of the aphasia from left and right injection, for each patient, was established by subtracting the total number of naming and series errors after right injection from the number after left injection and dividing by the sum of the two (i.e., L − R/L + R) and thus deriving an index whose value lay between +1.00 and −1.00. The resultant index for each individual is plotted in Fig. 1 according to whether the patient is right- or left- (non-right) handed. The eight patients who made errors only after left injection each have an index of +1.0; the one who made errors only after right injection has an index of −1.0. The other 14 each have an index falling between +1.0 and −1.0. It can be seen that these indices fall more or less on a continuum. Perhaps not surprisingly, left-handedness is significantly ($p < 0.05$) associated with a shift toward the right, that is, from +1.0 toward −1.0, indicating a greater relative effect of right injection. The side of operation (Fig. 2), and so presumably the side of pathology, does not seem to be a significant factor. All these 14 patients made naming errors after left injection. All but three also made series errors after left injection; the three who did not were the three with negative indices (−0.60, −0.66, −0.83) who clearly had predominantly right hemisphere dominance. After right injection, six made both series and naming errors, six made series errors only, and two made naming errors only. Five of the six with the lowest L − R/L + R indices (+0.41 to +0.08) had a dissociation of their performance on naming and series in that they made more naming errors after injection on one side and more series errors after injection on the other. Rasmussen and Milner (5) have previously reported a tendency to this dissociation among patients with bilateral language representation.

Some characteristics of the 10 right-handers who made aphasic errors after injection on each side are shown in Table 4. For clinical purposes, eight were classed as

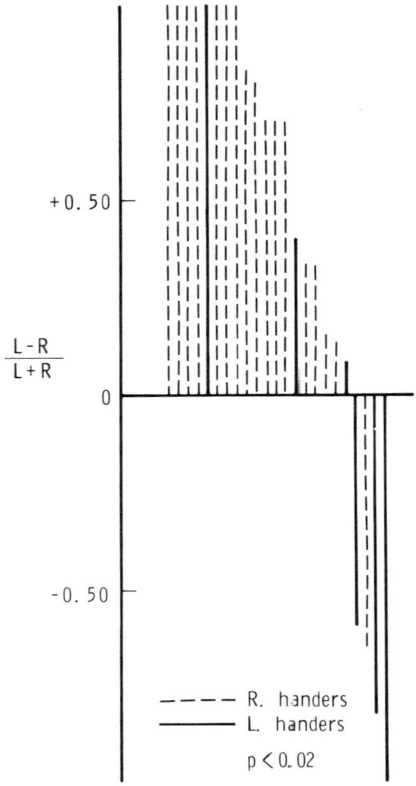

FIG. 1. Indices of each of the 23 patients according to handedness. Left-handedness is associated with a shift to the right, i.e., from +1.00 toward −1.00, suggesting greater right hemisphere involvement in language processes.

left hemisphere dominant, on the grounds that their language functions were predominantly subserved by their left hemispheres; the one with an index of −0.66 was classed as right hemisphere dominant on similar grounds. Only the girl with an index of +0.16 was regarded as "bilateral." After left injection, she had no speech arrest and made nine object naming errors and four series errors. After right injection, she had a brief speech arrest of 30 sec and made three naming and seven series errors. An analysis of our data based on clinical decisions about language dominance indicates that, of the 17 right-handers, 15 (88%) were left hemisphere dominant and two were other than left hemisphere dominant (one right dominant and one bilateral). Such figures correspond closely with those of Rasmussen and Milner (5). Our impression is that there is a continuous gradation from a very predominant effect of left injection to little difference between the two sides and to a predominant effect of right injection. Presumably, this gradation corresponds to increasing involvement of the right hemisphere in language function. If so, it then becomes a matter of definition as to who is left hemisphere dominant, who is right hemisphere dominant, and who is bilateral.

Five of the 10 patients had the histologic appearance of Ammon's horn sclerosis (severe neuronal loss from all zones of the hippocampus) on neuropathologic ex-

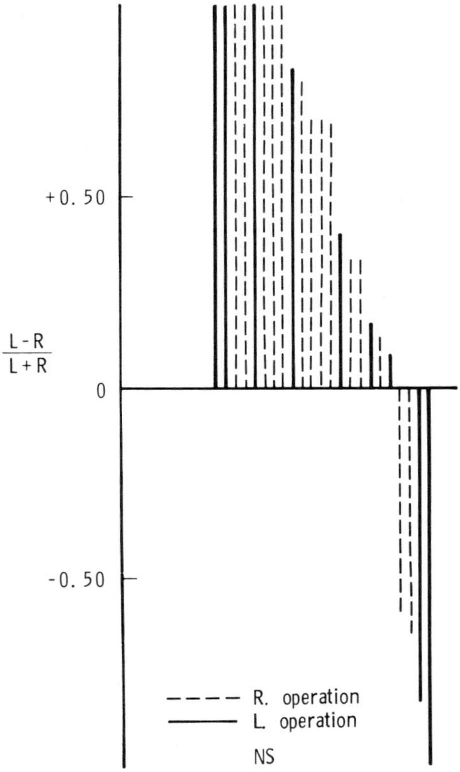

FIG. 2. Indices of each of the 23 patients according to side of temporal lobectomy; no significant difference.

TABLE 4. *Characteristics of 10 right-handed patients who made aphasic errors after amytal injection into each carotid artery*

L − R/L + R Index	Sex	Age (years) First seizure	Amytal	Preoperative IQ Verbal	Performance	Histology
+0.83	M	12	27	121	112	L, NS
+0.80	M	9	15	97	111	R, NS
+0.71	F	22	42	96	105	R, G
+0.71	M	<1	17	102	98	R, AHS
+0.69	M	3	17	95	100	R, AHS
+0.33	F	11	26	94	94	R, AHS
+0.33	M	18	24	117	120	R, AHS
+0.16	M	19	34	116	115	L, NS
+0.13	F	1	12	91	117	R, AHS
−0.66	F	7	19	78	109	R, NS

[a] AHS, Ammon's horn sclerosis; G, cryptic glioma; NS, nonspecific; L, left; R, right.

amination of their excised temporal lobes. This is the most common histologic finding in patients who have a temporal lobectomy performed at Oxford, and it is associated with a good prognosis for relief from seizures. Four others had only nonspecific findings on histologic examination. That is perhaps a higher incidence than would be expected, because such nonspecific findings occur in less than 15% of the total group of more than 50 patients in the temporal lobe series. There is no particular predominance of females [McGlone and Fox (2,3) have suggested that females may have a lesser degree of speech lateralization than males], left hemisphere pathology, or the onset of symptoms in early childhood, and most were of average intelligence. These results suggest that some degree of bilateral language representation might be quite common among right-handers, at least among those with long-standing temporal lobe epilepsy requiring surgical treatment.

It is necessary to consider the possibility that the bilateral representation is apparent rather than real, and that aphasic errors after injection ipsilateral to the nondominant hemisphere arise because amytal solution crosses to the dominant side through the circle of Willis. The anterior cerebral artery systems of the two hemispheres can arise from the same internal carotid system, but this pattern is not common. Blood can flow from one internal carotid system to the opposite side through the anterior communicating artery with a normal circle of Willis, but it is uncommon to see this during routine angiography in young people with normal cerebrovascular dynamics. The amytal solution is injected at considerably lower pressure than contrast medium during angiography, and that would make it even less likely to cross the midline. Thus the aphasic errors following injection of the nondominant side cannot be readily attributed to amytal solution crossing the midline, except on rare occasions. Furthermore, amytal solution crossing the midline should produce limb weakness ipsilateral to the injection, especially a weakness of the foot, and that does not happen.

If it is accepted that some degree of bilateral language representation occurs not uncommonly in people with long-standing temporal lobe epilepsy requiring surgical treatment, then the question arises of whether it occurs equally often in people without neurologic symptoms. This cannot be answered by the present data; some idea might be obtained from amytal examination carried out on patients requiring neurosurgical treatment for other conditions in situations where it was thought that the results of such examinations would facilitate treatment.

Our data do not confirm that incompletely lateralized cerebral dominance is associated with the onset of symptoms or cerebral pathology in particularly early life in the population who come to temporal lobectomy; nor do they suggest that it is particularly attributable to pathology in the left cerebral hemisphere. Such associations might appear with larger groups of patients, however, and the data of Rasmussen and Milner (5) indicate that left hemisphere pathology occurring early in life, but not confined to the temporal lobe, increases the extent of right hemisphere involvement in language processes. Our own data suggest that left temporal damage sustained early in childhood increases the incidence of left-handedness. Thus in the Oxford temporal lobectomy series, there were six patients who had prolonged convulsions under the age of 3 years and whose excised left temporal lobes showed Ammon's horn sclerosis; three of them were left-handed. The nine patients who had prolonged convulsions at the same age whose right temporal lobes showed the same pathology were all right-handed. The difference is significant beyond the $p < 0.05$ level, despite the small numbers.

ACKNOWLEDGMENTS

We acknowledge the great help that we have had from many members of the Oxford Neurosciences Departments while collecting these data, especially Mr. C. Adams, Dr. P. Sheldon, Dr. A. Molyneux, Dr. T. Hughes, Dr. H. Sagar, and Mrs. M. Crouch. Our thanks are also due to our patients for letting us examine them repeatedly over the years and for allowing us to gain some inkling of their cerebral organization. We also acknowledge gratefully the assistance of members of the Department of Medical Illustration at the John Radcliffe Hospital, especially that of Mr. D. Harwood.

REFERENCES

1. Brown, J. W., and Hécaen, H. (1976): Lateralisation and language representation. Observations on aphasia in children, left-handers, and "anomalous" dextrals. *Neurology,* 26:183–189.
2. McGlone, J. (1977): Sex differences in the cerebral organisation of verbal functions in patients with unilateral brain lesions. *Brain,* 100:775–793.
3. McGlone, J., and Fox, A. J. (1981): Evidence from sodium amytal studies of greater asymmetry of speech representation in men compared to women. Paper delivered at the Epilepsy International Congress, September 21, 1981, Kyoto, Japan.
4. Oldfield, R. C. (1971): The assessment and analysis of handedness. The Edinburgh inventory. *Neuropsychologia,* 9:97–113.
5. Rasmussen, T., and Milner, B. (1977): The role of early left-brain injury in determining lateralisation of cerebral speech functions. *Ann NY Acad. Sci.,* 299:355–369.
6. Satz, P. (1980): Incidence of aphasia in left-handers: A test of some hypothetical models of cerebral speech organisation. In: *Neuropsychology of Left-Handedness,* edited by J. Herron, pp. 189–198. Academic Press, New York.
7. Subirana, A. (1958): The prognosis in aphasia in relation to cerebral dominance and handedness. *Brain,* 81:415–425.

Advances in Neurology, Vol. 42: Progress in Aphasiology, edited by F. C. Rose.
Raven Press, New York © 1984.

Genetics of Handedness in Relation to Language Disorder

I. C. McManus

Department of Psychology, Bedford College, University of London; and Department of Psychiatry, St. Mary's Hospital Medical School, London, England

. . . nature's simple equations in the mind's precincts . . .
R. S. Thomas

In the second half of the 19th century, two major biologic discoveries were made. Broca described the dichotomous division of the population according to cerebral language dominance, and Mendel described the laws of the discrete, particulate inheritance of biologic characteristics and the "simple equations" governing them. Since that time, a number of attempts have been made at integrating these two discoveries. In this chapter, I describe a simple model for interpreting the available data.

A major intervening variable in the relationship between genes and language dominance is handedness. This is due in part to its moderate correlation with language dominance and its clear familial tendencies but also is a reflection of the inherent difficulties of studying language dominance *per se* within families. A genetic analysis of a characteristic is not possible unless chromosomal reassortment has occurred during meiosis, but such analysis necessarily entails a knowledge of the phenotypes of related individuals (parent/offspring or siblings); this is difficult to obtain. For instance, it is not easy to find cases of aphasia attributable to unilateral lesions for whom there is a relative with a similar lesion. As a result, phenotypic handedness, which is relatively easily and reliably assessible for whole families, acts as a surrogate or model of the far more interesting phenotype of language dominance. It is, therefore, a lateral step from most genetic models of handedness to a model of language dominance; usually only indirect (i.e., strictly nongenetic) evidence can be found for the genetic model of language dominance.

A consequence of the above is that much of the current chapter concentrates on handedness and will only eventually be extrapolated to language dominance and aphasia. Unless we have an adequate genetic model of the voluminous data available on handedness, genetic models of the sparse data on language dominance and aphasia probably are premature.

THE PHENOTYPE OF HANDEDNESS

The keystone of genetic analysis is an appropriate description of the phenotypes, as may be immediately realized by considering the problems that would have arisen in analyzing the genetic basis of the mental subnormality now known to be due to phenylketonuria, had the blonde hair of these children been taken as the primary phenotype for analysis.

In the case of handedness, two phenotypic approaches may be found in the literature. Early studies tended to take the stated handedness of individuals at face value, using simply the layman's criterion of the hand used for writing. The use of this description resulted in two awkward results for any simple genetic model: the incidence of left-handedness differed between studies (implying different allele frequencies in different populations), and the incidence differed within studies between parents and offspring (implying strong selective pressures, usually in favor of left-handedness). While neither implication is impossible, neither seemed to be reasonable.

A second approach originated in the doubts raised as to the utility of a simple dichotomization into right- and left-handers. Annett (1) explicitly suggested that a third category of mixed handers could be identified. It should be noted that these mixed handers were not the relatively rare ambidexters but rather a group of individuals who were neither pure right-handers nor pure left-handers; they represented some 32% of the population. Annett (2) developed this position, suggesting that handedness represented a continuum between pure right- and pure left-handedness, and that this continuum was seen in the distribution of skill asymmetries and in the distribution of grip strength asymmetry [a result based on Woo and Pearson's (31) analysis of Galton's anthropologic laboratory data of 1884].

According to Annett's (2) theory, it becomes impossible to classify individuals as being either right- or left-handed; rather, they are merely more or less right-handed. The incidence of apparent left-handedness in a population, therefore, depends on the particular threshold or criterion chosen, and the incidence thus can vary between studies, and can even vary within the same individuals in the same study if a different criterion is applied. Annett's approach solves the problem found in earlier studies of different incidences of sinistrality, but it subsequently fails itself, in that degree of handedness becomes an unmeasurable variable, manifesting only in the form of degree of skill asymmetry. Furthermore, it is necessary, for a number of reasons, to characterize the distribution as a mixture of several normal distributions (see, e.g., ref. 4). However, a statistical analysis of skill asymmetry data (21) finds that Annett's models of the skill distribution are inadequate as a description of actual data, and that the skill distributions are more compatible with a dichotomous description of the population (i.e., left- or right-hand writers), with a degree of variability introduced, due to either measurement errors or real individual differences, which give the superficial impression of a single continuous unimodal distribution.

My own interpretation of the phenotypic description of handedness follows the commonsense view in arguing that the clearest difference in skill between the hands is in writing ability, the vast majority of individuals being unable to write at all well with their nondominant hand. That a few individuals are not as clearly lateralized as the rest should not mean that we dispose of the conceptual advantages of a simple dichotomy; to do so would be to reproduce the "black-is-white" fallacy of Flew (10). Laterality researchers have continually searched for the elusive grail of the ideal measure of handedness [in part, as Bishop (6) has suggested, in the hope that clinically useful correlates would then emerge]. Nevertheless, it remains true that, of all the tasks that have been studied using either questionnaires or actual performance of skilled tasks, asymmetry of writing ability shows the greatest relative difference between hands: the least incidence of "either" responses on questionnaires (in approximately 2,000 laterality inventories, no subject has reported that he could write equally well with either hand) and the best test-retest reliability of all inventory or skill measures. The distribution of writing ability, therefore, is grossly bimodal, with minimal overlap between the distributions. Nevertheless, despite these strong features in its favor as a measure of handedness, writing hand suffers from several difficulties, which may be circumvented by careful statistical analysis:

1. Some individuals have been forced by teachers or parents to change from writing with the left hand to writing with the right hand [a practice that has now almost totally ceased in the West, although reports of it still occur from Russia (30) and Albania (9)]. This problem may be partially assessed in surveys by asking individuals whether or not they have ever been forced to change writing hand through either social pressure or injury, and reclassifying the positive responders.
2. For various reasons, individuals may conceal their true handedness in questionnaire surveys; in the earlier years of this century, left-handedness represented a social stigma; hence its incidence was lower than might be expected. In recent years, left handedness has come to be associated with creativity and hence is socially desirable.
3. Left- or right-handers may respond at a differential rate in questionnaire surveys either for similar reasons to those given above or because, in general, left-handers as a group seem to be interested in why they are different from the rest of the population.

As a result of these problems, we must distinguish an individual's manifest writing hand (i.e., as apparent in a survey) and his true writing hand. In a population, we must distinguish the manifest incidence and the true incidence of left-handedness. By assuming, in the first instance at least, that all populations have the same true incidence of left-handedness, and that parents and offspring also have the same true incidence of left-handedness, we may fit genetic models of handedness. Whether or not the fit of models is improved by allowing a secular increase in the incidence of left handedness then becomes an empirically answerable question.

It should be apparent that many of the difficulties associated with the classification of writing hand could be avoided if writing ability were assessed by performance rather than by inventory. However, since genetic studies are of necessity large, and

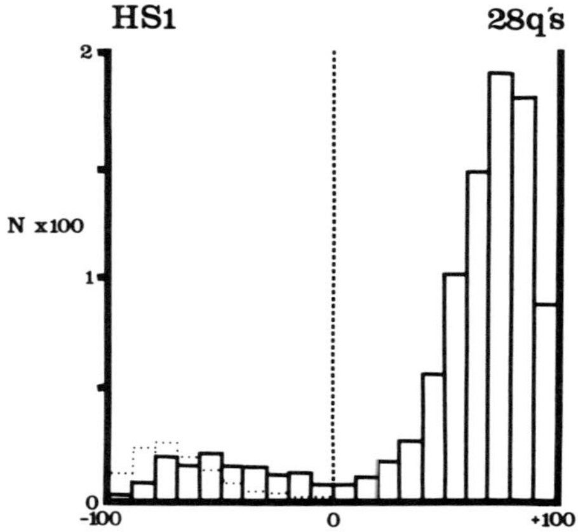

FIG. 1. Distribution of laterality scores of 948 undergraduates on a 28-item handedness inventory (15), each item being scored on a five-point scale. A score of −100 indicates that the subject responded "always left hand" on all items; a score of +100 indicates a response of "always right hand" on all items.

since genetically related individuals must be studied, this desirable feature is rarely attained.

This categorical approach to classification does not necessarily lack the desirable features of Annett's continuum of handedness. Figure 1 shows the responses of 948 subjects to a 28-item handedness inventory. Although the distribution is bimodal, within each mode there is a great amount of variability; indeed, it could be argued that there is a broad continuum across the whole distribution. It is important to note that the hand used for writing discriminates between the two modes almost perfectly (15), with almost no errors of classification. We may distinguish, therefore, between differences in direction of lateralization (right or left) and differences in degree of lateralization within each of the modes (Fig. 2); statistical methods for their differentiation in the case of overlapping distributions are described elsewhere (22). Since there is no correlation between the degree of handedness of parents and offspring (McManus, genetic model), and since degree of handedness within a direction group shows no relation to familial sinistrality (15), we may conclude that there is no inheritance of degree of handedness. In contrast, large numbers of studies have found strong familial trends in direction of handedness. It can be argued, therefore, that while Annett was right to stress that handedness is a continuum, that continuum is not itself homogenous. As a result, we may distinguish direction and degree of handedness. The former is dichotomous, has a familial component, and hence is of genetic interest, whereas degree of handedness is continuous, may represent either true individual differences or perhaps errors of measurement, and has no genetic component.

Finally, the distribution of Fig. 1 provides little support for the concept that the population contains a separate group who may be called ambidexters; if they do exist, they are sufficiently rare to mean they are unlikely to interfere with the genetic studies described.

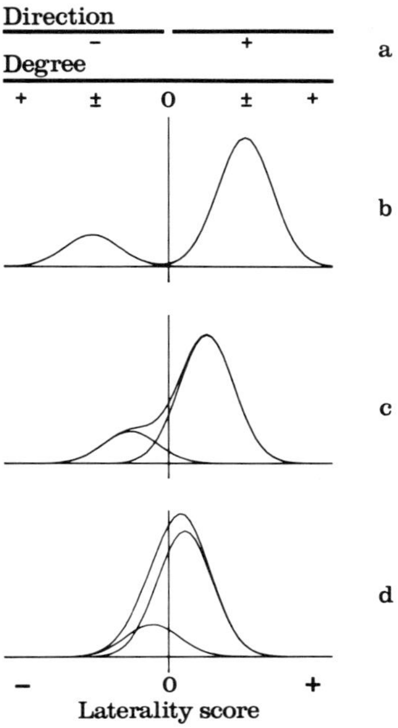

FIG. 2. The author's conception of the phenotypic description of handedness. Strongly lateralized scales (such as handedness inventories) show a bimodal distribution, in which the two modes are sufficiently far apart to mean that they hardly overlap at all (*b*). As a result, two independent measures, the direction of handedness (a categorical variable) and the degree of handedness (which is a continuous variable), may be derived (*a*). As the modes of the two distributions come closer together, it becomes more difficult to distinguish the two separate components in the overall distribution (*c* and *d*), such that *d* gives the superfical impression of being a single normal distribution.

A GENETIC MODEL OF HANDEDNESS

A genetic model of handedness has several biologic constraints, a more detailed account of which may be found elsewhere (19). In particular, the model must be compatible with the concept of fluctuating asymmetry, which says that the baseline for any lateralized biologic characteristic is a racemic mixture, in which 50% of a population are dominant on each side. Furthermore, any genetic model must be compatible with what I have called "Morgan's principle," which suggests that it is extremely unlikely that paired alleles can directly produce enantiomorphic phenotypes (25). Such a constraint rejects many of the earlier genetic models of handedness, such as those of Chamberlain (8), Rife (27), Ramaley (26), Trankell (28), and Annett (1). The detailed implications of the principle have been described by McManus and Mascie-Taylor (23). The only other genetic model compatible with Morgan's principle is Annett's second model (3), and I have argued elsewhere that it must be rejected on other grounds (21).

There are several problems with any genetic model of handedness:

1. Although almost all studies of handedness show significant familial trends, these are not as strong as might be expected under most simple Mendelian systems. Thus approximately 5% of the children of two right-handed parents are left-handed, and about 35% of the children of two left-handed parents are left-handed.

2. Studies of the handedness of twins show that while there is a slightly higher concordance for handedness in monozygotic (MZ) rather than in dizygotic (DZ)

twins, the overwhelming impression is of almost chance levels of concordance, for which conventional wisdom would suggest almost no genetic control of handedness. In passing, it should be noted that there is probably no clear evidence for twins having a higher incidence of sinistrality than singletons, or for the occurrence of the process known as mirror-imaging (for a review of handedness in twins, see ref. 16).

3. Many theorists have suggested that a relatively high proportion of left-handers may have become sinistral as a result of pathologic causes. Elsewhere, I have reviewed the historic basis and the evidence for the concept of pathologic left-handedness and have suggested that it has no empirical basis (20). In particular, I have found no evidence in two large studies for an association between left-handedness and birth trauma (18) or epilepsy (17). In fitting the genetic model, I have ignored such considerations, although it should be noted that the method of correction for differences in the incidence of left-handedness will generally take into account any such pathologic cases.

In this chapter, I present only the basic genetic model without providing the detailed justification for it, which may be found elsewhere (19). The model postulates that there are two alleles, D (for dextral) and C (for chance), which are at a single locus. Individuals who are of genotype DD are all right-handed [i.e., $p(L|DD) = 0$, a pure directional asymmetry]. Individuals who are of genotype CC exhibit pure fluctuating asymmetry; hence 50% of them are right-handed and 50% are left-handed [i.e., $p(L|CC) = 0.5$]. As such, the model is incompletely defined, since the phenotypic manifestation of the heterozygote, $p(L|DC)$, has not been given. This value cannot be defined *a priori* on theoretical grounds, however, and must be determined from the data. It is also necessary before fitting the model to know $p(C)$, the incidence of the C allele in the population [since this determines the true incidence of left-handedness, $p(L_t)$, which is assumed to be constant in all populations]. Neither $p(C)$ nor $p(L_t)$ can be determined in advance, and one or the other must be estimated from the data. Given particular values of $p(L_t)$ and $p(L|DC)$, any data set may be assessed for its fit to the model, a method of correcting for different manifest incidences of handedness having been described elsewhere (19). It is possible, therefore, by means of a computer, to assess the adequacy of fit of all data sets for all possible values of $p(L_t)$ and $p(L|DC)$ and hence to find the maximum likelihood estimates of those parameters. Such calculations suggest that $p(L|DC) = 0.25$ and $p(L_t) = 0.0775$. In other words, the genetic model is additive, rather than dominant or recessive, the heterozygous phenotype being midway between the two homozygotes. The true incidence of left-handedness is 7.75%; hence the frequency of the C allele is 0.155.

Table 1 summarizes the model which is a best fit to the data in the literature. Elsewhere (12), I have shown that this genetic model is a better fit to the available data than that of Rife (27) and Trankell (28) and is as good a fit as that of Annett (3), although that model fails on other grounds (21).

TABLE 1. *The proposed genetic model*[a]

Genotype	Phenotypes: Left	Phenotypes: Right	Population frequency	
DD	0.0	1.0	0.714	Directional asymmetry
DC	0.25	0.75	0.262	Additivity of heterozygote
CC	0.5	0.5	0.024	Fluctuating asymmetry

[a] Alleles: D, dextral; C, chance. $p(L_t) = 0.0775$; $p(C) = 0.155$.

Consideration of Table 1 shows why left-handedness runs so poorly in families; even if two left-handers are both of the CC genotype, their offspring have only a 50% chance of being left-handed (although they are, as it were, breeding true for the phenotype of fluctuating asymmetry). Table 2 shows the expected distributions of left-handed offspring in families of one and two children according to the handedness of the two parents.

The relatively low concordance of MZ twins is more interesting. Consider the 2.4% of the population who are of genotype CC. Each has his handedness phenotype determined by a chance process *in utero,* resulting in 50% of individuals becoming left-handed. Exactly the same process is assumed to occur in MZ twins, except that the two chance processes are assumed to occur independently in the two twins. As a result, 25% of CC MZ twins are both right-handed, 25% are both left-handed, and 50% are discordant, one being right-handed and the other being left-handed. Similarly, 37.5% of MZ twin pairs of the DC genotype will be discordant for handedness (although all DD pairs will be concordant). The result, as shown in Table 3, is that for the population as a whole, the MZ concordance rate is only slightly higher than that in DZ twins.

To summarize thus far, it is suggested that the genetic model of Table 1 is capable of fitting all the available family and twin data on handedness, appropriate correction having been made for differences between studies in the manifest incidence of left-handedness.

TABLE 2. *Probability of parents of known handedness having particular combinations of right- or left-handed children*

Parents[a]	One child: R	One child: L	Two children: RR	Two children: RL	Two children: LL
R × R	0.940	0.060	0.891	0.099	0.010
R × L	0.826	0.174	0.687	0.277	0.036
L × L	0.711	0.289	0.510	0.403	0.087

[a] R, right; L, left.

TABLE 3. *Predicted proportions of monozygotic (MZ) and diazygotic (DZ) twins of particular handedness combinations*[a]

Twins	R – R	R – L	L – L
MZ	0.867	0.110	0.022
DZ	0.859	0.127	0.014

[a] R, right; L, left.

A GENETIC MODEL OF LANGUAGE DOMINANCE AND APHASIA

A genetic model of language dominance must account for certain facts:

1. Tests of cerebral dominance by dichotic listening, unilateral electroconvulsive therapy (ECT), or intracarotid amytal suggest that between 8 and 20% of right-handers and 29 and 40% of left-handers show right-hemisphere dominance for language (7).
2. About 1 to 2% of right-handed aphasics and about 20 to 30% of left-handed aphasics have a right hemisphere lesion. The incidence of crossed dominance in right-handers, therefore, is estimated differently from clinical and laboratory data.
3. Left-handers are more likely to become aphasic after a cerebral lesion, are more likely to recover from that aphasia, and thus are less likely to suffer from aphasia (11,12).
4. Familial sinistrality seems to increase the likelihood of recovery from aphasia (12,32).

The following section outlines the extrapolation of the model of handedness to that of dominance and aphasia; once more, details of the statistical basis of the model fitting are omitted, and the interested reader is referred elsewhere (19).

Consider an individual of the CC genotype. During development, a random process determines whether or not he becomes right- or left-handed. If we allow the possibility in such individuals that a random process also determines whether or not they become right or left hemisphere dominant for language, and that the two random processes are statistically independent, then we would expect that 25% of CC individuals would be right-handed with right-language dominance, 25% right-handed with left language dominance, and so on.

Applying a similar process to individuals of DC and DD genotype (and of course all DD individuals must be right-handed and left-language dominant), then we can predict the incidence of right-hemisphere language dominance in right- and left-handers (Table 4). The incidence of right hemisphere dominance is compatible with that found in other studies, particularly after correction is made for differences in the manifest incidence of right dominance (due to nonspecificity or unreliability of the tests used). It is also clear from Table 4 that parental sinistrality relates to the likelihood of right hemisphere dominance, although the effect is far stronger in right-

TABLE 4. *Proportion of individuals who are expected to be right hemisphere dominant for language, as a function of handedness and parental handedness, under the simpler form of the model*

	Handedness	
Parents[a]	Right (%)	Left (%)
NK × NK	6.0	28.9
R × R	4.6	28.0
R × L	14.8	30.0
L × L	24.6	39.4

[a] NK, not known; R, right; L, left.

handers than left-handers. The only major problem with Table 4 is that the figure of 6.0% of right-handers showing crossed dominance is not compatible with the estimates of the incidence of crossed aphasia in the literature, which have an upper limit of about 2%.

Having allowed that two separate asymmetries may be independently controlled by the same gene, it is possible to extend the model in a purely formal manner by allowing three or more asymmetries to be determined by the same gene. Let there be two language dominances, which we may label LA and LB. We would then predict that one-eighth of CC individuals would be right-handed, with LA and LB both on the left, and so forth. At this point, it cannot be emphasized strongly enough that LA and LB do not correspond to Wernicke's and Broca's areas, or to any other established laterality system; they are merely a conceptual device for exploring the range of the model.

Considering LA and LB, it is clear that, since either may be right- or left-sided, three important groups of individuals can be distinguished: (a) LA and LB both left-sided, (b) LA and LB both right-sided, and (c) bilateral, in which case LA is on one side and LB on the other. If a lesion occurs in the right hemisphere, and if both LA and LB are right-sided, then the result will be an aphasia, since all linguistic capacity will have been removed. If LA and LB are both left sided, then a right-sided lesion will not cause any incapacity.

The interesting case arises if LA and LB are bilaterally distributed. A right-sided lesion will damage only one of the two language systems. Initially, we might expect this to cause aphasia or dysphasia, either because of the process of diaschisis or because in normal operation the two centers are integrated in their action and hence cannot function independently; the patient thus will be acutely aphasic. Since the patient still retains one language processing center, however, we may expect that in the long term he will recover functioning, using just his one remaining center. In the long run, the patient will not be permanently aphasic but will have recovered from his aphasia (Fig. 3).

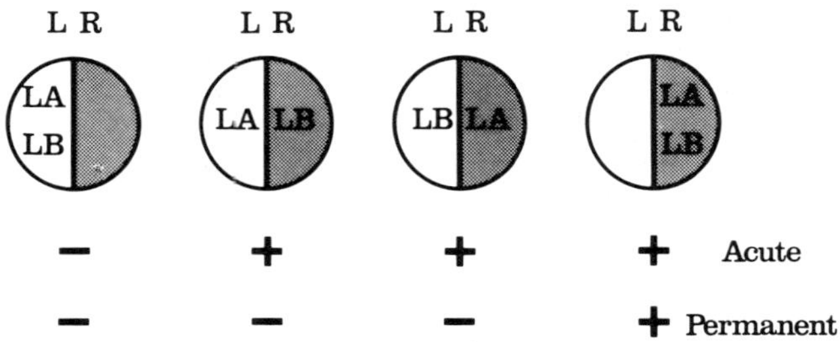

FIG. 3. Effects of a right-sided lesion on the four possible types of LA-LB organization, "+" indicating that a particular type of aphasia will occur and "−" indicating that it will not.

Under this extension of the model, it is necessary for a right hander to have LA and LB in the right hemisphere to suffer a permanent aphasia after a right-sided lesion. The usual estimates of the incidence of crossed aphasia are probably based on permanent aphasics, since these are the patients who are most likely to present for clinical psychologic assessment, and since studies of acute aphasia show a higher incidence of crossed aphasia than is usually reported.

Table 5 shows the expected incidence of the language dominance types by handedness. Table 6 shows the expected proportions of right- and left-handed aphasics who would be expected to have right-sided lesions, according to their parental handedness. It is clear that the incidence of permanent dextral crossed aphasia (1.8%) is now compatible with clinical data. It should also be noted from Table 6 that a parental history of sinistrality makes it more likely that a right-sided lesion has occurred. It might be thought at this point that the LA-LB model is incompatible with the simpler model described earlier (see Table 4), but this is not the case; if dominance as assessed by, e.g., dichotic tests is more dependent on one of LA and LB than on the other, then the LA-LB model reduces to the simpler model described above.

Table 7 shows the percentage of right- and left-handers who would be expected to be aphasic after a right- or left-sided lesion, or after a lesion on either side. Left-handers are more likely to be acutely aphasic after a cerebral lesion than are right-handers but are less likely to be permanently aphasic. Table 8 summarizes the probability of an acutely aphasic individual recovering language after a right- or left-sided lesion. Left-handers are more likely to recover than are right-handers, and the majority of this effect is with left-sided lesions. Parental handedness has an important

TABLE 5. *Expected proportions of right- and left-handers who would be expected to show right, left, or bilateral location of the LA and LB centers*

Handedness	Both left (%)	Bilateral (%)	Both right (%)
Right	89.7	8.6	1.7
Left	51.4	39.4	9.2

TABLE 6. *Expected proportion of aphasics who would have right-sided lesions by handedness and parental handedness*

	Right-handers (%)		Left-handers (%)	
Parental handedness[a]	Acute aphasia	Permanent aphasia	Acute aphasia	Permanent aphasia
R × R	7.4	1.3	34.2	13.9
R × L	20.9	5.3	35.7	16.6
L × L	30.6	13.2	42.7	30.9
NK × NK	9.5	1.8	34.8	15.1

[a] R, right; L, left; NK, now known.

influence on the likelihood of recovery, particularly in right-handers with left-sided lesions. A surprising prediction of the model is that a history of parental sinistrality makes recovery less likely after right-sided lesions, although the effect is small and primarily confined to those with two left-handed parents.

The above model has been fitted to a series of data sets from the literature and has generally been found to be compatible (see ref. 19). An interesting exception is that in fitting two series of data on aphasia after neurosurgical operation in patients with chronic epilepsy or temporal lobe glioma, it was found that the permanent model fitted the data better than the acute model, as was also the case in a series of non-operated patients with gliomata or meningiomata. It was argued that in both cases, the continual, chronic damage, be it recurrent ictal attacks or a slowly expanding tumor, had resulted in the abolition of diaschisis and the development of functional autonomy in the centers in the two hemispheres.

Once it has been suggested that several independent lateralized systems may be controlled by the same genetic mechanism, then the explanatory power of the model is rapidly increased; indeed, it rapidly exceeds that of the data available for testing it. Two possible cases can be briefly discussed. If the lateralization of visuospatial functions is also controlled by the same genetic locus as handedness and language dominance, then we might expect cases in which language and visuospatial ability are both in the same hemisphere. Such cases have been previously suggested, on

TABLE 7. *Expected incidence of aphasia after a unilateral lesion in right- and left-handers*

	Right-handers (%)		Left-handers (%)	
Lesion	Acute aphasia	Permanent aphasia	Acute aphasia	Permanent aphasia
Left	98.3	89.7	90.8	51.4
Right	10.3	1.7	48.6	9.2
All	54.3	45.7	69.7	30.3

TABLE 8. *Expected proportion of acutely aphasic individuals who would be expected to recover, as a function of handedness, lesion side, and parental handedness*

	Right-handers (%)		Left-handers (%)	
Parental handedness[a]	Left lesion	Right lesion	Left lesion	Right lesion
R × R	6.7	84.3	42.6	82.1
R × L	22.1	83.4	44.4	80.1
L × L	34.1	77.4	53.9	72.4
NK × NK	8.8	83.9	43.4	81.2

[a] R, right; L, left; NK, not known.

the basis of both tachistoscopic studies (14) and clinical cases (13). The number of such individuals is compatible with the predictions of the model. A more speculative possibility is that reading or writing skills may be lateralized independently, so that in some patients, a unilateral lesion will result in alexia without agraphia. As an example taken at random from the recent literature, consider the two cases described by Sevush et al. (29) of Wernicke's aphasia with intact oral reading after a left-sided lesion. The authors correctly point out the problems of interpreting these cases in conventional terms. If we suggest that some but not all of the typical processing of the left hemisphere is located in the right hemisphere in these individuals, however, then their defects become comprehensible.

Two other implications of the model are important for clinical and experimental purposes. First, if the present model is correct, then more than 10% of right-handed patients might have some linguistic ability in the right hemisphere, an incidence that is sufficiently high to make the interpretation of data from individual hemispherectomy, callosal section, or stroke patients difficult. Second, the present model allows for a certain rate of recovery from aphasia. No cognisance is taken in the model of the possible benefits of speech therapy, and it could be argued that the effects of therapy are primarily to speed recovery in those who would have recovered, rather than to change individuals from nonrecoverers to recoverers.

The model may also be extended to other areas in which laterality has been implicated. It is repeatedly claimed, both in stutterers and in those suffering from developmental dyslexia, that left-handedness is more common than in the general population [although McManus and Mascie-Taylor (24) failed to demonstrate any relationship between eye-hand dominance and a specific reading deficit, and Bishop (6) has found similar difficulties]. There are also suggestions that abnormal laterality is implicated in psychoses, particularly schizophrenia. If the present model is correct, then an implication is that all atypical forms of lateral organization (i.e., in which some or a majority of centers are not on their typical sides) should be more common in left-handers. If disorders such as dyslexia or stuttering involve failures of integration between, e.g., visuospatial and linguistic systems, because they are atypically arranged in the hemispheres, then the condition should be associated with sinistrality.

An atypical disposition of lateralized centers might require greater interhemispheric connections to produce functional integration and hence may explain the increased corpus callosum thickness that has been reported in schizophrenia (5).

CONCLUSIONS

This chapter briefly presents a genetic model that explains many of the features associated with the inheritance of handedness and of the association between handedness and language dominance and aphasia. Its major theoretical advantages are its conceptual simplicity (two alleles at a single locus and additivity) and its ability to be extended by the single gene controlling a number of independent lateralities. The resultant complexity is compatible with the complexity of the clinical phenomena. The major limitation of the model is a lack of adequate data for subjecting it to a rigorous test of its predictions.

REFERENCES

1. Annett, M. (1964): A model of the inheritance of handedness and cerebral dominance. *Nature,* 204:59–60.
2. Annett, M. (1972): The distribution of manual asymmetry. *Br. J. Psychol.,* 63:343–358.
3. Annett, M. (1978): *A Single Gene Explanation of Right and Left Handedness and Brainedness.* Lanchester Polytechnic, Coventry.
4. Annett, M., and Kilshaw, D. (1983): Right and left-hand skill. I: Estimating the parameters of the distribution of L-R differences in males and females. *Br. J. Psychol.,* 74:269–283.
5. Bigelow, L. B., Nasrallah, H. A., and Rauscher, F. P. (1983): Corpus callosum thickness in chronic schizophrenia. *Br. J. Psychiatry,* 142:284–287.
6. Bishop, D. V. M. (1983): How sinister is sinistrality? *J. R. Coll. Physicians Lond.,* 17:161–172.
7. Bradshaw, J. L., and Nettelton, N. C. (1983): *Human Cerebral Asymmetry.* Prentice Hall, New Jersey.
8. Chamberlain, H. D. (1928): The inheritance of left-handedness. *J. Hered.,* 19:557–559.
9. Dobbs, M. (1980): *The Sunday Times (London).* November 9, p. 9.
10. Flew, A. (1975): *Thinking about Thinking.* Fontana, London.
11. Hécaen, H., and Albert, M. L. (1978): *Human Neuropsychology.* Wiley, New York.
12. Hicks, R. E., and Kinsbourne, M. (1978): Human handedness. In: *Asymmetrical Function of the Brain,* edited by M. Kinsbourne, pp. 523–549. Cambridge University Press, Cambridge.
13. Kreindler, A., Fradis, A., and Sevastopol, N. (1966): La réparation des dominance hémisphériques. *Neuropsychologia,* 4:143–149.
14. McGlone, J., and Davidson, W. (1973): The relationships between cerebral speech laterality and spatial ability with special reference to sex and hand preference. *Neuropsychologia,* 11:105–113.
15. McManus, I. C. (1979): *Determinants of Laterality in Man.* Doctoral dissertation, University of Cambridge.
16. McManus, I. C. (1980): Handedness in twins: A critical review. *Neuropsychologia,* 18:347–355.
17. McManus, I. C. (1980): Left-handedness and epilepsy. *Cortex,* 16:487–492.
18. McManus, I. C. (1981): Handedness and birth stress. *Psychol. Med.,* 11:485–496.
19. McManus, I. C. (1983): Handedness, language dominance and aphasia: A genetic model. *Psychol. Med. [Monogr. Suppl.] (in press).*
20. McManus, I. C. (1983): Pathologic left-handedness: Does it exist? *J. Commun. Disord.,* 16:315–344.
21. McManus, I. C. (1983): Right and left-hand skill: Failure of the right-shift model. *Br. J. Psychol. (in press).*
22. McManus, I. C. (1983): The interpretation of laterality. *Cortex,* 19:187–214.
23. McManus, I. C., and Mascie-Taylor, C. G. N. (1979): Hand-clasping and arm-folding: A review and a genetic model. *Ann. Hum. Biol.,* 6:527–558.
24. McManus, I. C., and Mascie-Taylor, C. G. N. (1983): Biosocial correlates of cognitive abilities. *J. Biosoc. Sci.,* 15:289–306.

25. Morgan, M. J. (1976): Embryology and inheritance of asymmetry. In: *Lateralisation in the Nervous System,* edited by S. R. Harnad, R. W. Doty, J. Jaynes, and G. Krauthamer, pp. 173–194. Academic Press, New York.
26. Ramaley, F. (1913): Inheritance of left-handedness. *Am. Naturalist,* 47:730–738.
27. Rife, D. C. (1950): Application of gene-frequency analysis to the interpretation of data from twins. *Hum. Biol.* 22:136–145.
28. Trankell, A. (1955): Aspects of genetics in psychology. *Am. J. Hum. Genet.,* 47:730–738.
29. Sevush, S., Roeltgen, D. P., Campanella, D. J., and Heilman, K. M. (1983): Preserved oral reading in Wernicke's aphasia. *Neurology,* 33:916–920.
30. van der Post, L. (1965): *Journey into Russia.* Penguin Books, Harmondsworth.
31. Woo, T. L., and Pearson, K. (1927): Dextrality and sinistrality of hand and eye. *Biometrika,* 19:165–199.
32. Zangwill, O. L. (1960): *Cerebral Dominance and its Relation to Psychological Function.* Oliver and Boyd, London.

Advances in Neurology, Vol. 42: Progress in Aphasiology, edited by F. C. Rose.
Raven Press, New York © 1984.

Task- and Modality-Specific Aphasias

Freda Newcombe and John C. Marshall

Neuropsychology Unit, Neuroscience Group, The Radcliffe Infirmary, Oxford 0X2 6HE, England

Our general concern in this chapter is with the structural and functional fractionation of the language faculty as revealed by the behavioral consequences of brain damage in adult life. More specifically, we consider the extent to which the language faculty can be regarded as a modular component of cognitive capacity divorced from the sensory, perceptuomotor, and other performance mechanisms involved in the exercise of linguistic skills. In the simplest cases, the distinction between a pathology *of* language and a pathology that manifests itself *in* an impairment of language functioning is not problematic. There would be little point in describing a person with acquired peripheral deafness as dysphasic, despite the fact that he will manifest a severe comprehension impairment for spoken language; similarly, a man with a broken right arm should not be described as dysgraphic, despite the fact that his ability to write is impaired.

AGRAMMATISM

More problematic cases include the agrammatism of spontaneous speech seen in some patients with nonfluent aphasias (16). These patients have a selective tendency to leave out (in obligatory contexts) closed class items, both bound (markers of tense, case, and agreement) and free-standing (articles, prepositions, conjunctions, pronouns, and auxiliary verbs). It would be reasonable to think of this deficit as consequent on the (partial) destruction of some central grammatic module (either lexical, morphologic, or phonologic) that represented the class of so-called function words in question. If this were so, one would expect that those patients who manifest expressive agrammatism would also show receptive agrammatism. That is, they should fail to comprehend sentences (for example, passives) whose correct syntactic interpretation depends on the analysis of closed class vocabulary. Indeed, in *some* agrammatic patients, there is an analogous selective failure to appreciate the structure building aspects of closed class vocabulary in forced choice comprehension tasks (3,17). Furthermore, some of these expressive and receptive agrammatics also fail on tasks in which they are required to give grammaticality judgments that engage the role of closed class items in sentences (19).

Although agrammatism often reveals itself across a variety of different tasks, there are cases in which the phenomenon is manifest in one task, but there is no trace of a closed class deficit in another. For example, Miceli et al. (13) have recently published two cases of expressive agrammatism in Italian. Despite a striking tendency to omit function words and finite verb inflections in spontaneous speech, syntactic comprehension was within normal limits. Linebarger et al. (10) have reported four cases of Broca's aphasia in English with both agrammatic expression and comprehension. The patients are remarkably skilled nonetheless at making grammaticality judgments on sentences with correctly and incorrectly selected and placed function words. Goodglass (5) has reminded us that similar cases who "performed flawlessly in making grammaticality judgements" were reported in the classic German literature (7,8). *Prima facie,* these dissociations seem to argue against the notion of a central modality- and task-neutral module which is indiscriminately drawn upon in the exercise of distinct linguistic skills.

NAMING TO VISUAL AND TACTILE PRESENTATION

Von Eckardt Klein (18) suggests that the process of naming an object consists of (at least) four stages:

Stage 1. Computing a modality-specific representation of the object.
Stage 2. Computing a modality-neutral "conceptual" representation of the object.
Stage 3. Searching an internal lexicon for the name of the object on the basis of a conceptual access code.
Stage 4. Finding or compiling an articulatory motor program of the name and executing that program.

The point of calling the stage 2 code "modality-neutral" presumably is to indicate the unity of that representation across modalities. Thus Goodglass et al. (6) hypothesize that this stage involves "a process which is not bound to a specific afferent system [that] mediates between any stimulus and the evocation of the spoken word." This mediating process is the computation of a semantic or conceptual code, and the simplest hypothesis is that there is one mechanism within the brain that can compute such a code.

The line of argument is consistent with the fact that in most aphasic (as opposed to agnosic) patients, the approximate severity and the qualitative nature of naming difficulties are indeed comparable across modalities of stimulus presentation. Again, there are well-studied (albeit rare) cases in which a genuinely aphasic disturbance of naming is much more pronounced in one modality than another. Thus the studies of Lhermitte and his colleagues (9) have shown that semantic errors can occur in naming to visual confrontation (e.g., PICTURE OF A KNIFE→ "plate") in patients whose naming to tactile palpation (with either hand) is essentially intact. The very name of the syndrome (optic aphasia or visual anomia) indicates how poorly we can reconcile the phenomenon with the claim that aphasias are modality free (and agnosias modality specific).

Conversely, bilateral tactile aphasias have been described that are not immediately interpretable as an interhemispheric disconnection syndrome. The case of Beauvois and co-workers (1) made semantic naming errors to objects tactually presented to either the left or the right hand (e.g., CORK → "bottle"; TEACUP → "a plate . . . a spoon"). The naming of objects to visual confrontation was almost intact, however, and certainly did not show semantic paraphasias. It is difficult to see how these patterns of dissociation can be reconciled with the claim that a unitary "modality nonspecific process intervenes between stimulus presentation and naming" (6).

ACQUIRED DYSLEXIA AND DYSGRAPHIA

Our own work has been concerned with the fractionation of reading and orthographic skills. Studies of the acquired dyslexias show at least two distinct routes whereby the written word may be read aloud. One of these routes involves the indirect association of word forms with pronunciation via their respective semantic representations. Pathology within this route leads to the occurrence of numerous semantic paralexias when the patient reads aloud individual words (without context, time pressure, or stimulus degradation). Representative examples from our first case of "deep dyslexia" (11) include:

act → "play"
uncle → "cousin"
close → "shut"
truth → "honest"
test → "experiment"
XII → "B.C."

In other patients, access to sight vocabulary is impaired, and the patient must convert the constituents of letter strings into auditory form via grapheme-phoneme correspondence rules. In one particularly pure form of "surface dyslexia" (12), the patient assigns a phonetic value to each letter of a stimulus word, irrespective of the presence of digraphs, such as *ch, ea,* or *ow,* that should each be realized as a single phoneme. Representative errors from one such patient include:

tale → /tæ lij/
whip → /wə hIp/
feat → /fij æt/
suit → /su: It/
whom → /wə hɔm/
goes → /gɔ ɛs/

For each of these two patients, the pattern of error in writing to dictation matches qualitatively the character of reading aloud. Thus the deep dyslexic makes semantic paragraphias (15):

"boat" → SHIP
"glove" → LACE
"star" → MOON
"bun" → CAKE
"nephew" → UNCLE
"den" → HOUSE

The surface dyslexic consistently simplifies his writing to dictation and writes one orthographic symbol for one sound of the auditory stimulus:

"guess" → GES
"blood" → BLUD
"thumb" → FUM
"liquor" → LIKA
"phrase" → FRAZ
"goes" → GOZ

Do such cases imply that reading aloud and writing to dictation are mediated by two subsystems, such that for a given patient, "transcoding" in one direction (visual to auditory) will always match the pattern of performance in the reverse direction (auditory to visual)? Apparently not.

We recently studied a patient whose symptoms included an "auditory analogue to deep dyslexia," a rare syndrome first described by Goldstein (4) and thoroughly investigated by Michel (14). Our patient originally presented with a severe fluent aphasia consequent on an intraventricular meningioma situated mainly in the anterior horn of the left temporal lobe. Postoperatively, spontaneous speech was paragrammatic, with copious circumlocutions; object naming (to visual confrontation) was impaired, with many semantic circumlocutions that indicated correct identification of the object:

TREE → "nice and green plants"
TOOTHBRUSH → ". . . teeth . . . to brush your teeth"
WINDMILL → "the wind . . . the wind turn around"

Semantic circumlocutions and substitutions were also found in the immediate repetition of single words:

"book" → "from reading"
"nephew" → "father . . . mother"
"college" → "oh, yes . . . to learn"

Equivalent semantic paraphasias were also in evidence when writing to dictation:

"book" → READING
"tree" → PLANTS
"cousin" → SISTER

Reading aloud was also impaired (albeit not as seriously), but no semantic circumlocutions or substitutions were ever made in this task.

The patient reads by phonologic routes. She shows a strong "regularity effect" in reading aloud (that is, she is better at reading regularly than irregularly spelt words), and her errors include many regularizations and miscorrespondences of the type seen in surface dyslexia (e.g., *sew* → "sue"; *heir* → "here"). Testing with homophones frequently revealed misinterpretations, even when the word could be read aloud correctly. For example, the following glosses were produced:

eye → "I think"
sum → "some people . . . there are more than one"
oar → "I'll do the washing or the ironing"

The interpretation of written words is mediated by feedback from internal phonologic representations assembled or addressed prior to semantic access. By contrast, repetition of spoken words is mediated solely by their semantic representations in the absence of any peripheral route that can convert the auditory stimulus into phonologic and articulatory form. Similarly, in writing to dictation, the auditory stimulus can only contact its graphic equivalent *via* an intermediary semantic representation. In short, we see the co-occurrence of surface dyslexia with deep dysgraphia. A yet more striking dissociation has recently been reported by Bub and Kertesz (2): deep dysgraphia in the context of fully preserved reading aloud and oral repetition of single words.

CONCLUSION

This chapter looks briefly at three areas in which pathologies have been described that seem to implicate grammatic variables (morphologic, syntactic, or semantic) that are held in common across a variety of performance skills: (a) the manipulation of closed class vocabulary, (b) lexical access and retrieval in confrontation object naming, and (c) orthographic transcoding. But the realization of this linguistic competence can be differentially impaired across different overt tasks and modalities in ways that are not immediately interpretable as agnosic or apraxic deficits. Accordingly, one might want to consider the hypothesis that each performance module of the language faculty contains, in some sense, its own knowledge-base.

REFERENCES

1. Beauvois, M.-F., Saillant, B., Meininger, V., and Lhermitte, F. (1978): Bilateral tactile aphasia: A tacto-verbal dysfunction. *Brain,* 101:381–401.
2. Bub, D., and Kertesz, A. (1982): Deep agraphia. *Brain Lang.,* 17:146–165.
3. Caramazza, A., and Zurif, E. (1976): Dissociations of algorithmic and heuristic processes in language comprehension: Evidence from aphasia. *Brain Lang.,* 3:572–582.
4. Goldstein, K. (1948): *Language and Language Disturbances.* Grune & Stratton, New York.
5. Goodglass, H. (1983): Linguistic aspects of aphasia. *Trends Neurosci.,* 6:241–243.
6. Goodglass, H., Barton, M., and Kaplan, E. (1968): Sensory modality and object-naming in aphasia. *J. Speech Hear. Res.,* 11: 488–496.
7. Isserlin, M. (1922): Ueber Agrammatismus. *Z. Gesamte Neurol. Psychiatr.,* 75:332–410.
8. Kleist, K. (1934): *Gehirnpathologie.* Barth, Leipzig.
9. Lhermitte, F., Chedru, F., and Chain, F. (1973): A propos d'un cas d'agnosie visuelle. *Rev. Neurol.,* 128:301–322.
10. Linebarger, M. C., Schwartz, M. F., and Saffran, E. M. (1983): Sensitivity to grammatical structure in so-called agrammatic aphasics. *Cognition,* 13:361–392.
11. Marshall, J. C., and Newcombe, F. (1966): Syntactic and semantic errors in paralexia. *Neuropsychologia,* 4:169–176.
12. Marshall, J. C., and Newcombe, F. (1973): Patterns of paralexia: A psycholinguistic approach. *J. Psycholing. Res.,* 2:175–199.
13. Miceli, G., Mazzucchi, A., Menn, L., and Goodglass, H. (1983): Contrasting cases of Italian agrammatic aphasia without comprehension disorder. *Brain Lang.,* 19:65–97.
14. Michel, F. (1979): Préservation du langage écrit malgré un déficit majeur du langage oral (A propos d'un cas clinique). *Lyon Med.,* 241:141–149.
15. Newcombe, F., and Marshall, J. C. (1980): Transcoding and lexical stabilization in deep dyslexia. In: *Deep Dyslexia,* edited by M. Coltheart, K. E. Patterson, and J. C. Marshall, pp. 176–188. Routledge and Kegan Paul, London.

16. Pick, A. (1913): *Die agrammatischen Sprachstörungen*. Springer, Berlin.
17. Schwartz, M. F., Saffran, E. M., and Marin, O. S. M. (1980): The word order problem in agrammatism. 1: Comprehension. *Brain Lang.*, 10:249–262.
18. Von Eckardt Klein, B. (1978): Inferring functional localization from neurological evidence. In: *Explorations in the Biology of Language*, edited by E. Walker, pp. 27–66. Bradford Books, Montgomery, Vermont.
19. Zurif, E., Caramazza, A., and Myerson, R. (1972): Grammaticality judgements of agrammatic aphasics. *Neuropsychologia*, 10:405–419.

Advances in Neurology, Vol. 42: Progress in Aphasiology, edited by F. C. Rose.
Raven Press, New York © 1984.

Language Input Variables in Aphasia

David Crystal

Department of Linguistic Science, University of Reading, Reading RG6 2AA, England

THE SIGNIFICANCE OF LANGUAGE INPUT

"The first step [in aphasia research] is to compile a description of the patient's aphasic symptomatology." This statement, taken almost at random from the most recently published textbook on aphasia therapy (3, p. 145), is a truism that should not need stressing in the 1980s. Yet the full range of implications deriving from this statement have not yet been taken into account in either aphasia research or therapy. In a previous report (7), I emphasized the necessity of carrying out a complete description of the aphasic patient's (P) language in terms of some theory of linguistic levels, and argued that certain levels have been unjustifiably neglected: prosody and certain aspects of semantics, in particular (7). This chapter looks at a totally different dimension to the definition of aphasic symptoms, which has been even more neglected than the structural facets of P's language (it is given no systematic discussion in the textbook referred to above, for example): the nature of the therapist's (T) (or other investigating or managing adult's) input language.

It is not strange to discuss T's input language as constituting part of the definition of P's symptoms, considering that this is the field of language disorder. Language disability, as language ability, is canonically an interactive phenomenon. We do not typically talk when there is no one around to listen; we expect our talk to have an effect on others, and we are aware that others' talk will have an effect on us. Aphasic symptoms, then, will be manifest only in interaction, and in this respect they are unlike most other kinds of medical symptoms. A patient does not go home and nurse his aphasia, as he does a wounded knee. If P does not wish to communicate, or if no one wishes to communicate with P, there will be no aphasic symptoms. In like manner, the nature of these symptoms at least in part depends on the person P is talking to, and specifically on the kind of language he or she uses. For example, it would be easy to conclude that the following sequence of P sentences illustrated someone at a single clause element stage of grammatical development: *a car, a man, a bus, trees*. In fact, they were all used as responses in a drill in which T was asking "What can you see in the picture? What else can you see?" and represent a kind of single element sentence which is unrelated to developmental processes, as they are all elliptical. The sequence "*T* What can you see in the picture? *P* Trees." is a legitimate conversational turn. By contrast, the sequence "*T* Where's the man going?

P Trees." is not. P may be saying something relevant about the picture, but the linguistic relationship between *trees* and T's stimuli differs in these two sequences. In the first, P's utterance could be expanded into "I can see trees"; in the second, it cannot be expanded into "*The man is going trees." The second sentence is a cause for immediate concern; the first is not. We know this, however, only by considering the relationship between P's and T's sentences. It is in this way that the nature of T's input language forms part of the definition of P's disorder.

In other words, aphasic symptoms do not exist in isolation but are elicited; and the means of elicitation thus become part of the object of study. This becomes especially important when research is undertaken into therapeutics and management, where the ability to control or structure the linguistic interaction with P is considered to be a defining feature of T's professionalism and is a current focus of study, relating to the efficacy of speech therapy. The following set of quotations from Code and Müller (2) is illustrative of the need for foundational work in this area: "the majority of efficacy studies have shown methodological shortcomings and inconsistencies which give rise to difficulty in making comparisons between them" (11, p. 24) . . . "it is only by describing aims and methods precisely that the efficacy of speech therapy for aphasia can truly be evaluated. Too many papers gloss over the details of the therapeutic programme, so that objective judgement of its actual relevance to improvement in the patient's language function is virtually impossible" (14, p. 74) . . . treatment must "be described in sufficient detail to allow it to be exactly duplicated by other therapists teaching other patients" (3, pp. 198–199), which in effect means "a detailed account of every therapeutic step undertaken" (14, p. 74). Many variables are involved in this enormous task; but, whereas recent studies have become increasingly aware of the need to control such factors as the amount and duration of treatment, the crucial question of the nature of the treatment remains vague. In an account of the Bristol evaluation study, for example, precise details of amount and duration of treatment are followed by this account of the nature of the intervention: "The speech therapists treat the patient using such techniques as training and experience suggest to be appropriate" (11, p. 22).

In a recent comparative study of aphasic patients, in which I had an advisory role, I had to agree that the only way to proceed, in the present state of knowledge, was to instruct the participating therapists to interact as they normally would in carrying out their allocated tasks. This was reluctant agreement, however, for I knew some of the Ts involved and had analyzed samples of their work in other connections. I knew, therefore, that there were major differences of style and strategy in their use of language. One T, for example, said *good,* or an equivalent phrase, after almost every P response; another T was much more sparing in her praise. One T would repeat her action-cuing phrase as part of every stimulus (e.g., "Can you point to the blue pen? . . . Can you point to the red pencil? . . . Can you point to the . . ."); another T would rarely repeat the opening phrase and added many variations (e.g., "Can you point to the blue pen? . . . Now, the red pencil? . . . What about a green book? . . ."). It would be naive to assume that such stylistic differences would somehow "cancel each other out"; but there was no way of controlling for them without radically altering the proposed design of the study and vastly extending its length. As so often, more questions than answers were being generated.

It is difficult to know whether such research is ultimately a waste of time. After all, I could not honestly advise the researchers *not* to proceed, simply on the basis of my intuition that these stylistic differences are important. On the other hand, my quandary does illustrate the urgent need for further research into these differences, as an end in itself. In view of the widely expressed feeling that there are "few firm conclusions to be drawn from aphasia therapy evaluation to date" (11, p. 22), it would seem that my dissatisfaction with current procedures is not simply a private obsession.

An accurate description of T's input language, complementary to and in the same terms as that provided of P's language, is a *sine qua non* of progress in relation to the above areas. Only with such a description available can one begin to investigate systematically such central issues as the linguistic level of T's language in relation to the level at which P is functioning; the extent to which T is consistent in working with the same P or with different Ps; the role of different T strategies in working with P; and the variability that Ts manifest as a result of different kinds of training and experience.

We have become used to carrying out tests and other assessments on Ps' samples in recent years; it should also become routine to carry out no less stringent assessments on Ts' contributions to the interaction. As one looks at the various test forms, profile charts, and so on, it is rare to find space allocated for even the barest indication of T's input style; and when it is, it is often ignored by practising Ts. For instance, the Language Assessment Remediation and Screening Procedure (LARSP) chart (10) has a section B in which a simple but fundamental distinction is made between two kinds of T stimulus: whether or not T has used a grammatical question. The use of clearly defined questions, as opposed to the use of other stimuli (statements, commands, exclamations, prompt noises) is a major variable in therapeutic style. In brief, the more questions one introduces into an interaction, the more interrogating it becomes, and the less like natural conversation, where questions are not the dominant method of eliciting responses, as recent studies have shown (9,17). The LARSP distinction is a fairly basic measure; a more sophisticated classification of the grammatic functions of T stimuli is now practicable and certainly desirable. Even this basic distinction can be ignored, however, with Ts often using the LARSP approach without completing section B.

As a further example, we may consider the way in which the course of a particular P's aphasia is often studied, over a period of time, by obtaining tape recorded samples of the therapy sessions at specified times and of specified durations. Let us imagine a 30-min sample obtained 1 month after P's incident, and a second 30-min sample obtained 6 weeks later. The T is giving speech therapy to P twice a week. It is obvious that one of the most significant changes that will take place during this period is that T will become more used to P (and vice versa); as a consequence, T will not be talking to P in the same way. The conversation will become more informal; more information will be left unsaid; certain themes will become favorite topics; other themes will be a cause of upset; certain tasks will become routine—and all this will have specific linguistic consequences for T's choice of sounds, grammar, and vocabulary. It is inevitable that T's input language will change; and it is a sound therapeutic principle that it should change, as T keeps pace with (and, usually, aims to stay a little ahead of) the level of P's emerging language. If change is the expected state of affairs, care must be taken in any assessment of progress to ensure that like is being compared with like.

If, as a consequence of T becoming familiar with P's linguistic limitations, T develops language strategies to make P respond within these limitations, to make him feel at ease, and so on, it becomes unclear whether P's or T's progress is in fact being monitored. To say that P has made progress, in the sense that he is saying or understanding more, or is speaking more confidently, may be illusory.

Here is an illustration of the kind of stylistic change that can take place. In an early session (A), T used the following stimuli as part of her work on comprehension (transcription conventions are explained below):

A I 'just want you to 'point to the 'things that I sày/ OḰ/ . . . now I'm 'going to 'ask you some quèstions/ OḰ/ – and I 'just 'want you to say 'yes – or nò/
I've 'got some pìctures hére/ and I 'just 'want you to 'have a lóok/ – and 'tell me 'what you 'can aboùt it/ alríght/

Within two sessions, her style had altered markedly, primarily by reducing the length of these opening stimuli. She then used such sentences as the following:

B nòw/'here are some pìctures/ – réady/
'you 'point when I nàme 'something/ OḰ/
nòw/ 'say 'yes or 'no ònly/ OḰ/

This reduced (and almost telegrammatic, at times) style is presumably the result of T's growing awareness of P's limitations of comprehension, memory and attention—an awareness that one can actually observe in the course of development, in such "inverted pyramid" sequences (i.e., longer sentences above, shorter below) as the following, taken from session A:

when I 'ask you these quéstions/ I 'just 'want you to 'say yes or nò/
P looks blank
'you just say 'yes or nò/ OḰ/
'yes or nò Mister 'Smith/
'yes—or nò/
P grunts and nods
'nothing èlse/

It was fairly evident to all concerned that P was responding better to the questions in session B; he made fewer wrong responses, made more confident correct responses, and was generally less hesitant. To check whether it was genuine progress on P's part, it would be necessary to do one of several things, such as analyze P's behavior talking to people other than T, or see how P behaved if T reintroduced the longer stimuli of session A. It would not be enough to have recourse to formal testing in this kind of situation, as this would have little or nothing to say about the general conversational skills involved. The only way to determine the influence of these variables in T's behavior is to incorporate them into one's description of the session, relating them to the language used by P. It is then a matter of conscious decision whether to replicate an earlier interaction style for a new sample or to allow various changes. This decision must be based on detailed knowledge. It is worth recording that, in the above example, the skills displayed by T were not under conscious control; until this analysis was carried out several days later, she was not aware that she had changed her interaction style so drastically.

INPUT VARIABLES

If one wishes to control the nature of input language for purposes of diagnosis, assessment, or therapy, it is first necessary to be clear about the range of variables involved. Surprisingly, this basic awareness is not routine; fundamental aspects of language structure and use still are neglected, not only in everyday clinical work but even in research studies. The range of variables will be the same as that required for the specification of P linguistic behavior, but the descriptive statement will be inevitably more complex, as T's language (being "normal") will utilize more fully the resources available in the language. It should be pointed out, however, that not everything that T says is necessarily relevant for the description of input language. Clinical linguistic interaction is typically a three-part process, which has been described as a sequence of *stimulus, response,* and *reaction* (4,5). Usually, it is T who initiates an interaction with a *stimulus* utterance, as:

T 'point to the tàble/
T 'how are you fèeling to'day/
T 'tell me a'bout this pìcture/

P may then *respond,* and if he does, T may *react* to his response, with, e.g., agreement, praise, or amplification:

T 'what can you 'see in the pìcture/	*stimulus*
P a càr/	*response*
T yès/ it's a càr/ that's rìght/ . . .	*reaction*

Linguistic input refers primarily to T's stimulus and reaction language, i.e., language that is directed to P. Although T may say a great deal more than this in the course of a clinical session—he may answer the phone, talk to a relative, or talk to himself (not at all uncommon, especially when one is "organizing oneself" before a structured activity)—these kinds of utterance must be considered separately, if the notion of input is not to be rendered vacuous.

Following conventional linguistic accounts (5), input variables can be classified into variables of *structure* and *use*. *Structural* variables concern the form utterances take, described independently of the social situations in which they are used. *Use* variables specify the nature of these social situations and the functions performed by these utterances. In clinical linguistics, the traditional focus of attention has been on the structural specification of P language; only in recent years has there been a

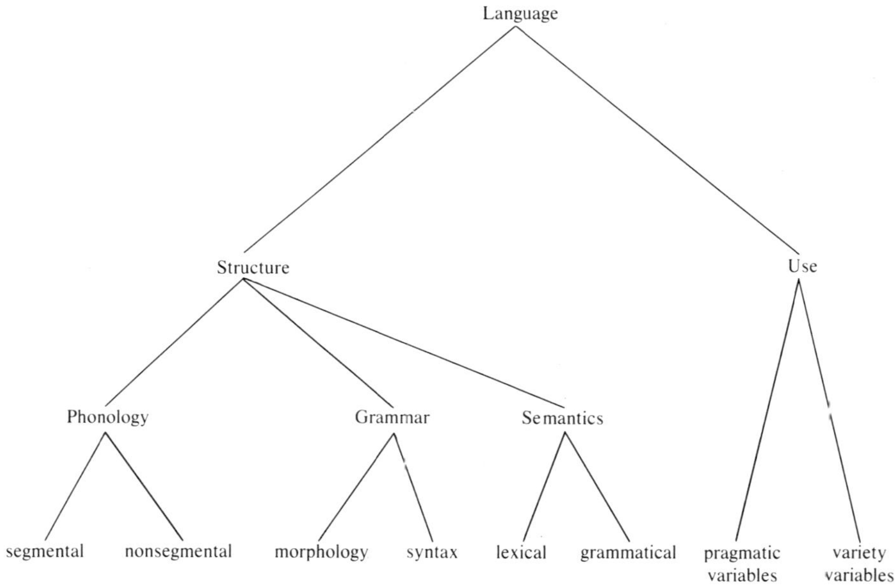

FIG. 1. Input variables in linguistic analysis.

complementary approach to the study of language in use. Current studies of input language, however, seem to be demonstrating a reverse neglect, focusing on utterance functions and situations at the expense of utterance forms. Thus, for example, several papers in language acquisition studies provide a classification of the functional reasons for an adult's child-directed utterances (such as agreeing, denying, directing, persuading), but few studies pay proper attention to the formal characteristics of the utterances that expound these functions (what kinds of ways are available in the language for the expression of agreement, denial, direction, persuasion). It would be unfortunate if clinical studies of T input demonstrated a similar lack of concern to preserve a balance between formal and functional dimensions of analysis, especially at the present time, when the research field is in need of delineation. The following model gives equal weight to the two major types of variable and to their subtypes, pending such time as their relative contribution to aphasic symptomatology can be determined.

Figure 1 outlines the main variables involved. Under the heading of structure, three levels of linguistic analysis are recognized: phonology, grammar, and semantics, the first and last of which are analyzed further into two sublevels. At the level of segmental phonology, one analyzes utterances into vowels, consonants, and their combinations as syllables. At the level of nonsegmental phonology, one analyzes the properties of utterance generally referred to by such labels as prosody, intonation, rhythm, and tone of voice. At the level of grammar, the structure of sentences and sentence sequences is analyzed in terms of syntax and morphology. At the level of lexical semantics, one analyzes the meaning and other properties of vocabulary.

At the level of grammatical semantics, one analyzes the meaning, or role, of the units (words, phrases, clauses) recognized by the study of grammar. The following sentence illustrates the kind of information that analysis at each of these levels would provide, using one particular approach (5).

The man's driving a car

Segmental phonological transcription: ða mænz draıvıŋ ə kɑ:

Nonsegmental phonological transcription: the 'man's 'driving a *càr*/
where / marks the end of an intonation/rhythm unit; italics marks the most prominent word in that unit; ` marks the direction of pitch movement (falling) on that word; and ' marks the occurrence of stressed syllables.

Grammatical analysis:

the man		's driving		a car	
Subject		Verb		Object	
Determiner	Noun	Auxiliary verb	Main verb	Determiner	Noun
		contracted auxiliary	*-ing* ending		

to which must be added grammatical information about the sentence type—a statement—and about the relationship between this sentence and others formally derivable from it, such as questions (*is the man driving a car?*) or the passive (*a car is being driven by man*).

Lexical semantic analysis: Each item would be analyzed in terms of the semantic field to which it belongs (e.g., *car* is a member of the field of *vehicles*) and of its relationship to other items in the language (e.g., one *drives* a *car* or *train*, but not a *bike* or *airplane*; with reference to the same object, one might be said to be driving a *car, auto, motor, jalopy*; *man* is in a certain sense the opposite of *woman*; and so on).

Grammatical semantic analysis: Each grammatical unit performs a semantic role. Thus, at the clause level, the subject performs the semantic role of *actor*; it is the element that carries out the action specified by the verb. At the phrase level, the semantic role of the determiner *the* is to specify that the *man* in question is identified, or definite; and so on.

Under the heading of *use*, several further dimensions of linguistic analysis must be recognized, which can be grouped into two main types: *pragmatic* and *variety* variables. Pragmatic variables refer to the factors governing the user's choice of utterance arising out of the social interaction in which he is involved, factors such as when someone chooses to speak, how much he says, whether the subject matter is appropriate to the situation, and so on. For example, the sentence "You'll be needing your coat, Mr. Jones," as said by T, would be appropriate, one imagines, only toward the end of a session, and if there was some reason for T to introduce the topic (e.g., if it were starting to rain, or if P has forgotten to pick it up); it is difficult to imagine a setting in which T used this sentence at the beginning of a clinical session. Pragmatic variables are currently attracting a great deal of interest in general linguistics and have received little application as yet in aphasiology (15,16). Variety variables refer to those features of an utterance that are situationally distinctive, in the sense that the linguistic features bring to mind a particular extralinguistic setting, and vice versa. Chief among these are the following (8):

Regional dialect features: signal where the speaker is from, in geographic terms, such as Scottish, American, or Liverpudlian.

Social dialect features: signal where the speaker is from, in terms of, e.g., class background and educability.

Temporal features: signal the historic period to which a speaker belongs, or his age (e.g., the use of old-fashioned parlance).

Province features: signal which specific occupational activity a speaker is engaged in, such as the "language" of a lawyer, a priest, or, for that matter, a speech therapist.

Status features: signal the nature of the social relationship that exists between the speaker and his interlocutors, such as whether it is friendly, formal, or polite.

Modality features: signal the purpose someone has in mind when conveying a message, by use of a particular format, such as the distinctions between telegram, letter, postcard, and memorandum, or, in clinical work, the various kinds of structuring given to a session.

Singularity features: signal a systematic idiosyncrasy on the part of the speaker, such as a particular turn of phrase (as in the regular use of *OK* by T in the examples above).

From time to time, stylistic analyses of language variety have recognized other variables. Terminology, moreover, is not stable in this domain, but the above list should suffice to illustrate the range and importance of this dimension of enquiry.

As this range of variables is less well-known in clinical work, a brief example of the kind of difficulty that might arise under each heading may be helpful:

Regional dialect: T, born and brought up in the South of England and trained in London, marries and finds herself working in Glasgow, with consequent problems of intelligibility between her and P.

Social dialect: T and P read different kinds of newspaper, are interested in different kinds of hobbies, can afford different kinds of things, use different kinds of social slang and exclamations, and so on.

Temporal: P may be 70; T may be 25. The language has changed enormously since the first quarter of this century (12).

Province: T uses medical or quasimedical terminology, which means nothing to P; or P assumes T knows technical terms belonging to P's previous profession.

Status: Personalities vary. Both Ts and Ps vary in the amount of informality they consider desirable in a session. The use of forms of address can vary from one extreme to another (*Mr. Smith, Mr. S, John, Johnny*). Age and sex of the participants are other obvious factors influencing the course of an interaction.

Modality: Likewise, both Ts and Ps vary in their readiness to be involved in format activities. Some Ts run a highly disciplined clinic; others run a more casual one. Some Ps want to be totally organized; others do not. The proportion of structured-to-nonstructured work in a session is also a significant variable when making comparisons between sessions.

Singularity: A habit of P's may be mistaken for a clinical symptom, e.g., a frequent use of *you know* or *really*.

Pragmatic variables: P fails to understand the nature of the turn-taking which T has attempted to explain in carrying out a task; P introduces a topic into the conversation without it being clear to what it relates; P goes on for too long in his reply to a simple question (as in much "fluent" speech); T's language is too complex for P to follow; T gives the impression of "speaking down" to P (the "Does he take sugar?" phenomenon); T uses materials (and thus language) which are of no interest to P or underestimate his maturity in some way (many clinical materials having been designed originally with children in mind).

A model of this kind raises many fascinating questions and hypotheses concerning the relative weighting of these variables in accounting for communicative failure in clinical sessions. T speaks; P fails to respond or responds inadequately. Which of these variables are implicated? It is often possible to eliminate some of the more obvious variety variables from the enquiry at the outset, e.g., if P and T are both speakers of the same regional dialect. It is never possible to eliminate the structural variables without careful study, however, and many pitfalls await the unwary T if insufficient attention is paid to the pragmatic variables. The analysis of a few real examples will illustrate these points and, incidentally, stress the need to adopt a balanced account of these variables in analysis of input language and to pay proper attention to their mutual dependence.

EXAMPLES OF INPUT FACTORS

With respect to the description of input factors in clinical sessions, all input variables have been neglected, but some more than others. Following the attention devoted to grammatical factors in recent years, this particular variable is now receiving some study (10,14), and the relatively discrete nature of segmental phonological and lexical semantic features of utterance has also promoted relevant research. The domains of grammatical semantics and nonsegmental phonology remain almost totally unexplored, however. In a previous publication (5), I gave some examples of the way in which the study of input in terms of grammatic/semantic roles could increase our understanding of the nature of T-P interaction; but that work gave no examples of the central influence of nonsegmental phonology in determining the character of T input language in aphasiology; hence the following illustrations.

That prosody has a role in influencing aphasic responses is well known since the work of Goodglass and others several years ago (1,13). Moreover, in some experimental work, and also in certain aphasia tests, it is standard practice to try to eliminate the effects of prosody by holding stimulus sentences constant in intonation and rhythm, as far as possible (although the naturalness of the subsequent stimuli, or the level of production consistency achieved by the investigator, is often questionable). So far uninvestigated is the role of the prosodic system in motivating and controlling P's responses, that is, the extent to which P is aware of the linguistic role of the different prosodic patterns available in the language. Of all the variables that affect P's ability to comprehend, recall, or repeat T's stimuli in this area, the role of tonicity seems most significant, i.e., the factor that determines which word (or words) in a tone unit carries greatest prominence. In the transcription used in this chapter, tonic words are shown by the presence of an accent mark above the vowel of their stressed syllable: if the accent is ˋ, the pitch movement which realizes this prominence is falling; ˊ is rising; ˉ signals a level pitch movement; ˆ a pitch movement that first rises and then falls within a syllable; and ˇ a pitch movement that first falls and then rises within a syllable.

The basic semantic principle involved in tonicity is that the word carrying the tonic accent is the one to which the speaker wishes to draw attention. Thus in the sentence "I can see an old red car," the tonic could be placed on any of the words, and different semantic implications would result, as the following glosses illustrate:

I can see an old red càr (as opposed to an old red bike, perhaps).
I can see an old rèd car (as opposed to an old blue car, perhaps).
I can see an òld red car (as opposed to a new red car, perhaps).
I can see àn old red car (not two such cars).

Some contexts are more likely than others, of course, but the underlying principle is constant, and it is one that aphasic Ps often have difficulty in grasping. They often assign a tonic syllable to a word that seems to have no special semantic significance in the discourse, as the following extract shows:

T 'what can you 'see in the pìcture/
P a rèd car/

As there was only one car in the picture, the focus on *red* was inappropriate. It would have been appropriate in this context, however:

T 'which 'car is 'near the shòp/
P the rèd car/

This pair of examples illustrates the way in which the adequacy of P's response, and in particular its prosodic character, is determined by T's input stimulus. Indeed, it is regularly the case that T will manipulate tonicity contrasts in order to draw P's attention to a significant word in her stimulus:

T can you 'give me the kéy/
P —[də]·kéys/ — P points to the keys
T can you gìve me the kéy/

P yés/ — P gives the keys
T thânk you/

When a sentence contains more than one important piece of information, it is normal practice to identify the information units by giving each its own tone unit. This is the principle that explains the contrast between:

there's a càt in the 'garage/

where the speaker is drawing attention to the cat but considers it routine that the cat is in the garage, and:

there's a càt/ in the gàrage/

where the speaker is surprised both that there is a cat, and that it is in the garage. In the following dialogue, T is making use of this principle in a comprehension exercise. A box and several small objects are on the table, and T is investigating P's awareness of prepositions. For the first instruction, both the object and the location are given separate tone units (line 1). Subsequent instructions using the same object are not split in this way (lines 7, 12, 18), however: the penny is now 'old news' and no longer requires a special tonic prominence. When a new object is introduced (line 22), however, the double-unit pattern reappears. (Other transcriptional symbols used in the examples are: . , –, —, ——, increasing degrees of pause length; ↑ , a step-up in pitch; ' ', speech uttered in a certain way (as glossed in the right-hand comment); [ ], enclose phonetic transcription; =, a lengthened segment; ( ), enclose unclear speech; **, overlapping speech.)

T 'can you 'put the pénny/ . 'in the bóx/
P —— thère/ —— puts penny in box
T gòod/
thànk you/
thàt's ríght/
P yéah/ (*coughs*) –
T 'can you 'put the 'penny . ↑ ùnder the bóx/
P —— puts penny under box
T ↑ gòod/ .
gòod/
P ḿ/
T – can you 'put the 'penny . be ↑ hìnd the bóx/
P —— 'm̀/' – 'weakly pronounced'
[tə̥ tə̥] ——
T gòod/
P ḿ/
T gòod/ ——
'can you 'put the 'penny . in ↑ frònt of the 'box/
P —— puts penny in front of box

T	gòod/ ——	
P	(*coughs*)	
T	'can you 'put the kèy/ . be ↑ sìde the bóx/	

What is interesting is to see what happens when T fails to control the prosodic structure of her input as successfully as on this occasion. In the following example, the same opening strategy is used (line 1), with an appropriate simplification in line 7; but in line 11, where the new object is being introduced, T fails to return to the double-unit structure. P follows the prosody, ignoring the lexical change, and must be corrected. Later in the session, a similar failure to make the new lexical item tonic (line 23) resulted in P having to rehearse the item to herself (line 24); it is interesting to note that she reintroduces the tonic syllable in the process.

T	'can you 'put the ↑ pěnny/ in the bòx/	
P	– pénny/	
	— well 'that's a pénny/ I suppóse/	
	(*laughs*) —	puts penny in box
T	'that's rìght/	
	gòod/ ——	
	can you 'put the 'pe̿nny . ↑ ùnder the 'box/	
P	—	puts penny under box
T	'that's ít/	
	gòod/ ——	
	'can you 'put̿ the key̿ . ↑ òn the 'box/ —	puts penny on box
P	—	puts penny on box
T	'that's the pènny 'on the 'box/	
P	òh/	
T	(we have)	
P	kèy/ .	
	kèy/ –	
	sǒrry/ (*laughs*)	puts key on box
T	gòod/	

. . . .

T	'can you 'put . the key̿ . in ↑ frònt of the 'box/	
P	—	puts key in front of box
T	gòod/ –	
	can you 'put the 'penny . be ↑ sìde the 'box/	
P	— pènny – be'side –	
	yèah/	
	besìde the 'box/	puts penny beside box

In discussing this example with T later, it emerged that she had made a conscious decision not to stress *penny* in line 23. She was trying to "catch P out" by not giving him the extra cue that the tonicity change would provide. Whether this is a desirable therapeutic strategy is debatable, but from a linguistic point of view, the stimulus involved must be regarded as deviant.

These examples also illustrate a general organizational principle in structured language work, whereby the prosodic structure of T's stimulus is the main linguistic crutch on which P can rely in order to determine what he must do. The following example has a clearly defined prosodic structure. T has been asking P to point to single objects and is now proceeding to two objects. In line 1, therefore, *two* is obligatorily tonic, as it is the main item of new information. In line 2, the two items are each given their own tone unit, again appropriate to their "new" status. The task proves initially complex for P, however, who fails to respond; hence in line 5, T repeats the stimulus but this time simplifies the stimulus by the process of reduction referred to above (her omission of the definite article before *table* is not relevant for the present discussion; in passing, it should be noted that this makes T's utterance ungrammatical). The simplification does not help, so T reintroduces the opening stimulus (line 8), this time giving it a strong prosodic demarcation. *Can you show me* is here acting as a kind of "pivot," as is common in drill work. P repeats the word *table* and uncertainly points to it, at which point T intervenes, aware that P is unlikely to complete the task successfully, and finishes the sentence (line 14), reintroducing the same prosodic parallelism as used in line 2.

T 'now can you 'show me twô 'things 'at a 'time/ –
"'where's the tāble/ – and the bòok/' — 'slow tempo'
P — (*coughs*)
[də – tɛm:] — er
T 'table and the bòok/
P m̀/
– [pə̥ . pə̥ . 'teibi] ——

T can you shòw mé/ – 'table and the bòok/
P [bɛ] . táble/ —
[pə̥ . pə̥ – bɛ . tə̥ . bɛ̀] — points to table

'yès/ — 'weak pronunciation'
*thère/'
T *that's ríght/
'there's the táble/ and 'there's the bòok/

CONCLUSION

Tonicity structure and function is but one aspect of intonation, which is only one dimension (albeit the most important) of nonsegmental phonology. It was chosen as an illustration because of its importance as a means of controlling and facilitating P's ability to comprehend and cooperate in clinical work. This chapter is deliberately selective in order to illustrate a particular issue, and thus ignores factors that would be considered in a more complete study. Primarily, in this connection, one should note: (a) the need to carry out comparable descriptions of interaction in settings other than the structured ones used above [there is some evidence that the same factors obtain in the unstructured parts of T sessions, but I have no information as to whether similar issues arise outside the clinic in general conversation; for work in these areas, the use of a prosody profile (see ref. 6) may prove helpful]; (b) the need to relate tonicity to other nonsegmental and communicative variables known to be important [rate of utterance and accompanying kinesic activity (e.g., head movement) in particular].

Despite these limitations, the illustration has some value, not simply because tonicity is a phenomenon of importance in its own right, but also because it shows the interdependence of the input variables outlined above. In addition to controlling P's awareness of semantic relevance, it also contributes directly to his understanding of the structure of the session (modality) and of the part he has to play in it (pragmatics). It is the interaction of these and other input variables that is especially significant when it comes to demonstrating the efficacy of aphasia therapy and explicating the notion of progress in the aphasic patient. Thus the further description of these variables, perhaps using profile techniques, is an important future goal of aphasiology.

REFERENCES

1. Blumstein, S., and Goodglass, H. (1972): The perception of stress as a semantic cue in aphasia. *J. Speech Hear. Res.*, 15:800–806.
2. Code, C., and Müller, D. J., editors (1983): *Aphasia Therapy*. Edward Arnold, London.
3. Coltheart, M. (1983): Aphasia therapy research: A single case-study approach. In: *Aphasia Therapy*, edited by C. Code and D. J. Müller, pp. 193–202. Edward Arnold, London.
4. Crystal, D. (1979): *Working With LARSP*. Edward Arnold, London.
5. Crystal, D. (1981): *Clinical Linguistics*. Springer-Verlag, Wien.
6. Crystal, D. (1982): *Profiling Linguistic Disability*. Edward Arnold, London.
7. Crystal, D. (1985): Linguistic levels in aphasia. In: *Aphasia*, edited by J. Oxbury, M. A. Wyke, M. Coltheart, and R. Whurr. Butterworth, London.
8. Crystal, D., and Davy, D. (1969): *Investigating English Style*. Longman, London.
9. Crystal, D., and Davy, D. (1975): *Advanced Conversational English*. Longman, London.
10. Crystal, D., Fletcher, P., and Garman, M. (1976): *The Grammatical Analysis of Language Disability*. Edward Arnold, London.
11. David, R. (1983): Researching into the efficacy of aphasia therapy. In: *Aphasia Therapy*, edited by C. Code and D. J. Müller, pp. 15–24. Edward Arnold, London.
12. Foster, B. (1970): *The Changing English Language*. Penguin, Harmondsworth.
13. Goodglass, F., Fodor, I. F., and Schulhoff, C. (1967): Prosodic factors in grammar: Evidence from aphasia. *J. Speech Hear. Res.*, 10:5–20.
14. Hatfield, F. M., and Shewell, C. (1983): Some applications of linguistics to aphasia therapy. In: *Aphasia Therapy*, edited by C. Code and D. J. Müller, pp. 61–75. Edward Arnold, London.
15. Leech, G. N. (1983): *Principles of Pragmatics*. Longman, London.
16. Levinson, S. C. (1983): *Pragmatics*. Cambridge University Press, Cambridge.
17. Stubbs, M. (1983): *Discourse Analysis*. Blackwell, Oxford.

Advances in Neurology, Vol. 42: Progress in Aphasiology, edited by F. C. Rose.
Raven Press, New York © 1984.

Word Order Processing in Aphasia: Effect of Verb Semantics

Eirian V. Jones

The City University, Centre for Clinical Communications Studies, London SE1, England

The work discussed in this chapter addresses the question of whether aphasic subjects show problems in processing grammatic relationships as marked by word order. The main study reports experimental work carried out on agrammatic subjects; on-going research, however, the preliminary results of which are also reported, involves the ability of Wernicke's type subjects to perform the same tasks.

Agrammatism is characterized chiefly by telegraphic utterances showing frequent omissions of bound and unbound morphemes, or functors, with a corresponding reliance on content words. It is considered to be characteristic of lesions involving frontotemporal areas of the brain and thus is more commonly associated with Broca's aphasia. It is a subject that has generated a great deal of research, particularly during the last decade, and discussion as to its cause(s) has been widely published. The question of whether agrammatic subjects show problems in processing word order has formed part of this discussion. Before examining this question, it is pertinent to give a brief outline of the development of thinking on agrammatism.

Agrammatism often coexists with distorted articulation and was originally thought to result from "economy of effort," the subject speaking asyntactically to reduce the strain of speaking (15,29). Such theory quickly gave ground to the more commonly held view that agrammatism reflected a problem at the syntactic level of language. On the basis of a number of studies, including analysis of spontaneous output, and in tasks designed to elicit specific syntactic structures, agrammatic subjects were shown to omit grammatic functors and inflectional affixes, to have difficulty in initiating utterances with any but stressed words, and to show a hierarchical ordering in terms of which morphemes and structures proved most difficult (9,10,12). Such problems, which were stated to exist in the presence of relatively good comprehension, suggested that the problem may be one of output alone. This view was disputed by later workers (4,25,38,40), who reported that the agrammatic subject's intuitions about his language and his ability to comprehend syntactic structures was as agrammatic as his output. Caramazza and Zurif (4) explained the seemingly normal comprehension of the agrammatic subject on the basis of his ability to use knowledge sources other than syntax when processing sentences (i.e., ability to comprehend semantically constrained, center-embedded sentences but not if these constraints were removed).

It is now generally agreed that these subjects can show problems in comprehending sentences if all other clues to interpretation are removed and they must rely on syntactic processing alone. The argument remains as to whether such failure results from loss of syntactic knowledge or difficulty in exploiting it in sentence comprehension tasks. Recently, Linebarger et al. (24) have argued that the good performance of agrammatic aphasics on grammaticality judgment tasks denies any loss of ability to analyze syntactic structures, thus suggesting significant sparing of syntactic knowledge. The authors put forward two possible explanations for the discrepancy between performance processing and grammaticality judgment: (a) problems lie not in constructing syntactic representations but in exploiting them for semantic interpretation; or (b) there is in agrammatism a trade-off between syntactic and semantic processing, so that subjects achieve their optimal performance in one domain only by sacrificing accuracy in the other.

The recognition that sentence processing involves the interactions of different levels of language was reinforced by the work of Kean (19–21), who suggested that the problems agrammatics show with bound and unbound morphemes in comprehension, production, and metalinguistic tasks can be explained best in terms of a phonologic and not a syntactic deficit. She states that major lexical items, which usually carry word stress, are fully attended to, but that function words and bound inflectional morphemes, which occur phonologically as clitics and which do not carry stress, are ignored.

Schwartz et al. (34) and Saffran et al. (30) contend that such an argument cannot fully explain agrammatic symptomatology. They point out that agrammatic aphasics can process such bound inflectional morphemes when they play a syntactic role; likewise, failure to map a simple NVN[1] string into a canonical structure—subject-verb-object (SVO)—in word order tasks cannot be explained by a phonologic deficit.

The question of the ability of agrammatic subjects to process word order is discussed further in terms of both clinical observations and the results of experimental studies. Black (1) claims that there is little evidence that agrammatic aphasics produce utterances that violate the standard word order of English. On the rare occasions when violations of canonical word order in a NP V NP clause did occur, she asserts they were limited to those times when lexical retrieval problems arose, delaying insertion or realization. Von Stockert and Bader (36), however, state that transposition of verb and noun phrase within the verb phrase is characteristic of Broca's aphasia in input and output. Although they quote the work of Zurif et al. (39) in support of this view, a study of that work does not support this claim. Subjects indeed violated the linguistic unity of both noun and verb phrases when asked to choose two words out of a triad which they felt went best together, but this appeared

[1]Abbreviations used throughout this chapter are as follows: N, noun; V, verb; S, subject; O, object; NP, noun phrase; IO, indirect object; DO, direct object; PP, prepositional phrase; A, animate; I, inanimate.

to be on the basis of failure to link function words to content words and was not related to constituent ordering.

In this writer's experience, violation of canonical word order is rare but does occur. One agrammatic subject produced: "Your holiday will extend your firm" ("Your firm will extend you holiday"), an error in which he fails to mark correctly the relationship of the noun arguments to the verb. On formal testing and informal observations, the word finding abilities of the subject were excellent, although output was marked by a severe articulatory apraxia. Such word order errors also occurred in written output.

Results of research studies are equally contradictory. Difficulties arise in evaluating them because so often they indicate only the relative difficulty of SVO type sentences in relation to other syntactic structures, and no error analysis is carried out. Goodglass (10), reviewing unpublished results of a study of a group of patients with Broca's aphasia, concluded that the best retained signal of grammatic relationships was word order as illustrated by the subject-object sequence in the active voice. Both Parisi and Pizzamiglio (28) and Lesser (23), using an English version of the former's test, showed that comprehension of word order contrasts were consistently difficult for both Broca's and Wernicke's patients. Word order was tested only incidentally by the studies cited so far, but others have attempted to address the question more closely.

In "dative" type sentences, word order can also be the only cue to grammatic relationships. Scholes (32) used such sentences to test the ability of aphasics to discriminate between sentences, such as

He showed her baby the pictures.
S V IO DO

versus

He showed her the baby pictures.
S V IO DO

Agrammatic aphasics performed no worse than did other aphasics. It should be noted, however, that such a task is not a test of the ability to interpret grammatic relationships, as correct interpretation depends only on the ability to use the cue provided by the determiner. At the same time, such sentences were pragmatically irreversible, and a better test would have involved a picture-pointing task with stimulus sentences of the type: "John showed the boy the women." Black (1), using such sentences as the latter, showed that agrammatic aphasics made a high number of errors, but analysis showed the errors not to be random but reflecting a strategy of interpreting the sentences in terms of S V DO IO, as if the preposition "to" was included. Interestingly, such a strategy cannot be taken as indicating a problem in processing grammatic relationships, because the same strategy was used frequently by normal subjects perhaps, as Black (1) suggests, reflecting a frequency of use effect. Such a finding does suggest that, with our present knowledge, word order is best tested in simple active reversible declarative sentences.

Comparatively recently, such a study was carried out by Schwartz et al. (34) and Saffran et al. (30). In a series of three picture-pointing tasks, Schwartz et al. showed that five agrammatic aphasics had difficulty in comprehending word order. Performance of individual subjects across the three tasks was inconsistent. The authors concluded that agrammatic subjects have difficulty in decoding grammatic relationships, suggesting a syntactic mapping defect that renders them unable to utilize a fixed and principled set of procedures to recover the relational structure of spoken sentences. Although this study attempted to overcome problems that had arisen in other studies, it is itself open to criticism on a number of points. The set of sentences used was not homogenous; four of 24 were of the structure NP V PP, while the remaining 20 were of the format NP V NP. The presence of the preposition could have had a contaminating effect, especially as the authors were attempting to argue against Kean's (20) hypothesis that a phonologic deficit can explain all agrammatic symptomatology. A two-picture choice format, as used in two of the tests, weakens their statistical argument. One subject, J.R., had an extensive posterior lesion, which makes his inclusion problematic; the very inconsistency of the results makes the authors' claims questionable.

In a parallel paper, Saffran et al. (30), using a sentence order task (SOT) originally devised by von Stockert (35), showed a similar problem in output and suggested that subjects used a strategy of treating the animate argument as the subject of the sentence. In the one experiment, target sentences were of the form:

NP (animate) v NP (inanimate) A/I condition
NP (animate) v NP (animate) A/A condition

In the second SOT task, there were four conditions:

1. A/A condition – verbs = follow, cut, carry.
2. I/I condition – verbs = pull, crash, hit.
3. A/I condition – verbs = all verbs above.
4. I/A condition – verbs = as above but reversed arguments.

As with the comprehension task, results across the five subjects were inconsistent. If indeed they were using such an animacy strategy, then performance in the A/A and I/I condition should have been at chance level. A closer look at the results, however, shows all subjects to have performed accurately under the I/I condition and four of five for the A/A condition. Results should have been considerably better than chance under the A/I condition and worse under the I/A condition; but again, this does not prove to be the case. In their conclusions, Saffran et al. (30) recognize some of these problems and alternatively hypothesize that what determines the placement of a NP in the subject position is the "potency or saliency" of its referent, saliency being an entity that is either animate or the source or cause of the action. The definition of saliency is not clear; in fact, it could be argued that results that present problems for the animacy hypothesis also do so for the saliency hypothesis.

Black (1) suggests that the work of Schwartz et al. (34) and Saffran et al. (30) does not provide conclusive evidence that agrammatic aphasics are unable to process grammatic relationships on the basis of word order alone. She goes further to suggest that problems that do arise in fact may occur due to problems with particular verbs. Although subjects are presented with the verb forms, semantic and syntactic information about them must be fully accessed if appropriate mapping of semantic and grammatic functions are to be achieved. Recognition that difficulty with the verbs may be at the root of the problem has come from Saffran et al. (31) themselves in a later work.

This focus of interest in verb processing in aphasics has come rather late, considering the vital role played in dictating sentence structure. Throughout the literature, only scant attention is paid to the ability of aphasics to process verb information. A number of studies report that nouns predominate in agrammatic output, and that verbs are underrepresented in spontaneous output (6,27). Goodglass (10) has stated that verbs, when they do occur, are often unmarked for person or tense or occur in the present participle form. He attributes this to a tendency to nominalize the verb, the *-ing* participle marking the gerundive rather than the progressive. The subjects are said to be using the verb to "name" the action rather than in a predicative sense. Saffran et al. (31), as stated, have recognized the importance of the verb and postulate that aphasics may have more problems with verbs that encode relationships between objects (chase, follow) than those which encode a property of the actor alone (smile, read). Verbs that mark relationships are exactly those involved in the question of word order. In simple active reversible declarative sentences, such as "The cat follows the dog," the only cue to semantic and grammatic relationships comes from the verb itself.

In English, there is generally no simple one-to-one correspondence between semantic and grammatic structure; the properties of verbs themselves determine the relationship between the two. Such mapping between semantics and syntax is considered in linguistic and psycholinguistic theories to be dependent on information attached to the lexical entries for the individual verbs (3,14,16). For example, according to Jackendoff (16), the lexical entry for "buy" is given as:

$$\text{Buy}\quad \begin{bmatrix} +\text{V} & \\ +\text{NP}_1 & \text{NP}_2\ (\text{from NP}_3)\ (\text{for NP}_4) \\ \text{CAUSE}\ (\text{NP}_1) & \begin{bmatrix} \text{CHANGE} \\ \text{possession} \\ \begin{bmatrix} \text{accompanied by} \\ \text{CHANGE}\ (\begin{bmatrix} \text{NP}_4 \\ \text{money} \end{bmatrix} \text{NP}_1,\ \text{NP}_3) \end{bmatrix} \end{bmatrix} \text{NP}_2\text{NP}_3\text{NP}_1 \end{bmatrix}$$

The entry specifies that the item(s) dominated by the NP_1 (the subject) is interpreted as the argument of the semantic function CAUSE (i.e., is interpreted as the AGENT), while the item(s) dominated by the NP_2 (the object) is interpreted as the argument of the semantic function CHANGE (i.e., interpreted as the THEME).

It could be hypothesized that if agrammatic subjects have problems in accessing some verbs more than others, or access only partial information, they might order the noun phrases at random and/or on the basis of some perceptual/cognitive strategy. It could also be hypothesized that they accessed the wrong lexical entry, e.g., the converse of the verb. For instance, the verb "follow" might be assigned as meaning equivalent to

$$\left[\begin{array}{ll} +V & \\ +NP_1\text{------------}NP_2 & \\ \left[\begin{array}{l} \text{MOTION} \\ NP_1 \text{ before } NP_2 \end{array}\right] & NP_1 \end{array}\right]$$

rather than

$$\left[\begin{array}{ll} +V & \\ +NP_1\text{------------}NP_2 & \\ \left[\begin{array}{l} \text{MOTION} \\ NP_1 \text{ after } NP_2 \end{array}\right] & NP_1 \end{array}\right]$$

It is of interest that substitution of a verb with its converse often occurs in slips of the tongue and tip of the tongue phenomena (7,8).

Black (*unpublished*) reported that one agrammatic subject, when tested for his ability to decode grammatic relationships in SVO type sentences, exhibited problems mainly in relation to verbs such as "push, pull, follow." These verbs did not differ from the other verbs used on grounds of frequency or syntactic characteristics but did so on the basis of semantic factors. The meaning of all three verbs does not only encode a particular action or relationship between two entities, but it also specifies that they must be in a particular spatial or directional relationship to each other. For instance, the meaning of "push" and "pull" can be represented in part as (see refs. 14 and 16):

$$\text{Push} \quad \left[\text{CAUSE } [NP_1 \left[\begin{array}{l} \text{MOTION} \\ NP_2 \text{ ahead } NP_1 \end{array}\right] \quad (NP_2)]\right]$$

$$\text{Pull} \quad \left[\text{CAUSE } [NP_1 \left[\begin{array}{l} \text{MOTION} \\ NP_2 \text{ behind } NP_1 \end{array}\right] \quad (NP_2)]\right]$$

It should be noted that these two verbs differ in only one aspect of their meaning. Both verbs express similar actions and, therefore, are identical with respect to this aspect of meaning; they differ, however, in terms of the embedded preposition and the way that thematic roles are mapped on to grammatic relationships. This difference is marked by the preposition considered to be inherent in such directional motion verbs (14,26). Unless this preposition was accessed, it would be difficult to process sentences such as "Mary pushes Jane" as opposed to "Mary pulls Jane." Black's findings with this one agrammatic aphasic deserve further consideration; should it prove to be the case that aphasics show more problems in decoding word order with these verbs, this would bear on the still unanswered problem regarding the existence of a word order deficit in agrammatic aphasics. It would also mean that the difficulties arose for lexical semantic, rather than syntactic, reasons. Such a finding would be particularly pertinent in view of the fact that directional motion verbs were used in some of the word order studies cited (30,34).

WORD ORDER PROCESSING IN AGRAMMATIC APHASIA

A series of experiments was carried out (17,18) to test whether directional motion verbs were more difficult for aphasics to process. Ten agrammatic subjects, all of whom had suffered a left cerebrovascular accident (CVA), were tested on their ability to process grammatic relationships in simple active reversible declarative sentences of the structure

Det N V Det N
NP V NP

containing three types of verbs: directional motion verbs, nondirectional motion verbs, and nonmotion verbs. The sentences were so designed that there was no pragmatic bias, and noun arguments were all animate. In the comprehension task, subjects had to select one of three pictures (target picture, reverse role picture, and a distractor in which the noun arguments were in the same relationship to the verb as in the target sentence but the verb was from a different category from the target verb) in response to an auditorily presented sentence. There were 10 verbs in each verb category, and each was inserted in two different sentences, making a total of 60 target sentences and 60 triadic sets. One of each pair of verbs was drawn with the characters going from L → R and the other drawn with the characters going from R → L. This was done in view of the findings of Déloche and Seron (5), who found aphasic subjects to use a strategy of relying on the L → R arrangement of the visual array in a picture selection task when unable to decode linguistically. All verbs used were of equal frequency (22).

The results of this test (Table 1) showed that, for these agrammatic aphasics, processing of sentences containing the directional motion verbs was significantly more difficult than processing sentences containing either the nondirectional motion verbs or the nonmotion verbs. There was no statistically significant difference between the number of errors made in these last two groups.

These same 10 agrammatic aphasics were also tested on their ability to produce the correct word order. Interpreting output from agrammatic subjects can be problematic because the intended word order is difficult to interpret due to the often omitted unbound morphemes and the frequently occurring articulatory deficit. Therefore, in this study, the subjects' ability to produce word order was tested in a SOT (35). In this paradigm, subjects are asked to arrange separately presented sentence constituents in linear order to describe a picture. The stimulus picture presented was the semantic reverse of the picture presented in the input experiment. The constituents of the sentence were separately presented as follows: Det N; V; Det N. The results (Table 2) showed that these subjects made significantly fewer errors in the production task than in the comprehension task, and the verb type effect seen in comprehension was not found in output. The significant finding that

TABLE 1. *Results obtained by ten agrammatic aphasic subjects in the comprehension task*

	Ten nonmotion verbs[a] (total no. errors, 41; mean, 4.1; SD, 2.64)		Ten nondirectional motion verbs[a] (total no. errors, 59; mean, 5.9; SD, 2.96)		Ten directional motion verbs[a] (total no. errors, 108; mean, 10.8; SD, 2.44)	
Error analysis	No.	%	No.	%	No.	%
No. times reverse role picture selected plus percent total errors	38	92.6	58	98.3	107	99
No. times distractor picture selected plus percent total errors	3	7.4	1	1.7	1	1

[a] No. stimulus items = 20.

in input, directional motion verbs were much more difficult to process deserves further consideration, as does the finding that the verb type effect was lost in the output task.

DISCUSSION

The findings of a word order problem in comprehension of simple active declarative sentences supports those reported by Schwartz et al. (34). In a parallel paper, Saffran et al. (30) suggested that, in processing word order in simple active voice sentences,

TABLE 2. *Results obtained by ten agrammatic aphasic subjects in the production task*

	Ten nonmotion verbs[b] (total no. errors, 32; mean, 3.2; SD, 2.25)		Ten nondirectional motion verbs[b] (total no. errors, 30; mean 3.0; SD, 2.83)		Ten directional motion verbs[b] (total no. errors, 46; mean, 4.6; SD, 3.14)	
Error analysis[a]	No.	%	No.	%	No.	%
No. times following structures appeared plus percent total errors						
OVS	32	100	29	96.6	45	97.7
OSV	0		0		1	2.3
SOV	0		1	3.4	0	

[a] OVS, object, verb, subject; OSV, object, subject, verb; SOV, subject, object, verb.
[b] No. stimulus items = 20.

subjects may use a strategy of assigning the actor role to the animate or more salient argument. In this study, there was no opportunity for the subjects to use such a strategy, as all noun arguments were animate. Saliency is not clearly defined by the latter authors, and it is difficult to decide on what criteria two animate noun arguments could be attributed relative saliency. Pragmatic bias was eliminated as far as possible by pairing noun arguments that had equal probability of playing an actor role in relation to a particular verb. In addition, the noun arguments used across all verb types were the same, although their distribution was such that no two noun arguments appeared together on more than one occasion. The chance that one noun argument was more salient than another was equally distributed across all target sentences. The possibility that errors may have occurred because subjects did not recognize the nouns or their pictorial representations was eliminated by the fact that identity of the noun arguments was made clear to each subject. Failure to identify the correct word order also may have occurred because of difficulty in comprehending the correct verb. If this were the case, errors made should have included choice of the distractor picture; however, although this involved the same noun arguments in the same relationship as the target sentence, it involved a different action.

Analysis of the results shows that the distractor was chosen on only five occasions (2.4% of all errors made), three of five distractor errors occurring on nonmotion verbs. The subjects' awareness of the correct verb was shown by their frequent rejection of the distractor picture. The finding that so few distractor pictures were chosen suggests that these subjects were at least able to decode some aspects of meaning of the verbs, that element which distinguishes one action from another (e.g., "push" from "approach"). If the noun arguments were recognized linguistically and visually and the correct verb chosen, the only explanation remaining for the high number of errors made is failure to process the grammatic relationships pertaining between the verb and the two noun arguments. This means that, although the subjects were able to access some elements of the verb meaning, they were unable to access that information which maps the predicate/argument structure onto the grammatic structure.

This conclusion is in agreement with that of Saffran et al. (30), who explain this failure in comprehending word order by proposing that agrammatic subjects lack "the mediating linguistic structures corresponding to the arguments of the relation leading to failure to extract from word order the directionality of the underlying relation." In a later report (31), the authors state that subjects have problems processing linguistic structures that encode relationships, such as verbs and prepositions. The findings of the current study would support this view in part, particularly with regard to verbs, but goes on to show that the degree of difficulty shown in processing the relationship between the noun arguments and the verb is dependent on the verb itself. Saffran et al. (31) indeed recognize that this may be the case when they suggest a different degree of difficulty between inherent verbs, which describe actions or states that are properties of the actor alone, and relational verbs, which encode relationships between entities.

In the current study, this question is addressed by testing comprehension across three types of verbs: nonmotion verbs, nondirectional motion verbs, and directional motion verbs. As predicted, the directional motion verbs were significantly more difficult to process for these subjects than the other two groups of verbs, but the reason for this is unclear.

In processing terms, there appears to be a fundamental difference between the verb groups when such verbs are placed in a NP-V-NP structure. Sentences used in this study can be analyzed in terms of the amount of processing needed to decode a "heard" sentence in relation to picture choice; this difference in the amount of processing needed relates largely to the verb. In some sentences (e.g., "The doctor shoots the vicar"), the subject of the sentence has a meaning relation to the verb that is independent of the object. The verb "shoots" encodes an action predicated of the actor alone. At the same time, this verb entails an instrument that is present in the target picture (a gun), which may further enhance the link between subject and verb in terms of selecting the correct picture. In processing such a sentence, the subject needs only to decode the first noun phrase plus the verb in order to select the correct picture from the target and its semantic reverse; there is no need to decode the object. In other sentences, however, there is no such tight relationship between the subject and the verb alone (e.g., "The fireman follows the policeman"). Correct interpretation is dependent on decoding the whole sentence in order to decode the meaning relationship between the nouns and the verb.

Examination of the three sets of verb group sentences used in this study shows the following: All the nonmotion verbs within the NP-V-NP structure, although marking a relationship between the two noun arguments, fall into the first category. In all, the verb is predicated of the actor alone; therefore, it is not necessary to decode the object in order to achieve correct interpretation. In seven of 10, the verb entails an instrument that was represented in the picture. Both the nondirectional and the directional motion verbs entail motion as a common factor in their meaning; but there is one fundamental difference between the two groups of verbs. The directional motion verbs also entail, as part of their meaning, a specification that the relationship between the noun arguments and the verb must be in a specific direction. The difference between these two groups of verbs can best be illustrated by comparing the semantic structure of "move," a nondirectional motion verb, and "push," a directional motion verb:

Move	[CAUSE (NP_1	MOTION	NP_2)]
Push	[CAUSE (NP_1	MOTION	NP_2)]
		[NP_2 ahead NP_1]	

It can be seen that the only differences between these two verbs in terms of predicate structure involve the presence of an inherent preposition in "push," marking the directionality of the relationship between the verb and the noun arguments.

In this study, it was shown that there was no significant difference between the nonmotion verbs and the nondirectional motion verbs in terms of processing difficulty. This could be predicted, as neither group of verbs has the added complexity of an embedded preposition marking directionality. The trend for nonmotion verbs to be easier could have been enhanced by the visually presented entailed instrument. As stated, the verb is predicated of the actor alone in the nonmotion verbs, and there is a suggestion that subjects may have processed the nondirectional motion verbs in the same way.

Of all errors made with this group of verbs, 39% were caused by failure in processing three of them: trips, shakes, and moves. If the subject and verb alone are processed in sentences containing these three verbs, then the meaning of the sentence changes as the verbs become intransitive. Subjects have a much greater problem in decoding the directional motion verbs, which must be attributable to the failure to access the prepositional information that is the only factor differentiating these verbs from the nondirectional motion verbs. If we examine the errors made in this group of verbs (Table 3), it will be noted that the greatest number of errors were made in the verbs push, pull, follow, lift, lower, and so on, in which retrieval of the prepositional information is vital if the converse of the verb is not to be accessed instead. It appears that the subjects could access some of the meaning of these verbs in view of their swift rejection of the distractor verbs but either failed to access that part of the semantic representation of the verb that involves the preposition and its two arguments or accessed its converse, both of which would result in selection of the reverse role picture. As seen from the semantic structure of a verb such as push, the inherent preposition results in one predicate—the prepositional predicate—being embedded in another—the verb predicate. It could be hypothesized that the presence of an embedded predicate increases the processing load of a verb considerably. As stated earlier, it is verbs such as push/pull and follow/pursue that are quoted in slips of the tongue literature (7,8), a factor that again suggests the complexity of these verbs in terms of processing. Although the normal subjects in this study obtained a 100% correct response in the comprehension task, it was the tester's subjective opinion that they were slower in decoding the sentences that contained the directional motion verbs. Given the fact that this task gave consistent ceiling effects for normal subjects, the impression of slower processing with directional motion verbs could be effectively ratified only by a reaction time analysis.

It was hypothesized that the subjects' much greater number of errors in processing directional motion verbs arose through failure to process the prepositional information inherent in the verb. An attempt was made, therefore, to test this further. If the preposition inherent in the verb was marked in the surface structure of the stimulus sentence, these same subjects would have far less difficulty in processing the directional motion verbs. Only a subset of the directional motion verb sentences could be used; with certain of these verbs, placing a preposition in the surface structure allows for two directions to be marked. This is best explained through consideration of the following sentence: In "The man pulls the girl," "pulls" encodes a preposition marking the direction of the movement of the girl relative to the man. In "The man pulls up the girl," "pulls" acts as before, but "up" encodes the movement of the girl relative to her original position. In this instance, "up" is playing the role of a particle and is adding new information rather than just marking redundant

TABLE 3. *Verbs used in all experiments together with the number of errors made for each verb in the comprehension task and the SOT*

Verbs	Comprehension task	SOT
Nonmotion verbs		
Shoots	4	0
Toasts	4	5
Paints	3	1
Weighs	4	3
Bandages	4	5
Pays	4	4
Photographs	3	2
Watches	5	6
Holds	5	3
Claps	5	3
Nondirectional motion verbs		
Throws	5	2
Moves	7	4
Kicks	5	1
Visits	6	2
Starts	5	4
Shakes	8	1
Rows	6	6
Trips	8	5
Carries	3	2
Drives	6	3
Directional motion verbs[a]		
Pulls	15	4
Pushes	14	4
Passes* (by)	11	11
Follows* (behind)	11	7
Drags	8	3
Lowers	9	3
Jumps* (over)	10	4
Approaches* (toward)	9	4
Lifts	11	3
Chases* (after)	11	3

[a] Asterisk denotes directional verb used in experiment 2 together with inherent preposition.

information. Use of these directional motion verbs with a surface marked preposition would not be merely assessing the subject's ability to access the prepositional information inherent in the verb.

A subset of five directional motion verbs was used, and there were two examples of each verb sentence; thus there was a total of 10 triadic sets. These were taken from the directional motion verb sentences used in the comprehension task. Methodology was exactly as in the comprehension task, except that on this occasion, the orally presented sentences included the prepositions inherent in the verbs chosen (14,26). Before carrying out this experiment, subjects were tested on their ability to comprehend the prepositions to be used. Each preposition was depicted in a line drawing by a spatial arrangement of figures. This picture formed one of a triad in which the other two pictures represented (a) its semantic opposite, and (b) another preposition. An example of such a triad would be

The man is behind the woman.
The man is in front of the woman.
The man is by the woman.

Only one subject made any errors in this task; he later corrected it spontaneously. The results of the experiment, set up to test whether surface marking of the preposition improved the subjects' abilities to decode word order in the directional motion verb sentences, show a near normal response, a result that requires consideration.

Placement of the preposition in the surface structure of the sentences indeed resulted in near normal processing of the verb, but there could be another explanation for this significantly improved performance. These subjects gave a normal response to the subtest with prepositions, contrary to the findings of Schwartz et al. (34), who found subjects in their series to be unable to decode grammatic relationships marked by prepositional predicates alone. It is unclear why this study should have given such contradictory results. Nevertheless, given the fact that subjects in this current study did so well in the preposition subtest, it could be argued that they decoded the sentences in experiment 2 correctly because they ignored the verb and processed the sentence on the basis of the prepositional information alone. Further investigation is needed; it would be interesting to see how these subjects perform when the distractor sentence contains the same locative preposition encoding the spatial arrangement alone; for example,

The fireman follows behind the policeman.
The policeman follows behind the fireman.
The fireman is behind the policeman.

If the subjects are relying on the preposition alone, then there should be an equal chance that they would pick the distractor picture. Such a test has not been completed to date, but three of these same subjects were tested on three triads such as that above; all three consistently chose the correct target picture.

The main comprehension task has shown that in these agrammatic subjects, comprehension of word order in simple active reversible declarative sentences is defective. More importantly, it has shown for the first time experimentally that the degree of difficulty is related to particular verbs, and that the difference seems to be related to the complexity of the predicate structure of these verbs. Directional motion verbs, which proved the most difficult in this work, were used in all four conditions of the report by Saffran et al. (30); this might explain the inconsistent results found in that study. Since the authors have not made a qualitative analysis, however, the theory cannot be verified. If, as appears to be the case, failure with the directional motion verbs arose because of failure to access vital prepositional information, the problem lies not at a syntactic level but at a lexical semantic level.

As agrammatic subjects are considered to be as agrammatic in input as in output (4,25,38,40), it could be argued that as the same knowledge sources would be used to decode grammatic relationships in both input and output, then agrammatic subjects should have similar problems in decoding word order. The results of the SOT show that this is not the case for these subjects, who made far fewer errors in the output task than in the comprehension task; and the verb type effect was not significant. This is hardly surprising, considering how different the two tasks were in terms of processing load, and it is worth considering how these differences might have influenced the results.

In the comprehension task, the subject was required to decode an auditorily presented sentence and to match it to one of three pictures depicting the target, its semantic reverse, and a distractor. In the SOT test, the subject was asked to place the three components of the sentence (NP V NP) in the correct order to match one target picture. The components were printed on three pieces of card and presented in vertical array alongside the picture. Thus it may be seen that in the comprehension task, subjects were immediately presented with confusion in terms of the target picture and its reverse role depiction. In the presence of problems in accessing verb information already discussed, the subjects were unable to resolve this confusion. In the SOT, no such conflict occurred instantly: only one picture faced the subject, and the sentence components were presented in vertical array. The subjects, therefore, were in a position to look at the picture and, with the relatively good content word retrieval found in such subjects (11), were able to start generating their own sentences. This was confirmed to some extent by the observation that most subjects started to verbalize a sentence before referring to or arranging the written components. Indeed, their unanimous strategy was to take the printed verb first, place it under the picture, and then try to place the noun phrases. It was observed that placement of the noun phrases was carried out with confidence initially; but after placement, doubts seemed to arise as the subjects became aware, for the first time, of a possible alternative. Nevertheless, although nonmotion verbs and nondirectional motion verbs seemed to be easier, the overall results were far superior to performance in the input task.

There are other differences between the two tasks that demand consideration. The input task also involves a greater cognitive load, in that subjects were required to hold a fleeting auditory input in memory while processing complex grammatic relationships. In output, the target sentence, in terms of its individual components, and the stimulus picture were permanently present, so that subjects were free to concentrate on the relationship between the individual components. No information was available on the short-term memory span of these 10 agrammatic aphasic subjects. Although repetition of the stimulus sentence on demand helps overcome any such problems, it does not affect processing load in terms of linguistic complexity.

An interesting finding in the SOT task was that when errors were made, they suggested that subjects were using a strategy of relying on the visual arrangement of the characters in the pictures. There was a marked increase in the number of errors when the characters were drawn from R → L. This was not seen in the comprehension task and perhaps can be explained by the nature of the instructions given to the subjects. They were asked to "make a sentence to *match* what you see happening in the picture''; thus they were encouraged to do just that when in difficulty linguistically. The use of such a strategy by aphasic subjects was suggested by Deloche and Seron (5), who found it used by Wernicke's type subjects in a picture selection task. In their experiment, Broca's type subjects were sensitive to the plausibility of the sentences and not to the visual array; in the current study they were unable to use any plausibility strategy. This fact suggests that in Broca's aphasia, the presence of the two alternatives inhibited such a strategy in the input study.

These differences between the two tasks, together with the fact that stimuli were presented in two different modalities and responses required were also different, make comparison between the input and output task problematic. This would still have been the case if oral output had been required in the output task, which adds to the difficulties in interpretation, as Saffran et al. (30) point out. They, too, considered the SOT to be the best way of measuring the ability of agrammatic aphasics to produce word order. Of great interest is examination of the within-subject responses across the two tasks: all except subject 1 made fewer errors in output than in input, and all except subject 10 made significantly more errors with directional motion verbs in the input task.

Five of the subjects made 75% or more of their total errors in the input task. This is particularly marked in one subject, who made a total of 27 errors in input but only three in output. Interestingly, this subject had one of the lowest grammaticality ratings on the Boston Diagnostic Aphasia Examination (BDAE). Likewise, another subject, who had the lowest grammaticality rating of all subjects (1.5), made only 25% of his errors in the output task.

Subject 1, who had the highest grammaticality rating score (5), which is just beyond the range for Broca's type subjects, was the only one to make more errors in the output (13 errors) than the input (12 errors) task. Three other subjects showed greater parity between the number of errors made in input and output; again, their performance does not correlate with the grammaticality rating scores, which were 4, 4, and 2. This lack of correlation between ability to process grammatic relationships and clinically defined agrammatism was also found by Schwartz et al. (34) and Saffran et al. (30).

There was some correlation between subjects' performance on the input task and their converted Z-score on the BDAE rating scale profile, in that the subject with the lowest auditory comprehension score of 0 made the highest number of errors (30), while the two subjects who had the highest auditory comprehension scores (+1) each made a total of 12 errors in input. There was not necessarily a correlation between the auditory comprehension scores on the BDAE and performance in the output task. Whereas the subject with the lowest auditory comprehension score did make 21 errors in output, another subject with an auditory comprehension score of +0.5 made 23 errors in output. This last subject used the visual array strategy most consistently in the output task, making 19/23 errors when the visual array went from R → L. In no subjects was there a marked verb type effect in the output task, although one subject did show a trend toward directional motion verbs being more difficult in output than input. This lack of a marked verb type effect in output is contrary to the finding in the input task, where all subjects except one found directional motion verbs to be more difficult than either of the other two verb groups.

Recently, Scholes (33) commented on the verb-right strategy purported to be characteristic of Broca's aphasia by von Stockert and Bader (36), who also used the SOT. Scholes suggests that when agrammatic aphasics use a verb-right strategy resulting in NNV construction, they may be utilizing a more natural, unmarked structure. Of the 600 possibilities for such a structure to emerge in the 10 subjects tested on the SOT, a NNV structure occurred on only two occasions. The results of this study provide additional information not only for our knowledge of word order processing in agrammatic aphasia but also for our understanding of agrammatism.

The subjects in this study showed a deficit in processing grammatic relationships in simple active reversible declarative sentences in both input and output; to that extent, the findings are in agreement with those of Schwartz et al. (34) and Saffran et al. (30). In the input task, however, it was shown that the subjects had much greater difficulty processing grammatic relationships in sentences containing the directional motion verbs than either of the other two groups of verbs. This effect of verb type was suggested but not statistically proven in the output task. It is possible that this difficulty seen with directional motion verbs arose because, unlike the verbs in the other two groups, they have a complex semantic structure in which one predicate, the preposition, is embedded in another, the verb predicate. Agrammatic subjects used in this study were able to access some part of the semantic representation of the verb; otherwise, they would have chosen more of the distractor pictures. The "action" element of the "meaning" of the verb was obviously accessible, but not that part which marks the directionality of the verbs: the preposition.

Saffran et al. (30) have stated that agrammatic subjects lack the linguistic structures that correspond to the arguments of the relationship, both abstract ones, e.g., the subject/predicate, and even semantic ones, e.g., agent/patient. They hypothesize that mapping into language occurs without the benefit of such abstractions. Although they conclude that the deficit is a syntactic one, their analysis already underlines the role of verb semantics and not syntax alone. Indeed, the problem in processing the directional motion verbs seen in this study can be interpreted only on a lexical semantic basis.

The fact that these directional motion verbs were so difficult for agrammatic subjects, that there was some suggestion that the normal group found them to be more difficult than the other two groups of verbs, that they are often referred to in slips of the tongue literature, and that there was little correlation between BDAE scores and the results in these experiments suggest that other Boston groups should also be investigated in this way. A similar series of experiments is being carried out with a group of Wernicke's type subjects. The study is on-going; therefore, only preliminary results can be reported.

WORD ORDER PROCESSING IN WERNICKE'S TYPE APHASIA

One of the diagnostic criteria of Wernicke's aphasia is a severe auditory comprehension deficit. It has been stated that the basis for such a deficit is semantic in

TABLE 4. *Results obtained by six Wernicke's aphasic subjects in comprehension task*

	Ten nonmotion verbs[a] (total no. errors, 24; mean, 4.0)		Ten nondirectional motion verbs[a] (total no. errors, 69; mean, 11.5)		Ten directional motion verbs[a] (total no. errors, 73; mean, 12.1)	
Error analysis	No.	%	No.	%	No.	%
No. times reverse role picture selected plus percent total errors	24	100	55	79.7	31	42.5
No. times distractor picture selected plus percent total errors	0		14	20.3	42	57.5

[a] No. stimulus items = 20.

nature and reflects a problem in the semantic organization of the lexicon (13,37,39). It could be hypothesized, therefore, that the verb type effect seen in the agrammatic subjects would not only be maintained but be of a greater severity in the Wernicke's subjects. This is attributable to the fact that the problem seen in the agrammatic subjects with the directional motion verbs was considered to have arisen because of a semantic deficit.

To test this hypothesis, six Wernicke's type aphasic subjects have been tested on the comprehension task given to the agrammatic subjects, as outlined above. Their responses are shown in Table 4. Statistical analysis has not yet been carried out; nor have statistical comparisons been made with the 10 agrammatic subjects, because the study is still in progress. Also, an additional four subjects have yet to be tested. It can be seen, however, in terms of total number of errors made, that these six Wernicke's subjects have proportionately more errors than the 10 agrammatic individuals. In the Wernicke's subjects, there is little difference in number of errors made between the nondirectional and the directional motion verbs. As found with the agrammatic subjects, there were far fewer errors with the nonmotion verbs. The finding that nondirectional and directional motion verbs were equally difficult for these Wernicke's subjects is contrary to the results from the agrammatic patients. Error analysis shows that all errors in processing the nonmotion verbs resulted in selection of the reverse picture. In processing the nondirectional motion verbs, 20.3% of errors resulted in selection of the distractor picture; in processing directional motion verbs, 57.5% errors were distractor choice.

Although no statistical comparison can yet be made between the results from the Wernicke's subjects and those from the agrammatic subjects, the differences not only are true for all the individual Wernicke's subjects but are of sufficient interest to warrant further discussion.

The finding that these six Wernicke's subjects made more errors than the 10 agrammatic subjects is not surprising in view of their severe comprehension problems. Of more interest is the spread and type of errors across verb types. The verb type effect, in terms of error numbers, is different from that seen in Broca's subjects; in the Wernicke's subjects, nondirectional and directional motion verbs seemed equally difficult.

None of the results can be explained on the basis of lack of understanding of the nouns or their pictorial representations. Again, these were made explicit to the subjects before testing. In these Wernicke's subjects, therefore, the only explanation for their failure comes from either lack of recognition of the verb or failure to process the grammatic relationships. In order to postulate which factor is the key to this failure, it is necessary to consider not only the total number of errors across the verb groups but also the type of error made in each verb group.

As with the agrammatic subjects, these individuals found nonmotion verbs to be the easiest verb group to decode. No distractor choices were made with these verbs; therefore, the Wernicke's subjects must have been able to access that part of the semantic representation which denotes the action element of the meaning. Failure must have resulted from inability to access that part of the semantic representation which maps semantic and grammatic information. The fact remains that the number of errors made with these verbs was considerably less than with the nondirectional motion verbs, whereas in the Broca's agrammatic subjects, these two groups of verbs were statistically of equal difficulty. It was hypothesized that, with respect to the Broca's type subjects, nonmotion verbs were easier because, in these sentences, the verb is predicated of the actor alone, and the instrument is visually represented in the picture. There is no reason to assume that these same factors are not influential in the Wernicke's subjects. It appears that the presence of the visually presented instrument had a facilitatory effect for both groups of subjects.

The fact that nondirectional and directional motion verbs were equally affected in the Wernicke's group (this is true for all individual subjects) is of particular interest. It was hypothesized that in agrammatic subjects, directional motion verbs were significantly harder to process than nondirectional motion verbs because the former had a more complex semantic structure, involving an embedded predicate. Why, then, should these two groups of verbs appear to be of equal difficulty for Wernicke's subjects? The results of the error analysis may provide an explanation, if only that they show that there was a substantial difference across these two verb groups in terms of type of error made. In the nondirectional motion verbs, these six Wernicke's subjects made only 20.3% distractor choices; in the directional motion verbs, 57.5% of errors made were the distractor. Such findings suggest that nondirectional and directional motion verbs were not equally difficult to process.

In the case of the directional motion verbs, the six Wernicke's subjects were unable to access any of the semantic representation of the verb, with the result that they chose a different action depicted by the distractor picture. With respect to the nondirectional motion verbs, they were able to access the action element of the verb meaning on many occasions; because they were unable to access that information which codes the grammatic relationships, however, they chose the reverse role picture. This suggests that directional motion verbs were more difficult to process, as seen with the agrammatic subjects. The complexity of these verbs, in relation to the processing load imposed by the double embedded predicate, may have inhibited these Wernicke's subjects from accessing any of the verb information. Their failure arose because they could not comprehend the verb and relied only on comprehension of the two noun arguments which were in the same relation to the verb in the distractor picture as in the target sentence. The question of whether these subjects had lost the semantic representation of these verbs because of lexical disorganization is addressed below.

The problem remains of why these Wernicke's subjects found the nondirectional motion verbs to be more difficult than the nonmotion verbs. In the latter group, no distractors were chosen, but 20.3% of the errors in the nondirectional motion verbs were distractors. As pointed out, seven of 10 nonmotion verb pictures contained an instrument in the hand of the actor, thus facilitating the link between the actor and the verb. In the nonmotion verbs, however, there was no instrument in seven of 10 pictures. Therefore, in processing terms, the nondirectional motion verbs were more difficult, as they lacked any pictorial information to aid processing; subjects had to rely solely on linguistic processing. The fact that 79.7% of the errors made with the nondirectional motion verbs were reverse role errors suggests that the subjects were at least accessing the action element of the meaning of the verb.

It appears that in this comprehension task, the responses of Wernicke's subjects reflected across the verb types how much the complexity of the verb allowed for accessibility of the semantic information attached to the verb. Nonmotion verbs were considerably easier to process, because they are predicated of the actor alone; their nature allows for the visual depiction of the instrument to facilitate the link between subject and verb. Nondirectional motion verbs were harder to process because they lack this pictorially presented instrument. Error analysis showed that the directional motion verbs were the most difficult, as with the agrammatic subjects, because in these Wernicke's subjects, more distractor errors were produced, suggesting that the verb complexity made it impossible for the subject to access any of the verb information. The pattern of error types across the verb groups in the Wernicke's subjects correlated with the number of errors across the verb groups in the Broca's subjects. The question still remains as to whether this failure of the Wernicke's subjects to access any of the semantic representation of the directional motion verbs reflects a problem in the semantic organization of the lexicon.

It has often been stated that the comprehension abilities of these Wernicke's type subjects improve considerably in a more functional communication setting, where they are said to be able to bypass in depth linguistic processing by relying on other cues, e.g., pragmatic knowledge, gestural cues, and contextual information. It would be of interest to know whether it is merely a case of bypassing or whether in fact other knowledge sources can interact with linguistic knowledge to make vital information more accessible.

To test this, the same Wernicke's subjects were given a picture selection task. Stimuli consisted of the same directional motion verbs used in the previous task, and methodology remained exactly the same. This time, however, the noun arguments were chosen in order to provide a pragmatic bias. The arrangement of the noun arguments was such that although the sentences were reversible in terms of each noun argument being possible as the actor, there was, from world knowledge, a built-in expectancy that one of the noun arguments would be the more plausible actor, e.g., "The policeman chased the thief." As with the previous task, animacy was held constant. The eight directional motion verbs used were incorporated in such a pragmatically biased sentence, and there were two sentences for each verb. Thus there was a total of 16 triadic sets. The results of this experiment showed a 100% correct response. It could be conjectured that the subjects' success in this task reflected only reliance on pragmatic knowledge in terms of knowing the plausibility of the two noun arguments being in a particular relationship. This cannot have been the total answer, however, because in eight of the triads, in the distractor picture in which the same noun arguments were represented, there was an equal amount of pragmatic bias. This was a deliberate design of the study in order to try and "trap" the subjects. An example of such a triad would be as follows:

The policeman chases the thief	Target
The thief chases the policeman	Reverse
The policeman handcuffs the thief	Distractor

If the subjects were relying on pragmatic bias alone, there would have been equal chance that they would have chosen the distractor picture. The fact that they did not do so suggests that they were able to access the verb information in the target sentence and reliably process its different action element from that in the equally plausible verb in the distractor. It also means that they must have processed the prepositional element in the verb meaning; otherwise they would not have been correct in choosing between the target picture and its reverse role depiction.

The results of this test suggest that the pragmatic information did not merely allow the subject to bypass linguistic processing but, more important, interacted with semantic/syntactic information to have allowed the subject to process the sentence in full. In relation to these Wernicke's subjects, there appeared to be no correlation between the degree of neologistic jargon present in an individual subject and the results of the main comprehension task. Indeed, the two subjects who presented with the most jargon in spontaneous output showed the lowest overall error scores.

The results of these experiments, in both groups of subjects, emphasize the psychologic reality of differences in processing load of the three types of verbs tested. In both the agrammatic and the Wernicke's subjects, the directional motion verbs proved to be the most difficult to process. This seemed to be related to their complex semantic structure in which one predicate, the prepositional predicate, is embedded in another, the verb predicate.

The agrammatic subjects certainly showed a word order deficit, which was much more marked in relation to the directional motion verbs. Their failure with these verbs seemed to be attributable not to total failure to access some element of the semantic representation of the verb but to a particular problem in accessing the prepositional information; therefore, there is a semantic deficit in relation to these verbs.

Although there were fewer Wernicke's type subjects than agrammatics, the former made proportionately more errors in processing grammatic relationships marked by word order alone; analysis of the errors made by this group shows once again that directional motion verbs were the most difficult. The complexity of the these verbs appears to have inhibited retrieval of any verb information in view of the number of distractors chosen.

The results of the second experiment with the Wernicke's subjects suggest that pragmatic knowledge interacts with, rather than merely bypasses, semantic/syntactic information. This finding also suggests that, particularly in Wernicke's subjects, comprehension problems seen in formal tests may be incorrectly interpreted as loss of semantic knowledge. These results suggest that the meaning of verbs themselves may not be lost but only inaccessible, depending on the influence of the structures in which they appear, what a particular task entails, and whether different knowledge sources can be brought into play to release knowledge. These results support the view of Blumstein et al. (2), who showed semantic facilitation effects in a lexical decision task in Wernicke's subjects. Those authors also concluded that comprehension deficits seen in these subjects may not be due to problems of semantic organization per se but more to problems in one of the processes involved in access to that information.

The fact that within identical syntactic structures certain verbs are easier than others has import for therapeutic strategies in terms of devising hierarchies of difficulty. Furthermore, knowledge of other influencing factors allows for more pertinent manipulation of variables to ease comprehension and to provide strategies for the patient. At the same time, too much emphasis has been placed in therapy on working on syntactic structure, particularly in terms of person and tense agreement without any real awareness of the importance of other aspects of verb information that dictate structure. Since verbs in isolation bear only minimal resemblance to their import within a sentence structure, it is important for us to be more aware of what aspects of verb information are required for particular tasks.

The results of the pragmatically biased picture selection task with the Wernicke's type subjects reinforce the view that functional communication situations allow for greater interaction of different knowledge sources and therefore enhance comprehension and probably production of language. This emphasis on functional communication is to be welcomed, but only if its significance is understood in terms of analyzing the variables in it to allow subjects to perform better. Unless these variables can be understood and manipulated, the subject will be able to perform better only under certain circumstances, which would be undefined and therefore uncontrollable and closed to replication.

We must investigate further what the differences are between the groups and between individuals within the groups. While most clinicians who work daily with aphasics recognize the heterogeneity of these broad groupings, we must look deeper into differences that may lie outside linguistic knowledge. Such pointers for future work emphasize that aphasia can no longer be looked at by one discipline, but must be viewed more in terms of psycholinguistic processing, defining what knowledge sources are used in processing language for either input or output, how and under what circumstances these sources interact, and what factors lead to breakdown or enhancement in processing. It is hoped that such an approach would not only tell us more about individual problems and their possible remediation but might suggest how normal subjects process language, particularly if, as should always be the case, they are included in such investigations.

REFERENCES

1. Black, M.: The processing of grammatical relations in agrammatism. Unpublished manuscript. University College, London.
2. Blumstein, S., Milberg, W., and Shrier, R. (1982): Semantic processing in aphasia: Evidence from an auditory lexical decision task. *Brain Lang.*, 17:301–315.
3. Bresnan, J. (1978): A realistic transformational grammar. In: *Linguistic Theory and Psychological Reality*, edited by M. Halle, J. Bresnan, and G. A. Miller, pp. 1–59. M.I.T. Press, Cambridge, Massachusetts.
4. Caramazza, A., and Zurif, E. B. (1976): Dissociation of algorithmic and heuristic processes in language comprehension. *Brain Lang.*, 3:572–582.
5. Deloche, G., and Seron, X. (1981): Sentence understanding and knowledge of the world: Evidences from a sentence-picture matching task performed by aphasic patients. *Brain Lang.*, 14:57–69.
6. Fillenbaum, S., Jones, L. V., and Wepman, J. M. (1961): Some linguistic features of speech from aphasic patients. *Lang. Speech*, 4:91–108.
7. Garrett, M. (1975): The analysis of sentence production. In: *Psychology of Learning and Motivation, Vol 9*, edited by G. Bower, pp. 133–177. Academic Press, New York.
8. Garrett, M. (1976): Syntactic processes in sentence production. In: *New Approaches to Language Mechanisms*, edited by E. Walker and R. Wales. North Holland, Amsterdam.
9. Gleason, J. B., Goodglass, H., Green, E., Ackerman, N., and Hyde, M. R. (1975): The retrieval of syntax in Broca's aphasia. *Brain Lang.*, 2:451–471.
10. Goodglass, H. (1968): Studies on the grammar of aphasics. In: *Developments in Applied Psycholinguistics Research*, edited by S. Rosenberg and J. Kaplin. Macmillan, New York.
11. Goodglass, H., and Kaplan, E. (1972): *The Assessment of Aphasia and Related Disorders*. Lea & Febiger, Philadelphia.
12. Goodglass, H., Gleason, J. B., Bernholtz, N. A., and Hyde, M. R. (1972): Some linguistic structures in the speech of a Broca's aphasic. *Cortex*, VIII:191–212.
13. Goodglass, H., and Baker, E. (1976): Semantic field, naming and auditory comprehension in aphasia. *Brain Lang.*, 3:359–374.
14. Gruber, J. (1976): *Lexical Structures in Syntax and Semantics*. North Holland, New York.
15. Isserlin, M. (1922): Uber Agrammatismus. *Z. Gesamte Neurol. Psychiatr.*, 75:332–410.
16. Jackendoff, R. S. (1972): *Semantic Interpretation in Generative Grammar*. M.I.T. Press, Cambridge, Massachusetts.
17. Jones, E. V. (1984): *Submitted for publication*.
18. Jones, E. V. (1982): *Word Order Processing in Agrammatism*. M.Sc. project, University College, London.
19. Kean, M. L. (1977): The linguistic interpretation of aphasic syndromes: Agrammatism in Broca's aphasia, an example. *Cognition*, 5:9–46.
20. Kean, M. L. (1978): The linguistic interpretation of aphasic syndromes. In: *Explorations in the Biology of Language. Report of the M.I.T. Work Group on the Biology of Language*, edited by E. Walker. Bradford Books, Montgomery, Vermont.
21. Kean, M. L. (1979): Agrammatism: A phonological deficit? *Cognition*, 7:69–84.
22. Kucera, H., and Francis, W. N. (1967): *Computational Analysis of Everyday American English*. Brown University Press, Providence, Rhode Island.
23. Lesser, R. (1974): Verbal comprehension in aphasia. *Cortex*, X:247–263.

24. Linebarger, M. C., Schwartz, M. F., and Saffran, E. (1983): Sensitivity to grammatical structure in so-called agrammatic aphasics. *Cognition*, 13:361–392.
25. Marin, O. S. M., Saffran, E. M., and Schwartz, M. F. (1976): Dissociations of language in aphasia: Implications for normal function. *Ann. NY Acad. Sci.*, 280:868–884.
26. Miller, G. (1972): English verbs of motion: A case study in semantics and lexical memory. In: *Coding Processes in Human Memory*, edited by A. W. Melton and E. Martin. Winston, Washington, D.C.
27. Myerson, R., and Goodglass, H. (1972): Transformational grammars of three agrammatic patients. *Lang. Speech*, 15:40–50.
28. Parisi, D., and Pizzamiglio, L. (1970): Syntactic comprehension in aphasia. *Cortex*, VI:204–215.
29. Pick, A. (1913): *Die Agrammatischen Sprach Storungen*. Springer-Verlag, Berlin.
30. Saffran, E. M., Schwartz, M. F., and Marin, O. S. (1980): The word order problem in agrammatism. II. Production. *Brain Lang.*, 10:263–280.
31. Saffran, E. M., Schwartz, M. F., and Marin, O. S. (1980): Evidence from aphasia: Isolating the components of a production model. In: *Language Production*, edited by B. Butterworth. Academic Press, London.
32. Scholes, R. (1978): Syntactic and lexical components of sentence comprehension. In: *The Acquisition and Breakdown of Language: Parallels and Divergencies*, edited by A. Caramazza and E. Zurif. Johns Hopkins Press, Baltimore.
33. Scholes, R. (1982): The verb-right strategy in agrammatic aphasia. *Neuropsychologia*, 20:361–363.
34. Schwartz, M. F., Saffran, E. M., and Marin, O. S. (1980): The word order problem in agrammatism. I. Comprehension. *Brain Lang.*, 10:249–262.
35. von Stockert, T. (1972): Recognition of syntactic structure in aphasic patients. *Cortex*, VIII:323–334.
36. von Stockert, T., and Bader, L. (1976): Some relations of grammar and lexicon in aphasia. *Cortex*, XII:49–60.
37. Whitehouse, P., Caramazza, A., and Zurif, E. B. (1978): Naming in aphasia: Interacting effects of form and function. *Brain Lang.*, 6:63–74.
38. Zurif, E. B., Caramazza, A., and Myerson, R. (1972): Grammatical judgements of agrammatic aphasics. *Neuropsychologia*, 10:405–418.
39. Zurif, E. B., Caramazza, A., Myerson, R., and Galvin, J. (1974): Semantic feature representations for normal and aphasic language. *Brain Lang.*, 1:167–187.
40. Zurif, E. B., Green, E., Caramazza, A., and Goodenough, C. (1976): Grammatical judgements of aphasic patients: Sensitivity to functors, *Cortex*, XII:183–186.

Advances in Neurology, Vol. 42: Progress in Aphasiology, edited by F. C. Rose.
Raven Press, New York © 1984.

Interpretation of Spelling Disorders in Aphasia: Impact of Recent Developments in Cognitive Psychology

Frances M. Hatfield and Karalyn E. Patterson

MRC Applied Psychology Unit, Cambridge CB2 2EF, England

A PROCESS MODEL DERIVED FROM DYSGRAPHIC AND NORMAL SPELLING BEHAVIOR

In cognitive psychology, the study of aphasia generally takes the form of developing process models of relevant behavior. Figure 1, which presents a processing model for the major routines involved in input and output for spoken and written words, is based on Morton's logogen model (9,10) and also shares major similarities with models presented by Marshall and Newcombe (8), Shallice (14), Coltheart (3), and others. The model is organized around two major sets of distinctions: (a) the separation between spoken and written words (which spatially in the diagram is a left-right separation), and (b) the separation between input and output procedures (which here is an up-down separation). Since this sort of model is discussed frequently in the literature, it needs no detailed description here.

In this chapter, our concern is spelling, more explicitly, the operation of written spelling to dictation. In Fig. 1, this means proceeding from auditory analysis of the spoken word to a written response. The model shows two primary routines for spelling to dictation. One involves segmental translation from phonology to orthography. For simplicity, this has been represented in the figure as one process, although in fact it must involve at least three procedures. The spoken word must be analyzed or parsed into phonologic segments. Orthographic representations then must be assigned to these individual segments on the basis of the speller's knowledge about correspondences between sound and spelling in his/her language. Finally, the orthographic segments must be assembled so that a single whole word can be produced as response. The procedures on such segmental translation can be applied by anyone knowing the spelling conventions of the language to any speech sound, whether or not it is a real lexical item. Thus by using these procedures, a normal speller can produce some spelling of an unfamiliar word or name.

The second major routine (indicated by dashed lines) involves recognizing the spoken word as a familiar item, accessing its semantic representation, and then consulting an orthographic output lexicon, which contains the spelling of known words.

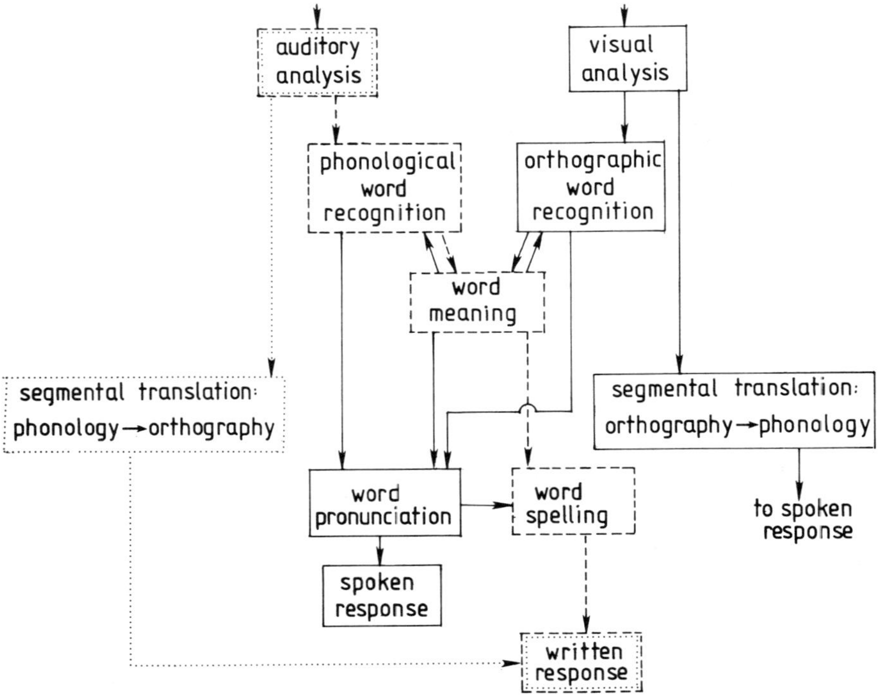

FIG. 1. Process model showing two major routines involved in input and output for spoken and written words. *Dotted lines*: Routine involves segmental translation from phonology to orthography. *Dashed lines:* Routine involves recognizing spoken word as a familiar item, accessing its semantic representation, and then consulting an orthographic lexicon, which contains the spelling of known words.

The procedures in this routine are obviously appropriate only for real words; moreover, these must be real words for which a semantic representation is available. It should be noted that this routine is in no sense parasitic on speech or phonologic processes, whereas some earlier models (7,16) had suggested that spelling obligatorily involves phonology.

There are a variety of ways for utilizing this kind of approach in research. First, one can study spelling in normal subjects; for example, one can devise tasks which stress one of the routines and thus force normal subjects to make spelling errors. Indeed, one of the satisfying aspects of spelling as a skill to study is that normals do make frequent errors, even without stress. This means that both neurologically normal and impaired subjects provide sources of evidence which can be checked for convergence. That a single process model can account for performance by both normal and brain-damaged populations enhances our confidence in the model. The second major realization of this approach, and the one more relevant to this exposition, is the study of these routines as demonstrated by aphasic patients whose

TABLE 1. *Three contrasts in stimulus dimensions*

Word/nonword (e.g., *state*/shate)
Content word/function word (e.g., *flat*/*that*)
Spelling regularity (or predictability) versus irregularity (e.g., lunch/yacht; /lʌntʃ/ /jɔt/)

impairments selectively disrupt the use of one routine, forcing the patient to rely on the more-or-less spared alternative procedure.

Two major techniques have been used in the context of single case studies. (A full description of these two techniques in the study of reading disorders is given in ref. 12.) The first technique is error analysis. Two of our Cambridge patients were recently dictated the word "narrow" to spell: one patient's written response was *naro*; the other's was *thin*. It seems clear that the response *thin* could not arise from the routine involving segmental translation from phonology to orthography but must instead arise from the second routine. The spoken word has been correctly recognized by the phonologic word recognition system and has furthermore accessed at least a partially correct semantic representation. The error presumably arises either because the exact meaning has not been computed, the spelling of "narrow" could not be retrieved from the orthographic output lexicon (word spelling), or there is imperfect communication from word meaning to word spelling.

Conversely, the response *naro* derives from the first routine. The logic is different here: it would be indefensible to argue that such a response could not arise from the second routine. After all, if the representations in the orthographic output lexicon are not fully intact, then one might expect to find responses from this routine which are incorrect but orthographically similar to the target word; and *naro* fits this description. However, there is no particular reason why such partial orthographic knowledge should generate phonologically plausible responses. Thus if one looks not at one but at hundreds of the patient's errors, essentially all of which are phonologically plausible (and some indeed not orthographically similar, e.g., "injury" → *ingerry*), one begins to suspect that spelling is reliant on the first routine (6). Additional examples of this kind of error analysis are presented in connection with the case studies described below.

CRITICAL DIMENSIONS IN IDENTIFYING ROUTINE FOLLOWED AND IN CLASSIFICATION OF SUBJECTS

The other major technique involves the design of spelling tests around certain crucial stimulus dimensions which implicate particular components or routines in the model. Table 1 illustrates three contrasts upon which such tests are based.

Word/Nonword

The letter string *state* is a legitimate lexical item; the letter string *shate*, although it obeys both the orthographic and phonologic conventions of English, happens not to be a word. Someone spelling by the second routine should be maximally affected by this contrast, since these spelling procedures require recognition of the item as a familiar word. For someone spelling primarily by the first routine, on the other hand, there should be essentially no difference between /steit/ and /ʃeit/ in terms of the ease of segmental translation from phonology to orthography.

Content Word/Function Word

The word *flat* is an open class item or content word, whereas the word *that* is a closed class, grammatic function word. If either (a) these two word classes are differentially represented in terms of semantics, or (b) the second routine is influenced by another process (not shown here), such as the syntactic function of words, then someone spelling by the second routine will be influenced by this contrast. For segmental translation, on the other hand, /flæt/ and /ðæt/ should be equally easy to convert to orthographic equivalents.

Spelling Regularity or Predictability Versus Lack of Predictability

This contrast is not a dichotomy but a continuum, the extremes of which might be represented by the words *lunch* and *yacht*. Anyone who did not know these words and tried to spell them by segmental translation would probably do well with /lʌntʃ/ → *lunch* but badly with /jɔt/ → *yacht*. By the second routine, on the other hand, since the spelling of a familiar word is merely addressed or "looked up," spelling regularity should be irrelevant.

A certain number of patients with acquired spelling disorders have been described in the past decade whose characteristic responses seem to assign them to two broad categories, although there are within-category differences. By analogy with the terminology recently adopted for the dyslexias (4,8) these two groups have been called deep and surface dysgraphics. As an example of the first kind, the patient J.C., described by Bub and Kertesz (2), can be cited: Following a stroke which left her aphasic, J.C. made many semantic paragraphias in writing, of the type "time" → *clock*, and had severe difficulty in writing four-letter pronounceable nonwords. Similarly, Hatfield (5) gives an account of three patients who made a large proportion of so-called visual, derivational, and semantic errors. Other researchers, e.g., Marshall and Newcombe (8,11), have described similar cases. A subvariety has been called phonologic agraphia by Shallice (15), where the patient's difficulty manifested itself principally in writing nonwords to dictation. For the deep dysgraphics, it is inferred from their characteristic performance in writing to dictation that the segmental routine for translating phonology to orthography is malfunctioning or inactive, and that the semantic routine is better spared, although not intact.

The group called surface dysgraphics makes different kinds of errors. Characteristically, they make phonologically plausible responses; instances are cited above (namely, "narrow" → *naro*; "injury" → *ingerry*). Semantic paragraphias do not occur or are very rare. Examples of this kind of patient have been provided in studies by Hatfield (5), Hatfield and Patterson (6), and Beauvois and Derouesné (1), who

TABLE 2. *Patients' performance on three tests of writing to dictation*[a]

Dysgraphics	Content words (*N* = 60)	Function words (*N* = 60)	Real words (*N* = 20)	Nonsense words (*N* = 20)	Regularly spelled words (*N* = 28)	Irregularly spelled words (*N* = 28)
Deep						
B.B.[b]	20	4	2	0	3	5
D.E.	25	6	10	0	5	5
Surface						
T.P.[b]	57	48	18	18	24	19
S.C.	25	29	14	6	11	7

[a] Figures are correct responses.
[b] These are the subjects discussed in the text.

prefer the label lexical or orthographic agraphia. In these cases, it is inferred that the phonologic routine is spared, at least at an elementary level, and that it is the lexical-semantic process that is defective.

Our investigation of the spelling problems of individual patients involves both the approaches outlined above, namely, the use of specific tests and analysis of errors. A small number of subjects have been selected to represent the two broad varieties of deep and surface dysgraphia; of these, two subjects are discussed in some detail. Although these two patients have quite different forms of aphasia, it is submitted that their writing problems can be more clearly understood by looking directly at which features, or processes, in their writing system are better preserved and which are more severely impaired than by looking at their aphasic symptoms. The basic assessment of our patients' writing includes, in addition to assessment of visual perception and ability to copy letters, tests designed to highlight fundamental qualitative distinctions at the level of written spelling. Three such tests are described above.

Table 2 shows the contrast in performance between deep and surface dysgraphics, two of each kind, on these three tests of writing to dictation. The two cases under discussion are footnoted. From the results of the first test, which examines word semantics, particularly the factor of concreteness, it can be seen that B.B., a deep dysgraphic representative, had specific difficulty with grammatic function words (for example, prepositions, pronouns, and other closed class words) compared with content words. From the second test (real words versus nonwords), it can be seen that he was unable to write even the simplest nonwords, or nonsense words (and was indeed never observed to write these during this period). The figures for the second deep dysgraphic patient, D.E., for this test are even more convincing. The inference to be drawn for these two patients is that they are unable to use a phoneme-to-grapheme routine in writing to dictation; this subskill is represented in the model by the box labeled "segmental translation of phonology to orthography." Instead, they are relying on direct recall of semantically rich whole words. This twofold inference is reinforced by the results of the third test (examining the effect of regularity of spelling), which show no facilitatory effect of regularity, as indeed one would expect from recourse to the semantic routine, by which the spelling of a familiar word is addressed *in toto*.

The spelling of the surface dysgraphic patients, on the other hand, was unaffected by semantic factors; words with little content were transcribed as easily as those with much more. The patient T.P. had virtually no difficulty in transcribing nonsense words, which by definition have no semantic content and can be transcribed only by means of a segmental translation from phonology to orthography. Unlike the deep dysgraphics, the two surface dysgraphic patients show a superiority with regularly spelled words, which was even more marked at an earlier stage.

Even more striking are the types of errors. In common with other deep dysgraphics, B.B. made visual, semantic, and derivational errors. Visual errors (sometimes simply called spelling errors) are those bearing a strong visual similarity to the stimulus word; as they often contain a number of letters shared with the stimulus, there may be a partial phonologic similarity. Derivational errors are those in which the word root is correctly spelled, but there is an error in the suffix, e.g., "called" → *calling*, "sees" → *seen*. Patient B.B.'s semantic paragraphias, for example, "little" → *small*, "stove" → *shiver* (in both cases the stimulus word was repeated correctly and without difficulty), provide further support for his putative reliance on semantic factors in the stimulus as a spelling strategy. Figure 2 shows B.B.'s responses to part of the content-versus-function word test referred to above. Formerly right-handed, B.B. was now forced by his right hemiparesis to write with his nonpreferred left hand.

An important feature in B.B.'s spelling is his particularly poor response to the function words. Some are not attempted at all; others are responded to by forms bearing little phonologic, visual, or semantic resemblance to the stimulus, except that they are often items of a large set which includes prepositions, conjunctions, and other "little words." Thus "too" is written as *all* and "how" as *why*; "off," "has," and "yet" are not attempted. A few extra items were slipped in, which were homophonic to the failed function word items and were themselves content words. (These are in square brackets in Fig 2.) Although B.B. failed on the adverb *too*, he was successful with the number *two*; although unable to attempt the pronoun (possessive adjective) *our*, he had no difficulty in spelling the noun *hour* (both correct items having, incidentally, irregular spelling). He was unsuccessful both with the pronoun *him* and with the noun *hymn*, but on subsequent occasions was often able to write the noun (but not the pronoun) correctly. Other cases of greater success with certain content words than with homophonic function words were observed with this patient. This phenomenon was exploited in the therapy that followed the testing.

In marked contrast were the errors made by the surface dysgraphic patient T.P. These were characteristically phonologically plausible. Formerly a good speller and a senior member of her profession, she wrote, for the word "major," *mager*, and for the word "ghost," *goast*. She also made many errors of homophone confusion of the type of *peal* instead of *peel* for the peel of an orange. Figure 3 shows T.P.'s

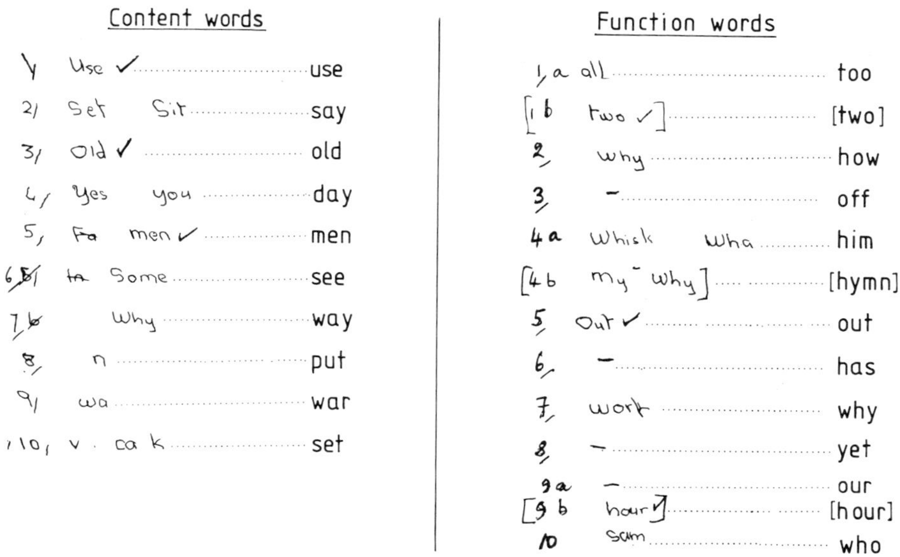

FIG. 2. Responses of patient B.B. to part of a single word dictation test, comparing content and function words.

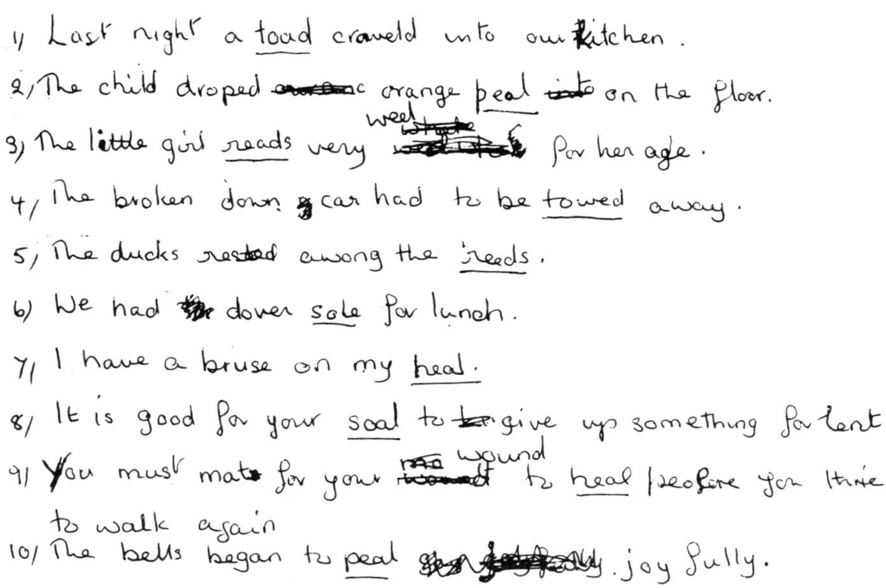

FIG. 3. Responses of patient T.P. to a test of dictation of sentences.

performance on a task of writing sentences to dictation a few months prior to the other tests. This patient had no motor impairment and was still able to write with her preferred right hand.

Among typical errors are T.P.'s phonologically plausible rendering of the word *bruise* as *bruse* and a homophonic error in the word *heel*, both in sentence 7. Sentence 8 contains a phonologically plausible spelling of the word *soul*, possibly by analogy with *coal*. Thus her spelling errors show a relatively well-preserved ability to transcribe heard words by a phoneme-to-grapheme routine, although at a fairly elementary level; she failed at the level of more complicated orthographic rules, such as "final 'e' rule" and the consonant-doubling rule, as shown in the word *droped* (intended for *dropped*) in sentence 2. At this stage, she made frequent letter inversions, confusing *m* and *w*, *p* and *b*, but errors of inversion decreased with time. Unlike B.B., she made no semantic paragraphias. The character of T.P.'s errors confirms that, on the whole, the segmental phonologic routine is preserved in writing to dictation, but the knowledge of specific orthography of whole individual words has seriously suffered.

Background Information

Patient B.B., a deep dysgraphic, had a massive cerebrovascular insult at the age of 41, 2½ years before this study. He was formerly a wholesale grocer, of average education. The computerized axial tomography scan revealed extensive damage in the left middle cerebral artery territory, implicating the frontal, temporal, and parietal lobes and extending vertically to a depth of 66 mm. His expressive speech was labored and mainly confined to single word utterances, especially of nouns. There was a mild articulatory dyspraxia. Auditory comprehension of single words was quite good, but comprehension at sentence level was moderately impaired. There was a short auditory memory span and a digit repetition span of only two (forward). Reading was of the deep dyslexic variety, with specific deficits on abstract and function words and an abundance of visual, derivational, and semantic errors characteristic of this group; in other words, it essentially mirrored the profile of his writing impairment.

Patient T.P., a surface dysgraphic, was formerly a senior radiographer. She was 50 years old when she suffered a subarachnoid hemorrhage from a left temporooccipital angioma 18 months before the study. Surgery was carried out for removal of a left temporoparietal hematoma and for the angiomatous malformation. She was left with a right homonymous hemianopia and a fluent, anomic aphasia with some auditory comprehension loss. Digit repetition was six digits (forward). Her reading aloud improved with time and therapy. She favored two strategies, reading the letters sound by sound (and then trying to fit the string of phonemes to a familiar word) and pronouncing the letter names.

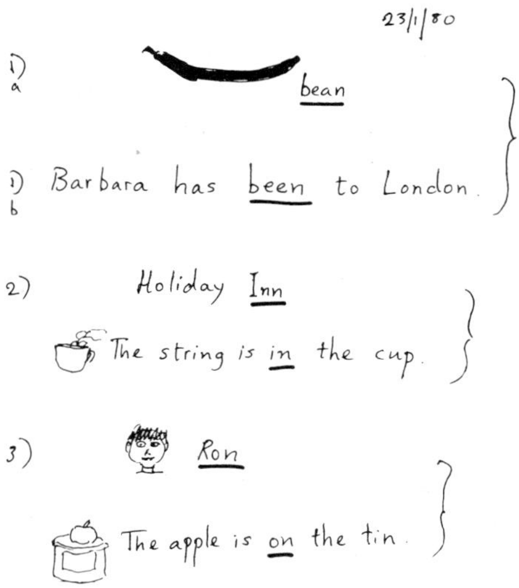

FIG. 4. A page from B.B.'s practice book near the start of his retraining in writing function words. (From Hatfield, ref. 5, with permission.)

DERIVATION OF REEDUCATIONAL STRATEGIES FROM THE MODEL

Use of the above kind of process model to interpret spelling behavior indicated the need for a completely separate reeducational approach for written spelling for the two patients, based on two different types of impairment.

For B.B., the deep dysgraphic in whom the process for converting phonology to orthography in an analytic, segmental way was the more impaired of the two fundamental processes of writing, therapy was based on his much better preserved alternative system, that which utilizes word meaning and whole word spelling (the semantic routine). The first step was to exploit his better performance on content words, with their relatively rich semantics, to reteach spelling of the elusive function words. Figure 4 reproduces a page from his practice book and illustrates how function words were trained by linking them with content words, which were either homophones or near homophones. The strategy of first writing the content word and then retrieving the function word from it was gradually phased out until this was done internally or omitted altogether. (Fuller details of the therapy are given in ref. 5.) This approach to reeducation of impaired skills in aphasia essentially constitutes a reorganization of function at a deep level, rather than an attempt to restore an impaired function in its former form by direct training of that function (see also ref.13). The same type of therapy was used for two other patients with similar problems.

For T.P., the surface dysgraphic, therapy was based on her partial preservation of a phonologic process. Her knowledge of phonology-to-orthography conversion was consolidated, and practice was given in more advanced rules of spelling, such as "final 'e' rule," consonant-doubling rule, and similar rules. Pairs and triads of homophones were also given for reacquisition, with various mnemonics. She had to be helped to know when to write the sound *ay* with *ai*, as, for instance, in the word *plain*, meaning simple, flat, or level, and when with *a* and *e* after the consonant, as in the *plane* tree. In this case, the unforgettable line, "The rain in Spain falls mainly on the plain" helped. The individual strategies for specific items were often suggested by the patients themselves or by the therapist in consultation with the patient.

In both cases, this initial step in reeducation of spelling produced satisfactory improvement within its modest aim. Thus an approach has been adopted by the two authors which integrates the theory outlined in the first section of this chapter, the model, the spelling problems of a small number of contrasting patients studied in depth, and, finally, their rehabilitation.

ACKNOWLEDGMENTS

The authors are grateful to Dr. O. M. Edwards and Mr. A. Holmes, two of the consultants at Addenbrooke's Hospital, Cambridge, for facilities to study their patients and for permission to report clinical data. This study was supported, in the case of Mrs. Hatfield, by a grant from the Medical Research Council, to whom thanks are expressed.

REFERENCES

1. Beauvois, M. F., and Derouesné, J. (1981): Lexical or orthographic agraphia. *Brain*, 104:21–49.
2. Bub, D., and Kertesz, A. (1982): Deep agraphia. *Brain Lang.*, 17:146–165.
3. Coltheart, M. (1981): Disorders of reading and their implications for models of normal reading. *Visible Lang.*, 15:245–286.
4. Coltheart, M., Patterson, K., and Marshall, J. (1980): *Deep Dyslexia*. Routledge and Kegan Paul, London.
5. Hatfield, F. M. (1982): Diverses formes de désintégration du langage écrit et implications pour la rééducation. In: *Rééduquer le Cerveau*, edited by X. Seron and C. Laterre, pp. 135–156. Mardaga, Brussels.
6. Hatfield, F. M., and Patterson, K. (1983): Phonological spelling. *Q. J. Exp. Psychol.*, 35A:451–468.
7. Leischner, A. (1957): *Die Störungen der Schriftsprache*. George Thieme, Stuttgart.
8. Marshall, J., and Newcombe, F. (1973): Patterns of paralexia: A psycholinguistic approach. *J. Psycholinguist. Res.*, 2:175–199.
9. Morton, J. (1980): The logogen model and orthographic structure. In: *Cognitive Processes in Spelling*, edited by U. Frith, pp. 117–183. Academic Press, London.
10. Morton, J., and Patterson, K. (1980): A new attempt at an interpretation, or, an attempt at a new interpretation. In: *Deep Dyslexia*, edited by M. Coltheart, K. Patterson, and J. Marshall, pp. 91–118. Routledge and Kegan Paul, London.
11. Newcombe, F., and Marshall, J. (1980): Transcoding and lexical stabilization in deep dyslexia. In: *Deep Dyslexia*, edited by M. Coltheart, K. Patterson, and J. Marshall, pp. 176–188. Routledge and Kegan Paul, London.
12. Patterson, K. (1981): Neurological approaches to the study of reading. *Br. J. Psychol.*, 72:151–174.
13. Seron, X. (1982): Les choix de stratégies: rétablir, réorganiser ou amenager l'environnement? In: *Rééduquer le Cerveau*, edited by X. Seron and C. Laterre, pp. 63–76. Mardaga, Brussels.
14. Shallice, T. (1981): Neurological impairment of cognitive processes. *Br. Med. Bull.*, 37:187–192.
15. Shallice, T. (1981): Phonological agraphia and the lexical route in writing. *Brain*, 104:21–49.
16. Wernicke, C. (1874): *Der aphasische Symptomencomplex*. Cohn & Weigert, Breslau.

Advances in Neurology, Vol. 42: Progress in Aphasiology, edited by F. C. Rose.
Raven Press, New York © 1984.

Sentence Comprehension and Production in Aphasia: An Application of Lexical Grammar

Ruth Lesser

Department of Speech, The University, Newcastle upon Tyne NE1 7RU, England

The distinction between Broca's and Wernicke's aphasia, which had been considered as reflecting predominantly expressive or predominantly receptive difficulties, has been redefined in terms of supramodal linguistic processing. Broca's aphasic patients are now considered to be impaired in those aspects of both language production and comprehension which involve syntax and Wernicke's aphasic patients in those aspects which involve the lexicon, i.e., the semantics and phonologic shapes of words (5,12). Anomic patients who score relatively well on tests of auditory verbal comprehension have also been classed with other patients with posterior lesions as having a fuzziness of lexical semantics as well as difficulty in projecting word meaning onto word sound.

There are grounds, however, for questioning whether this new dichotomy of syntactic versus lexical does not itself suffer from the oversimplification of the expressive-receptive one it superseded. Changes in prosody have been described in Wernicke's aphasia, which suggest that syntax is not necessarily unaffected in this syndrome (6). The lexical deficit may also not be as radical as has been supposed in these patients. The study by Blumstein et al. (1) of semantic priming in a lexical decision task indicates that recognition of words in patients with Wernicke's aphasia is facilitated by semantic priming, even though these patients may not be able to make correct semantic judgments about the relatedness of the pairs of words used. Similarly, some of the evidence concerning the supramodal loss of a specialized processor for grammatic words in Broca's aphasia (17) has been questioned. This notion was promoted largely by a reaction time study of lexical decision by Bradley et al. (2), which compared closed class (grammatic) and open class (substantive) words. Gordon and Caramazza's (8) repetition of this study did not find that agrammatic patients performed differently from other aphasic patients. Jones' experiment (reported in the preceding chapter of this volume) also indicates that patients considered to be agrammatic are significantly influenced in their comprehension of sentences by lexical factors.

Saffran et al. (12) have suggested that agrammatism may be of at least two types, morphologic and constructional. In the former, grammatic words and inflections are unavailable, although basic grammatic relationships are preserved. In the latter, the morphologic aspects of grammar which were impaired in the former are preserved, but the basic phrase constituents of a sentence, such as subject-verb-object, cannot be assembled for the production or comprehension of speech. Inasmuch as the latter deficit can be reliably examined through tests of comprehension of reversible sentences, it is notable that individuals from all categories of aphasia make more errors with reversible than with nonreversible sentences; this is not restricted to the agrammatic. This does not in itself mean that different types of patients do not have difficulties with different aspects of such sentences, lexical or syntactic.

There is a major problem in examining these questions. Although it may be legitimate to speak of lexical impairment when considering tasks that use substantive words in isolation, when we discuss syntactic impairment in connected language, we must ask in what way a principled distinction can be made between lexical and syntactic aspects of the on-line processing of sentences. So far, distinctions made between lexical and syntactic deficits in the comprehension of sentences have assumed that lexical items can be treated as distinct from their syntactic manipulation [see, for example, Peuser's three figure test (10)]. Some recently proposed theories of grammar make such an assumption questionable. These are the lexicalist interpretive grammars, which claim that much of the information about sentence structure that was accounted for by syntactic transformations in the earlier versions of transformational grammar is in fact inherent in the lexical entries for words. Production of sentences in the passive, for example, is explained by the existence of passive forms of verbs in the lexicon rather than by the transformation of a base sentence in deep structure into a passive one in surface structure.

The most elaborated recent exposition of such a lexical grammar is that of Bresnan (3,4). In justifying lexical functional grammar, the author claims that it is psychologically real and therefore provides a valid basis for a model of the mental representation of language. Bresnan argues that the extreme rapidity of language comprehension implies that psycholinguistic models should minimize the amount of grammatic processing needed and maximize the amount that can be interpreted through lexical information. The capacity of the brain for long-term lexical storage seems to be extremely large, and Bresnan points out that it is much easier to look up than to compute information. This lexical grammar has been supported by Pinker (11) as a foundation for a psychologically plausible theory of language acquisition. Ford (7) has also tested the predictions it makes about where pauses occur in natural speech.

LEXICAL FUNCTIONAL GRAMMAR

A brief account of lexical functional grammar may show how some predictions derived from it could be used to clarify the nature of the syntactic or lexical deficit in aphasia. Lexical functional grammar makes a distinction between the constituent structure of a sentence (its phrase structure and parts of speech, such as noun and verb) and its functional structure (the grammatic relationships of subject, object, and complement, and such aspects as tense, number, and gender). Functional structure combines grammatic functions with logical argument structures. The lexical entry for each verb or other predicative word specifies both its permissible syntactic contexts and its functional structure. The distinctiveness of the specification for constituent structure context and for functional structure can be illustrated with the verb "eat." In its intransitive form ("The cat is eating"), it retains a logical object in its functional structure, even though this is not realized in the syntactic context. This notion of functional structures is used to describe how passive verbs exist in their own right as lexical entries rather than through transformations from the active. "The cat was eaten" has a functional structure of $(\exists x)x\text{EAT NP}_1$, compared with that of $(\exists y)\ \text{NP}_1\ \text{EAT}\ y$ for "The cat was eating."

The functional structure assigned to each word relates only to such logical arguments as can be assigned a limited number of basic syntactic functions, such as subject, object, complement. It does not include logical or semantic entailments. Bresnan gives the example of "escape (from prison)," which logically entails a time, place, and manner, but she notes that temporal, locative, and manner adjuncts are not part of the functional structure of "escape." Nor is the functional structure isomorphic with semantic or thematic roles, such as source, theme, and goal. For example, "give," which has the three logical arguments in its structure corresponding to subject, object 1, and object 2, has entries for two separate functional structures, according to whether it is usable in a double-object constituent structure ("John gave the baby a toy") or a to-object structure ("John gave a toy to the baby").

In summary, lexical functional grammar makes a distinction that can be usefully applied in reexamining the supposed syntactic-lexical contrast in aphasic impairment. Apart from the semantic aspects of words, which are outside their grammatic roles, it incorporates an aspect of grammar into the lexicon through the functional structures of predicative words and distinguishes this from constituent structure. If lexical functional grammar indeed is psychologically real, the interesting question for a neurolinguistic dissociation of syntax and the lexicon is whether operations that involve functional structures are to be aligned with syntax or with the lexicon. Put more concretely, does the lexical impairment attributed to Wernicke's and anomic patients incorporate a reduction in knowledge or use of the functional structures associated with lexical items, or is it restricted to lexical semantics? Is the syntactic impairment in Broca's aphasia restricted to constituent structure, or does it include the functional structures of lexical items?

We have undertaken two experiments in an attempt to shed light on the role of functional structure. Both used sentences incorporating to-complements.

Experiment 1

The first experiment, undertaken in association with Richard Zatorski (15,16), tested the prediction that patients who had difficulty in accessing words in the lexicon should have more difficulty in generating sentences which used verbs with to-complement functional structures than they had in generating sentences with question structures. Bresnan's theory of lexical grammar accepts that the latter are achieved through a transformational movement, and they may be considered an operation at constituent structure level. An example of a to-complement verb is "persuade," which has as one of its possible functional structures NP_1 persuade NP_2 and NP_2 V (as in "John persuaded Ted to stop"). The subjects were four aphasic patients with word-finding difficulties in conversational speech but evidence of relatively good grammatic ability, and who had parietal or temporoparietal damage. They each heard six brief incomplete stories designed to elicit a specific type of verb complement in their completion and six extensions of these stories designed to elicit questions. Each eliciting trial for to-complements or questions was followed by repetition of similar sentences in imitation of the experimenter, after which the stories were presented again for elicitation. The entire procedure was repeated after an interval of 4 to 7 days. All subjects were more successful in producing questions than to-complement sentences through elicitation. Two subjects were also more successful in repeating questions than to-complement sentences, the other two performing at or near ceiling level on both.

The results of this small-scale study were consistent with the prediction made by lexical functional grammar, in that patients with difficulties in lexical retrieval had more difficulty in producing constructions that depend on the realization of a complex functional structure than in producing those which require a constituent structure movement. The study did not address whether Broca's aphasics might show the reverse pattern or be equally impaired on both tasks.

Experiment 2

The second experiment, undertaken with Rosemary Varley in 1981 (14), attempted to compare the role played by verb semantics with that played by the functional structures of predicative adjectives in both auditory comprehension and elicited production and in two types of aphasia. The format used for the comprehension task was picture choice and for the production task again elicitation through completion of a brief story. Since lexical semantic impairment with spared syntax has been hypothesized to occur in nonaphasic patients with right brain damage, a group of such patients was used. The control group consisted of neurologically intact subjects of the same ages and socioeconomic classes as the aphasic patients.

Each sentence used was six words in length and was illustrated by pairs of black and white line drawings showing a correct version and an incorrect version in which subject and object roles were reversed. Twenty were reversible simple active declarative sentences using verbs expressing aggressive action of some kind (e.g., "The horse is kicking the girl"); 20 were similar sentences which used verbs of directional motion similar to those in Jones' study (e.g., "The dog is dragging the man"); and 20 were sentences with predicative adjectives followed by to-complements (e.g., "The donkey is fun to kick"). In half of the last type of sentences, the adjective was such that the grammatic subject of the sentence was the functional subject of the to-complement; and in half, the grammatic subject of the sentence was the functional object of the complement.

The contrast between the sentences with verbs used in a context of aggression and those with verbs of directional motion was a contrast of verb semantics; syntactically they were the same. Since both types required word order in constituent structure to be processed, according to the hypothesis of Saffron et al. they should present particular difficulties for agrammatic patients. The to-complement sentences contrasted with them in that the interpretation depended on the functional structures inherent in the lexical entries for the predicative adjectives rather than on the ordered constituent structure. If this syntactic disorder of Broca's aphasic patients is at constituent-structure level, they should make more errors with the sentences requiring processing of word order than with to-complement sentences and should be little affected by the contrast of verb semantics. If their syntactic disorder is also at the higher level of functional relationships, they would experience difficulties also with the to-complement sentences but still be little affected by verb semantics. In contrast, for posterior patients, verbs of directional motion should be harder than verbs of aggression; if their lexical impairment also included the functional structures associated with the predicative adjectives, they should also find the to-complement sentences more difficult than the verbs of aggression.

The aphasic patients were classified by their speech therapists on the basis of their profiles on the Boston Diagnostic Aphasia Examination and other observations as nonfluent or fluent. Patients with severe comprehension problems (i.e., failing to identify any of 10 items pictured) were excluded. The fluent group included members who could be classified as anomic or with residual deficits during recovery from Wernicke's aphasia. The nonfluent group included patients who still showed some restrictions on the ability to produce grammatic constructions, although at the time of testing the degree of agrammatism in some of them was not severe.

Each subject in each of the four groups was tested first for auditory comprehension of the set of 60 sentences by choosing top or bottom picture for each sentence spoken twice by the tester. The subject was then asked to produce 30 of the sentences as completion of a brief story, such as "Wasps are always quick to strike. The wasp is in the kitchen and stings the girl. She agrees . . . ?" After the first attempt at elicitation, the target sentence was spoken by the tester, and the story was presented a second time. Responses were classed as correct or not in accordance with the following criteria: errors were failures to respond, or utterances in which subject-object roles were reversed, which were insufficient for the roles to be identified, or which showed inappropriate perseveration of a lexical item from an earlier response. Any utterance from which the thematic roles could be derived was considered correct, however incomplete, or even if it incorporated a semantic paraphasia, such as "bee" for "wasp." Self-corrections were accepted.

The results of the experiment are summarized in Table 1. The normal control subjects experienced significantly more difficulty with the to-complement sentences in the comprehension task. This was attributable to greater difficulty with those sentences in which the functional structure imposed an object role on the grammatic subject; e.g., there were five errors in selecting "The donkey is fun to kick" but

TABLE 1. *Mean number of errors in different sentence types*[a]

Subjects	Comprehension A	Comprehension D	Comprehension T	Production A	Production D	Production T
Fluent aphasics	3.0 (2.9)[b]	4.7 (3.4)	6.9 (3.2)	5.4 (3.2)	5.7 (3.5)	6.8 (3.0)
Nonfluent aphasics	2.3 (1.8)	3.1 (2.8)	3.7 (1.5)	5.2 (3.3)	6.0 (2.9)	7.4 (4.1)
Right brain damaged	1.5 (1.3)	1.4 (1.8)	3.5 (2.9)	2.2 (3.1)	3.3 (3.3)	3.9 (4.2)
Normal controls	0.4 (1.0)	0.7 (1.2)	1.7 (2.1)	1.3 (2.1)	1.4 (1.8)	2.0 (2.5)

[a] A, sentences with verb of aggressive action; D, sentences with verb of directional motion; T, sentences with to-complement.

[b] Numbers in parentheses are standard deviations.

none in selecting "The donkey is inclined to kick." Elicitation showed the same order of difficulty as comprehension.

Patients with right brain damage made more errors than the nonbrain-damaged subjects, but not to a significant degree. Although they also had more difficulty with the to-complement sentences in the comprehension task, those patients made slightly fewer errors on the sentences with verbs of directional motion than on those with verbs of aggression. All the right brain-damaged patients had made at least two errors on a 10-item version of Warrington's test of the recognition of objects photographed from unusual angles (mean error rate, 4.9). It is interesting that, despite the possible visuoperceptive deficit this suggests, they showed no sign of impairment on a linguistic task using words that imply directional positions.

For the nonfluent aphasic patients, the elicitation task proved significantly harder than the comprehension task. In comprehension, their pattern of errors was similar to that of normal controls, although at a higher level: there was no evidence that the to-complement structures presented particular difficulties. Indeed, on the latter, they made about the same number of errors as did the right brain-damaged patients on to-complement structures. When these sentences were examined further, it was noted that they made fewer errors than the right brain-damaged patients on the subject-function forms of these sentences (see Table 2). Given the evidence from the nonbrain-damaged controls that the sentences with verbs of directional motion were slightly harder to understand than those with verbs of aggressive actions, there is no basis to suggest that the nonfluent aphasic patients were particularly influenced by verb semantics or by lexical functional structures over and above their general impairment in coping with constituent structure.

The fluent patients, although significantly more impaired than the nonfluent on the comprehension task, scored slightly better on the elicitation task. Where they differed particularly from the nonfluent was in comprehension of the to-complement sentence (Fig. 1). Their overall baseline for the simple reversible sentences was

TABLE 2. *Errors on comprehension of to-complement sentences*[a]

Subjects	Grammatic subject is functional subject of complement (e.g., "x is happy to —")	Grammatic subject is functional object of complement (e.g., "x is fun to —")
Fluent aphasics	26	43
Nonfluent aphasics	6	31
Right brain damaged	8	27
Nonbrain damaged	3	14

[a] Maximum possible = 100.

worse, but they appeared to be proportionately more impaired by the requirement to interpret directional motion and to process the functional structures of the to-complement sentences. Unlike all the other groups, this was not attributable primarily to the object-function sentences: only 62% of their errors were on these sentences, compared with 77 to 84% in the other groups.

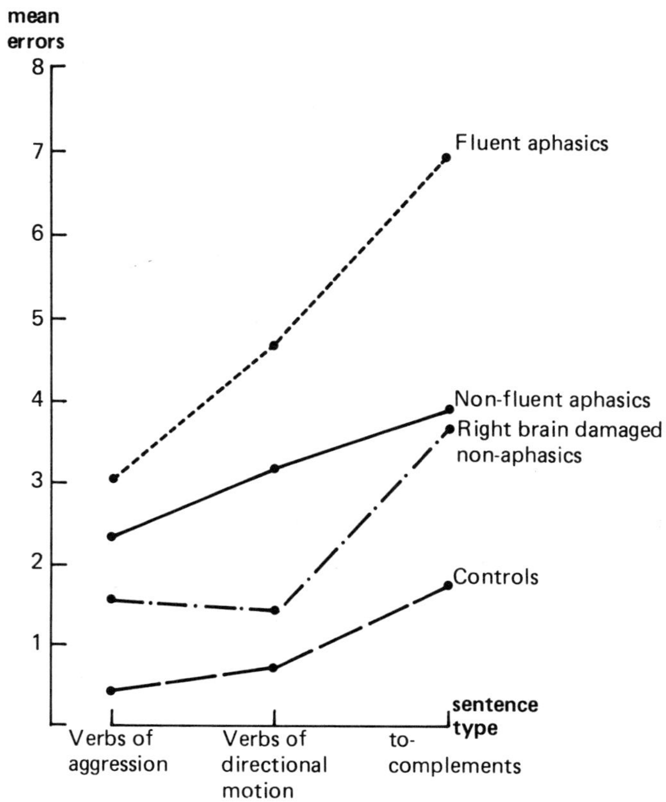

FIG. 1. Mean errors of comprehension. Comparison of performance across the groups.

CONCLUSION

There are limitations to the interpretation that can be made of these results. The classification of aphasic patients had been made from clinical observations over a period of time but was without neuroanatomic confirmation; the individuals did not necessarily represent the pure "syntactic" or "lexical" syndromes. The fluent group did not include patients with severe lexical deficits, in that they were able to recognize drawings by name; their relatively good performance on the reversible sentences with verbs of aggression confirms this. Their disproportionate impairment on comprehension of the to-complement sentences could not have been due to a frank lexical-semantic deficit in denotation. Moreover, using pictures to examine the comprehension of to-complement sentences requires more of an exercise of metalinguistic judgment than do reversible sentences, in that an act is illustrated while the sentence only refers to the intention that the act shall be performed. The fluent aphasic patients could have been more impaired in their capacity to make such metalinguistic judgments rather than to understand the linguistic form of the sentences. Nevertheless, the differential difficulty of the object and subject functional structures of the to-complement sentences does suggest that the most important influence on the results was linguistic.

At face value, the results suggest that it is fluent rather than nonfluent patients who experience difficulties in comprehending the functional structures of predicative words used in sentences. In comprehension, we found no evidence that these nonfluent patients experience particular difficulties at this deep level of syntactic representation. In producing constructions, their ability to convey the basic relationships between subject and object was almost on a par with that of the fluent aphasics, although the former had slightly more difficulty with the to-complements. Nevertheless, it was only aphasic subjects, of both types, who made errors in production in which noun phrases were not ordered around the verb. The fluent showed more of a tendency than the nonfluent to reduce the verbs of directional motion to simpler verbs of action or state.

The results suggest that basic predicative relationships are likely to be preserved in Broca's aphasia in comprehension. Those patients who show the greatest impairment of the ability to understand functional structures predicatively are the fluent patients. Such a conclusion would be consistent with Luria's (9) observation that patients with posterior lesions have difficulty accessing logical relationships in sentences. It also agrees with Schnitzer's (13) claim that Wernicke's area handles semantics and basic predicational functions, and that this is the area in which the brain puts "cognitive matter" into lexical predicational form.

If the lexicon indeed includes specifications for functional and syntactic structures, as lexical functional grammar claims, a lexical impairment might legitimately be conceived of as incorporating a reduction in the ability to use such predicative functions in comprehending and producing sentences. This observation both supports and modifies the dissociation between syntax and the lexicon in the brain and suggests a way in which lexical impairment may itself have consequences on the production and comprehension of grammar.

REFERENCES

1. Blumstein, S. E., Milberg, W., and Shrier, R. (1982): Semantic processing in aphasia: Evidence from an auditory lexical decision task. *Brain Lang.*, 17:301–315.
2. Bradley, D. C., Garrett, M. E., and Zurif, E. B. (1980): Syntactic deficits in Broca's aphasia. In: *Biological Studies of Mental Processes*, edited by D. Caplan. M.I.T. Press, Cambridge, Massachusetts.
3. Bresnan, J. (1978): A realistic transformational grammar. In: *Linguistic Theory and Psychological Reality*, edited by M. Halle, J. Bresnan, and G. A. Miller. M.I.T. Press, Cambridge, Massachusetts.
4. Bresnan, J., editor (1982): *The Mental Representation of Grammatical Relations.* M.I.T. Press, Cambridge, Massachusetts.
5. Caramazza, A., and Berndt, R. S. (1978): Semantic and syntactic processes in aphasia: A review of the literature. *Psychol. Bull.*, 85:898–918.
6. Danly, M., Cooper, W. E., and Shapiro, B. (1983): Fundamental frequency, language processing and linguistic structure in Wernicke's aphasia. *Brain Lang.*, 19:1–24.
7. Ford, M. (1982): Sentence planning units: Implications for the speaker's representation of meaningful relations underlying sentences. In: *The Mental Representation of Grammatical Relations*, edited by J. Bresnan. M.I.T. Press, Cambridge, Massachusetts.
8. Gordon, B., and Caramazza, A. (1983): Closed- and open-class lexical access in agrammatic and fluent aphasics. *Brain Lang.*, 19:335–345.
9. Luria, A. R. (1975): Two kinds of disorders in the comprehension of grammatical function. *Linguistics,* 154/155:47–56.
10. Peuser, G. (1976): Der Drei-Figuren-Test. In: *Interdisziplinäre Aspekte der Aphasieforschung*, edited by G. Peuser. Rheinland-Verlag, Cologne.
11. Pinker, S. (1982): A theory of the acquisition of lexical interpretive grammars. In: *The Mental Representation of Grammatical Relations*, edited by J. Bresnan. M.I.T. Press, Cambridge, Massachusetts.
12. Saffran, E. M., Schwartz, M. F., and Marin, O. S. M. (1980): Evidence from aphasia: Isolating the components of a production model. In: *Language Production, Vol. 1, Speech and Talk*, edited by B. Butterworth. Academic Press, New York.
13. Schnitzer, M. L. (1982): The translational hierarchy of language. In: *Neural Models of Language Processes*, edited by M. A. Arbib, D. Caplan, and J. C. Marshall. Academic Press, New York.
14. Varley, R. A. (1981): A study of differential impairments of syntactic and lexical operations in aphasia and right brain damage. University of Newcastle upon Tyne. Unpublished B.Sc. dissertation.
15. Zatorski, R., and Lesser, R. (1980): The lexicon and sentence generation in aphasia. *Working Papers in Linguistics, University of Melbourne*, 6:1–20.
16. Zatorski, R., and Lesser, R. (1981): Notes and discussion: The lexicon and sentence generation in aphasia. *Brain Lang.*, 13:185–190.
17. Zurif, E. B. (1980): Language mechanisms: A neuropsychological perspective. *Am. Sci.*, 68:305–311.

Advances in Neurology, Vol. 42: Progress in Aphasiology, edited by F. C. Rose.
Raven Press, New York © 1984.

Phonologic Disturbances in Aphasia: Is There a "Markedness Effect" in Aphasic Phonetic Errors?

*,**Jean-Luc Nespoulous, **,†Yves Joanette, **Renée Béland, **,‡David Caplan, and **,†André Roch Lecours

**Départment de Linguistique et Philologie, Université de Montréal; **Laboratoire Théophile-Alajouanine, Centre de Recherche, Centre Hospitalier Côte-des-Neiges; †Faculté de Médecine, Université de Montréal; and ‡Faculty of Medicine, McGill University and Montreal Neurological Institute, Montréal, Québec, Canada*

From the outset, psycholinguists and neurolinguists have constantly looked within the linguistic theory for plausible explanations of such phenomena as children's chronologic acquisition of the phonological system of their mother tongue and aphasics' impairment of some components (or subcomponents) of language, while others are totally unimpaired. Similarly, as long as they accepted external evidence, linguists have tried to integrate such observations within their theoretical framework in order to build up more powerful models of language structure and function (9). Among the myriad of operational concepts fostered by linguists, "markedness" has been a focus for both psycholinguists and neurolinguists. The latter hope to find in it the reason why some linguistic elements or properties would be more labile than others in both child language development and aphasia.

MARKEDNESS: DEFINITIONS

The notion of markedness was first developed by the Prague School (34) to account for the neutralization phenomena within the context of "privative oppositions":

> . . . privative oppositions are those in which one term of the opposition is marked and the other unmarked . . . *Logically* privative oppositions [i.e., those contrasts which could be privative] become *effectively* privative oppositions [i.e., actually receive marked and unmarked terms] through the process of neutralization, which puts the distinction between marked and unmarked terms on an objective basis. [translated by the authors]

Thus in German, /p.t.k/ and /b.d.g/ are neutralized in word-final position. Since it is usually the opposition member which lacks some phonetic property (here "voicing"), which is to be found in the position of neutralization, it is suggested that such a member be labeled "unmarked." Within the context of Troubetskoy's phonology, as well as in many other phonological frameworks (5,15,23), marked and unmarked values are attributed to segments from evidence internal to synchronic properties of the phonologic system.

Subsequently, other criteria have been used to determine the marked and unmarked values for phonemes and features, thus giving to the markedness notion a somewhat heterogeneous flavor, with frequent overlaps: (a) evidence from historic linguistics [with "loss of the marked values"(13)], (b) evidence from physiological and perceptual investigations [marked values present added complexity to production and perception (13)], (c) evidence based on frequency factors within the language system [unmarked phonemes tending to be more frequent than marked phonemes (23)], (d) evidence from linguistic "universals" [features more common to most languages being the unmarked values (10)], and (e) evidence from child language development studies [unmarked phonemes and features tending to be learned earlier than marked ones (4,13)].

Other terms have been coined by different authors with the common above-mentioned aim to organize, in a hierarchical way, the different elements or properties constituting the structure of a linguistic system, e.g., naturalness (12,32) and strength (31). With the development of more modern phonological theories attempting to integrate the previously neglected "syllable" within their framework, markedness was again emphasized, and syllabic structures were thus seen as being distributed on a markedness continuum scaled from less marked to more marked syllables: CV, V, CCV, CVC . . . (8,11,12,17,21,35).

It follows from the above that there is not one definition of markedness. Some definitions concern internal structural properties of the phonological system; they have been made up by linguists. Other definitions, particularly ones emanating from psycholinguists, are based on evidence external to the phonological system per se, such as frequency of occurrence and—of paramount interest for our present purpose—processing complexity. The borderline between both types of above-mentioned definitions is unclear, the more so if one considers that what is structurally more complex in abstract phonological representations might be at the same time more complex in terms of processing.

MARKEDNESS AND APHASIA

Jakobson (13) was probably the first to contend that, in aphasia (as well as in language development), there was a tendency for marked values to be replaced by unmarked values. Blumstein (2), in her doctoral dissertation, similarly claims that substitution errors observed in aphasics, regardless of their clinical category, tend to occur from marked to unmarked phonemes. All patients are considered to perform better on "more basic or natural phonemes" than on phonemes in which a "marked value adds a new specification or complexity to the system" (2): "Regardless of the area of brain damage, the most complexly organized structures are impaired in contrast to the relative preservation of the less complex phonological structures" (p. 25). Thus the error patterns of aphasics are believed to be inherent to properties of the linguistic code itself.

Using French-speaking subjects, we carried out a study (25–27) similar to that of Blumstein (2). In this chapter, results from these studies are reinterpreted in the light of the markedness framework; new data and interpretations are also provided on consonantal cluster production in aphasia, another domain in which the existence of a markedness effect might be substantiated.

SUBJECTS

Subjects were eight aphasics with evidence of phonetic (arthric) and/or phonemic disturbances. Four were clinically labeled as Broca's aphasics, that is, according to Lecours et al. (20), nonfluent aphasics with (a) no (or minimal) comprehension deficits, (b) word-finding difficulties, (c) agrammatism (although nonconstantly[1]), and (d) arthric disturbances [''phonetic disintegration'' in the terms of Alajouanine et al. (1)]. The other four patients were clinically labeled as conduction aphasics, that is, again according to Lecours et al. (20), fluent aphasics with (a) no (or minimal) comprehension deficits, (b) word-finding difficulties, (c) no arthric disorder, and (d) producing numerous phonemic paraphasias (most typically in repetition tasks) as well as some verbal paraphasias.

METHODOLOGY

Subjects were submitted to a repetition test comprising 300 words differing as to length (from one to four syllables) and phonemic structure (words with or without consonantal clusters). All selected items were presented in a randomized fashion at the time of testing. All subjects' responses and attempts at producing the correct target words were tape recorded and afterward transcribed using the International Phonetic Alphabet. Data were computerized for statistical analyses.

ERRORS AT THE PHONEMIC LEVEL AND MARKEDNESS

In our earlier studies (25–27), both a featural and a contextual analysis evidenced that, contrary to what Blumstein (2) had found, the two groups of patients presented different error patterns:

1. Conduction aphasics produced significantly more contextually determined errors, particularly displacements of phonemes, than did Broca's aphasics.
2. Substitutions at interphonemic distance 1 (2,19) were significantly more frequent in Broca's aphasia than in conduction aphasia (Fig. 1), the patients in the latter group generating many substitutions at interphonemic distance >2.
3. Whereas no preferential error patterns were evidenced in phonemic substitutions produced by conduction aphasics, Broca's aphasics' error trends appeared to be coherent (Figs. 2 and 3), with a devoicing tendency being observed when target phonemes were voiced and a change in place of articulation when target phonemes were unvoiced.

[1]In fact, none of our four Broca's aphasics was agrammatic.

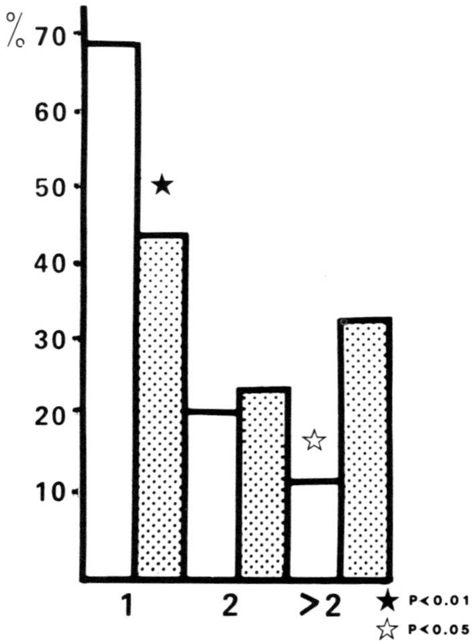

FIG. 1. Percentages of substitutions at interphonemic distances 1, 2, and >2 for subjects with Broca's (*open columns*) and conduction (*dotted columns*) aphasia.

On the basis of such results, it was reasonable to assume that there existed, at least in part, a somewhat different trend in the basic underlying causality and determinism of deviations generated by the two groups of patients. Since 70% of the substitutions produced by Broca's aphasics were close approximations to the target (with rather clearcut preferential deviation trends), it was possible to state that their basic problem, in terms of speech production, stood at the feature level (28). Since conduction aphasics produced as many substitutions at interphonemic distance 1 as at interphonemic distance >2, and considering the higher percentage of displacement errors observed in these patients, their deficit was interpreted as a difficulty in the monitoring of the dynamic organization of phonemic strings (25,28).

With respect to markedness, if the absence of coherence and stability in conduction aphasics' errors makes it clear that no markedness effect plays a role in the pathogenesis of these patients' deviations, it does not follow from the presence of coherence and stability in Broca's aphasics' errors that the preferential deviations of the latter are the outcome of a markedness effect. Even if their coherent deviation patterns can be interpreted as simplification strategies, the necessity to resort to markedness to account for such a simplification process remains to be assessed. Other alternatives do exist to apprehend the determinism of their deficit, such as the simplification of motor (or phonetic) patterns in speech production (16,22) or the reduction of articulatory gestures (16).

If an interpretation of the pathogenesis of Broca's aphasics' errors were set forth in terms of markedness, one would need to specify which of the above-mentioned definitions of markedness one would resort to. In other words, if there were some

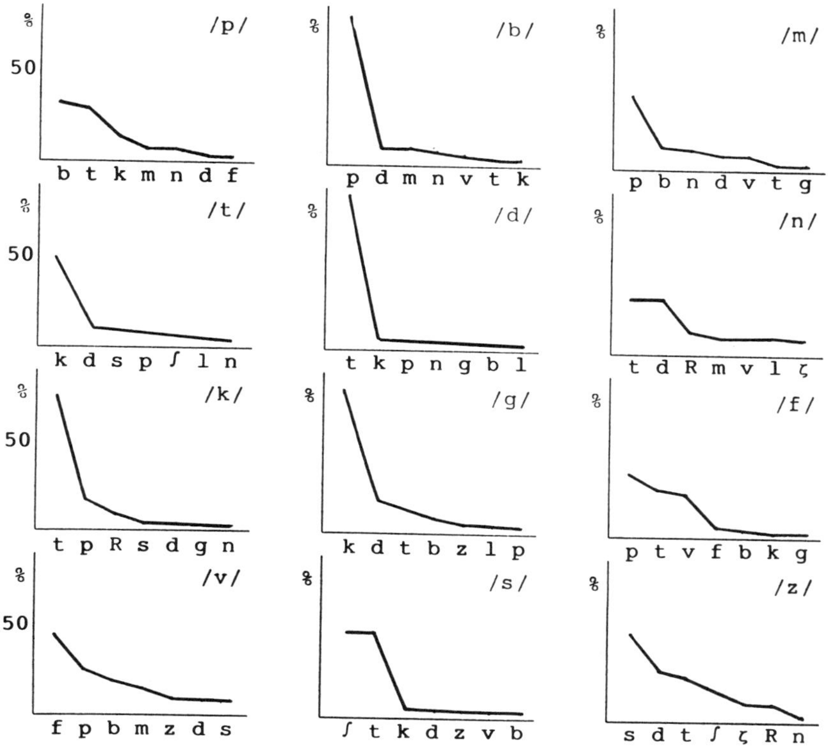

FIG. 2. Pattern of preferential substitution of phonemes /p/, /b/, /m/, /t/, /d/, /n/, /k/, /g/, /f/, /v/, /s/, and /z/ for subjects with Broca's aphasia.

markedness effect at stake in the genesis of the errors characteristic of Broca's aphasia, would such an effect be interpreted as deriving from abstract structural properties of the phonological system, such as accounted for by linguists, or would it derive more directly from production and/or perception processing complexity?

CONSONANTAL CLUSTER PRODUCTION AND MARKEDNESS

Our original pathological data, collected in Montréal and France 10 years ago, did not allow us to carry out specific investigations at the syllabic level in a way that would be fully compatible with modern phonological approaches to syllabic structure. Nevertheless, our corpus did offer a way that made it possible for us to study, albeit indirectly, syllabic structure: consonantal cluster production.

In the present work, any sequence of at least two consonants (CC) was considered to constitute a cluster, regardless of its locus within the word, which could be intrasyllabic (as in "grand" /gRɑ̃/) or intersyllabic (as in "action" /aksjɔ̃/). The reason we carried out our analysis in such a way is that, in both cases, cluster destructions

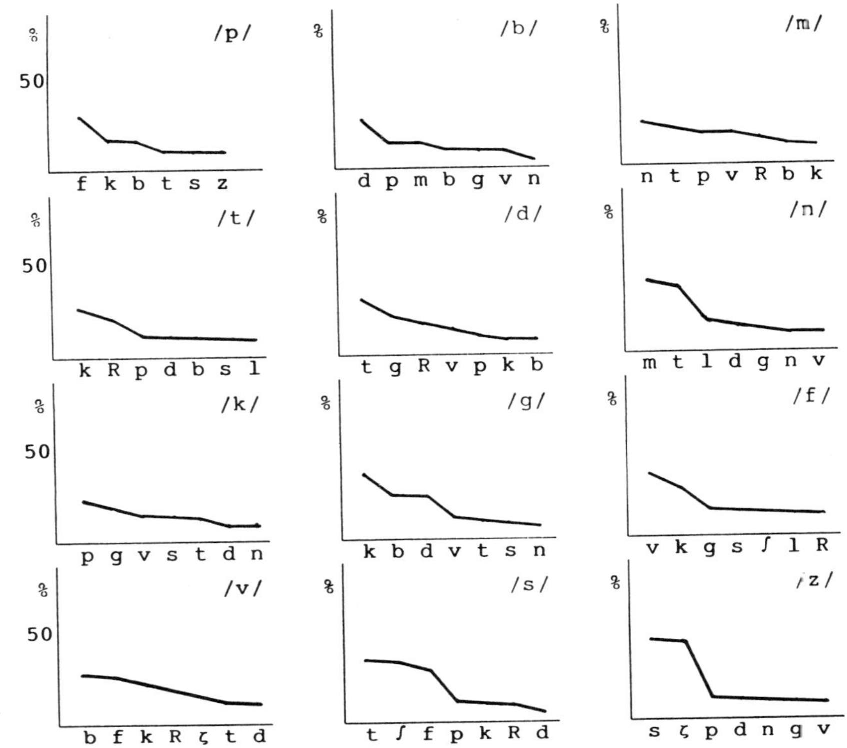

FIG. 3. Pattern of preferential substitution of phonemes /p/, /b/, /m/, /t/, /d/, /n/ /k/, /g/, /f/, /v/, /s/, and /z/ for subjects with conduction aphasia.

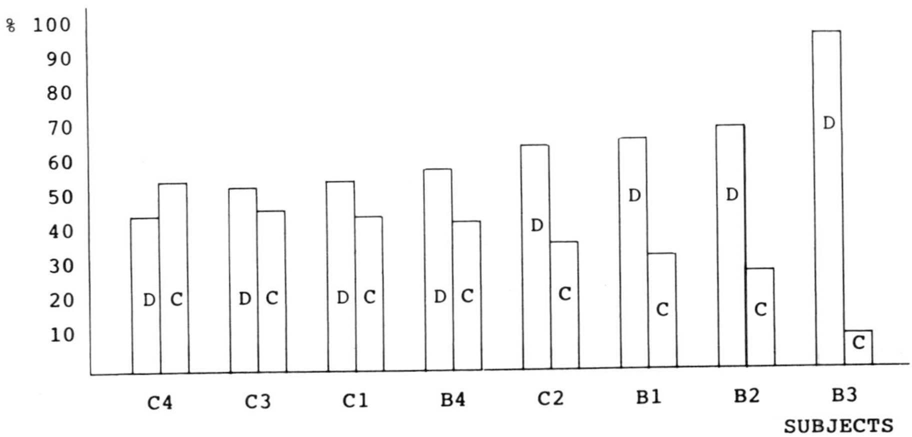

FIG. 4. Percentages of consonantal cluster destruction (D) and creation (C) for subjects with conduction aphasia (C1 to C4) and Broca's aphasia (B1 to B4).

TABLE 1. *Percentages of destruction and creation of consonantal clusters for subjects with Broca's aphasia (Broca 1 to 4) and with conduction aphasia (conduction 1 to 4)*

	N	Destruction	Creation	D/C Ratio
Broca 1	83	62.6	37.4	1.67
Broca 2	95	67.5	32.4	2.06
Broca 3	77	92.2	7.8	11.80
Broca 4	57	54.3	45.7	1.19
Conduction 1	137	53.3	46.7	1.14
Conduction 2	82	62.1	37.9	1.64
Conduction 3	33	51.5	48.5	1.06
Conduction 4	94	47.8	52.2	0.91

tend to generate phonemic strings of a lesser degree of complexity, with CV and V syllabic structures being the rule:

/gRɑ̃/→ /gɑ̃/.

/ak—sjɔ̃/→ /a—sɔ̃/.

Another analysis of these data, taking into consideration the intrasyllabic/intersyllabic distinction, is now underway in Montréal (29).

Two complementary hypotheses were submitted to investigation in our study: (a) with respect to consonantal cluster production, is there a significant difference between Broca's and conduction aphasics? (b) Is such a difference (if present) interpretable in terms similar to the ones we used at the strictly segmental level, i.e., presence of a simplification strategy (markedness effect?) in Broca's aphasia versus absence of such a strategy in conduction aphasia?

In order to test both hypotheses, we analyzed destruction versus creation of consonantal clusters (as defined above) in both groups of patients. Cluster destructions were significantly ($p < 0.02$) more frequent than cluster creations in Broca's aphasics, whereas no such tendency was observed in conduction aphasics (Table 1) (for similar findings, see ref. 16).

On the basis of destruction/creation (D/C) ratios, a Mann-Whitney test yielded a significant difference between both groups of patients. Figure 4 represents the percentages of cluster destructions (D) and cluster creations (C) for each patient (all subjects being arranged in ascending order of D/C ratio). Therefore, the simplification already observed at the segmental level in Broca's aphasics' errors can be evidenced when one considers consonantal cluster production. Again, conduction aphasics present a different pattern, with almost as many cluster creations as cluster destructions, thus emphasizing the fact that such patients do not seem to be looking for a simplification of verbal output.

Qualitative examination of the internal nature of the consonantal clusters "destroyed" versus "created" by both groups of patients (Table 2) leads to the following conclusions:

TABLE 2. *Percentages of consonantal cluster destruction and creation for subjects with Broca's and conduction aphasias according to the nature of the consonantal cluster*

	Broca				Conduction			
Consonantal cluster[a]	*N*	Destruction (%)	Creation (%)	D/C Ratio	*N*	Destruction (%)	Creation (%)	D/C Ratio
Plosives + /R/	58	43.0	57.0	0.7	84	29.7	70.3	0.4
/l/	39	94.8	5.2	18.5	30	66.6	33.4	2.0
/j/	0	—	—	—	0	—	—	—
Plosives + other C	33	84.8	15.2	5.6	49	48.9	51.1	1.0
Fricatives + /R/	8	12.5	87.5	0.1	11	9.0	91.0	0.1
/l/	7	57.0	43.0	1.3	5	80.0	20.0	4.0
/j/	14	93.0	7.0	13.0	10	70.0	30.0	2.3
Fricatives + other C	58	77.5	22.5	3.4	45	77.7	32.3	3.5
Other CC	70	82.8	17.2	4.8	102	58.8	41.2	1.4

[a] C, consonant; CC, consonantal cluster.

1. Only one[2] type of [consonant-consonant] sequence seems to be created more often than destroyed, i.e., [Plosive + R], with the plosive being most of the time a /t/. Such a tendency is greater in conduction than in Broca's aphasics. Apart from this single case, an overall tendency toward cluster destruction is evidenced in both groups.
2. A closer look at the data shows some important contrasts between both groups of patients:
   a. [Plosive + l]: Destructions are more frequent than creations in both groups, but the D/C ratio is significantly greater in Broca's aphasics than in conduction aphasics.
   b. [Plosive + other consonant[3]]: Destructions are more frequent than creations only in Broca's aphasics; conduction aphasics create and destroy such clusters in equivalent proportion.
   c. [Fricative + other consonant[3]]: Destructions are more frequent than creations, with about the same D/C ratio in both groups of patients.
   d. [Other clusters]: Apart from a few intrasyllabic clusters, such as /spR/, many complex intersyllabic consonantal sequences may be found. Interestingly, Broca's aphasics distinguish themselves again in that they often destroy such clusters (with a D/C ratio of 4.8), whereas conduction aphasics manage to create many of these (with a D/C ratio of only 1.4). Thus it is possible to assume that Broca's aphasics do not only simplify consonantal sequences when all consonants belong to the same syllable; they go as far as simplifying such sequences at syllabic junctures (6). Conduction aphasics, on the contrary, are capable of creating consonantal clusters in any locus, thus emphasizing the fact that these patients' errors cannot be interpreted as the manifestation of a simplification strategy.

DISCUSSION

The data reported in this chapter make it clear that there is no unitary tendency in the error patterns observed in both groups of patients. These results, in contrast to those of Blumstein (2), are akin to those of Trost and Canter (33), Burns and Canter (3), Keller (16), and Stachowiach (*personal communication*); they have been recently corroborated in French-speaking patients by Martory and Messerli (24). Thus it may be assumed that, contrary to what Blumstein has claimed, the pathogenesis of errors is different in Broca's than in conduction aphasia.[4]

To what extent is the notion of markedness of use in accounting for the underlying determinism of deviant patterns evidenced by patients of one and/or the other type?

---

[2]The same apparently holds true for fricative /R/, but data were insufficient here ($N = 8$ in Broca's aphasics, $N = 11$ in conduction aphasics).

[3]Other than /R/, /l/, and /j/.

[4]It is noted that, in Blumstein's (2) work, while there was a significant contrast in both Broca's and Wernicke's aphasics between both types of substitutions (from marked to unmarked versus from unmarked to marked, the former tendency being more frequent than the latter), such a trend was not found to be significant for the conduction aphasics.

In other words, is the cause of the errors observed in both groups of patients to be looked for among abstract structural properties of the phonological system or in the disruption of one, or several, of the psycholinguistic processing mechanisms that are assumed to play a role in language production?

The absence of coherence and stability in deviation patterns of conduction aphasics (at least at the level of analysis used here) makes it possible to discard the interference of any markedness effect in their generation of errors. Such an observation is consistent with that of Shattuck-Hufnagel and Klatt (31), according to whom consonant substitution errors gathered among normal subjects ("slips of the tongue") do not show any markedness effect. Thus we hypothesize that consonant substitutions produced by conduction aphasics and normal subjects (both "fluent" speakers) might have something in common. This hypothesis is all the more plausible when one considers the fact that, both in conduction aphasics and in normals, many errors appear to originate in the disruption of what Shattuck-Hufnagel (30) calls, after Lashley (18), a serial-ordering mechanism, a mechanism that assigns each candidate segment (in a target word) to one particular slot in the structural syllabic framework required for that specific lexical item.

By emphasizing the plausible existence of such a processing disturbance in conduction aphasia, we do not mean that all errors generated by these patients can be adequately accounted for in such a way. We only suggest that the disruption of such a serial-ordering mechanism can yield a reasonable explanation for three of the semiological characteristics found in these patients: (a) the absence of clearcut feature preferences in consonant substitution (such as those observed in Broca's aphasics); (b) the production of complicating as well as simplifying errors; and (c) the frequent occurrence of phonemic displacements in oral production.

Such an interpretation supports the original model of Lecours and Lhermitte (19), according to which the problem, for conduction aphasics, lies at a premotoric "phonemic" level, where phonemes are taken as unitary production segments, and not at a motor featural level (in their terms), a level which would only be disturbed in Broca's aphasia. It obviously leaves unanswered other important issues, such as, for instance, the production by these patients of verbal paraphasias that indicate the existence of a lexicosemantic problem in the pathogenesis of their errors.

With respect to Broca's aphasics, the presence of stable, coherent, preferential, simplifying errors might be appealing to those who advocate the role of a markedness effect in these patients' erroneous productions (2,7). Undoubtedly, such an interpretation would be most plausible if Broca's aphasics did not have massive arthric disturbances. Then one could be led to consider that pathological phenomena would find their origin in abstract (universal?) phonological properties of the phonological system. Nevertheless, since most Broca's aphasics do have arthric impairments, it remains to be determined to what extent there might be a motor component in their speech errors.

Such an enterprise was carried out by MacNeilage (22) in his attempt to account for devoicing errors found in Broca's aphasics (and not in conduction aphasics) in corpora borrowed from Johns and Darley (14) and Trost and Canter (33). These corpora yielded results similar to our own. In his study, MacNeilage (22) demonstrated (a) why voicing was physiologically more difficult to achieve during obstruents (fricatives and stop consonants) as compared with vowels; and (b) how such a devoicing simplifying effect could be correlated with the slow rate of speech of Broca's aphasics (27) and categorical perception artifacts from the transcribers. He was led to the conclusion that nonfluent aphasics "who are considered to have motor deficits . . . also show what we consider to be motor difficulties in their substitution error patterns," an interpretation similar to that of Alajouanine et al. (1). Thus he rejected any interpretation of such deviations in terms of abstract phonological markedness effect.

It is reasonable to assume that there is indeed a motor component in the pathogenesis of errors in Broca's aphasia. Whether such an interpretation enables us to account for all simplificatory errors, observed in both consonantal segments and clusters, generated by these patients remains to be further assessed. If, as can be reasonably claimed, motor simplicity and complexity closely parallel abstract phonological simplicity and complexity, the task of distinguishing the respective roles of both potential determinisms in Broca's aphasics' error production might turn out to be a bottomless chasm and, conceivably, an irrelevant venture. Both approaches, at least for Broca's aphasics, are worthwhile.

If we decide to resort to the notion of markedness while expanding its scope as many authors (mainly psycholinguists) have done before us, then the interpretation of our results might be reworded in the following way: If we assume that conduction aphasics produce errors (at least in part) through a disturbance of a serial-ordering mechanism, and that the phonological representations relevant to this mechanism are a relatively abstract characterization of phonological structures, we may conclude that markedness effects stated for this relatively abstract level of structure do not influence error generation in these patients. Granting this conclusion, we can attribute the markedness effects in Broca's aphasia to a later stage in motor speech planning and thus conclude that it is the motor aspects of markedness which produce the effect.

In general, we hypothesize that aspects of markedness pertaining to relatively peripheral, late stages of motor speech planning and execution affect (Broca's) aphasic distortions of speech, while aspects of markedness of phonemes that pertain to more abstract characterizations of phonological segments do not.

ACKNOWLEDGMENTS

This work was supported by Program Grant PG-28 from the Medical Research Council of Canada.

REFERENCES

1. Alajouanine, T., Ombredane, A., and Durand, M. (1939): *Le Syndrome de Désintégration Phonétique dans l'Aphasie*. Masson, Paris.
2. Blumstein, S. (1973): *A Phonological Investigation of Aphasic Speech*. Mouton, The Hague.
3. Burns, M., and Canter, G. (1977): Phonemic behavior of aphasic patients with posterior cerebral lesions. *Brain Lang*, 4:492–507.
4. Cairns, H. S., Cairns, C. E., and Williams, F. (1974): Some theoretical considerations of articulation substitution phenomena. *Lang. Speech*, 17:160–173.

5. Chomsky, N., and Halle, M. (1968): *The Sound Pattern of English*. Harper & Row, New York.
6. Denny-Brown, D. (1963): The physiological basis of perception and speech. In: *Problems of Dynamic Neurology*, edited by L. Halpern, Jerusalem Post Press, Jerusalem.
7. Dressler, W. (1982): A classification of phonological paraphasias. *Wien. Linguist. Gazette*, 29:3–16.
8. Feinstein, M. H. (1979): Prenasalization and syllable structure. *Linguist. Inquiry*, 10(2):245–278.
9. Ford, A., and Singh, R. (1978): L'importance théorique de la linguistique appliquée. In: *Models of Grammar, Descriptive Linguistics and Pedagogical Grammar*, edited by G. Nickel and D. Nehls. Julius Groos Verlag, Heidelberg.
10. Greenberg, J. H. (1966): Synchronic and diachronic universals in phonology. *Language*, 42:508–517.
11. Halle, M. (1978): Metrical structure in phonology. (*Unpublished.*)
12. Hooper, J. B. (1976): *An Introduction to Natural Generative Phonology*. Academic Press, New York.
13. Jakobson, R. (1942): Kindersprache, aphasie und allgemeine lautgesetze. *Uppsala Univ. Arsskr.*, 9.
14. Johns, D., and Darley, F. (1970): Phonemic variability in apraxia of speech. *J. Speech Hear. Res.*, 13:556–583.
15. Kean, M.-L. (1980): *The Theory of Markedness in Generative Grammar*. Indiana University Linguistics Club, Bloomington.
16. Keller, E. (1984): Simplification and gesture reduction in phonological disorders of apraxia and aphasia. In: *Apraxia of Speech: Physiology, Acoustics, Linguistics, Management*, edited by J. C. Rosenbek, M. R. McNeil, and A. E. Aronson. College-Hill Press, San Diego, California.
17. Kiparsky, P. (1979): Metrical structure assignment is cyclic. *Linguist. Inquiry*, 10(3):421–441.
18. Lashley, K. S. (1951): The problem of serial order in behavior. In: *Cerebral Mechanisms in Behavior*, edited by L. A. Jeffress. Wiley, New York.
19. Lecours, A. R., and Lhermitte, F. (1969): Phonemic paraphasias: Linguistic structures and tentative hypotheses. *Cortex*, 5(3):193–228.
20. Lecours, A. R., and Lhermitte, F. (1979): *L'aphasie*. Flammarion, Paris.
21. Lowenstamm, J. (1979): *Topics in Syllabic Phonology*. University of Massachusetts Graduate Linguistic Student Association, Amherst.
22. MacNeilage, P. (1982): Speech production mechanisms in aphasia. In: *Speech Motor Control*, edited by S. Grillner, B. Lindblom, J. Lubker, and A. Persson. Pergamon, London.
23. Martinet, A. (1956): *La Linguistique Synchronique*. Presses Universitaires de France, Paris.
24. Martory, M. D., and Messerli, P. (1983): Analyse phonologique comparée des troubles de l'expression orale. In: *Neuropsychologie de l'Expression Orale*, edited by P. Messerli, P.-M. Lavorel, and J.-L. Nespoulous. Les éditions du C.N.R.S., Paris.
25. Nespoulous, J.-L., Lecours, A. R., and Joanette, Y. (1982): Stabilité et instabilité des déviations phonétiques et/ou phonémiques des aphasiques. *La Linguist.*, 18(2):85–97.
26. Nespoulous, J.-L., Lecours, A. R., Deloche, G., Joanette, Y., and Lhermitte, F. (1982): On the non-oneness of phonemic deviations of aphasic patients with and without phonetic disintegration. Paper presented at the I.N.S. European Meeting, Deauville, France (*unpublished*).
27. Nespoulous, J.-L., Lecours, A. R., and Joanette, Y. (1983): La dichotomie phonétique/phonémique a-t-elle une valeur nosologique? In: *Neuropsychologie de l'Expression Orale*, edited by P. Messerli, P.-M. Lavorel, and J.-L. Nespoulous. Les éditions du C.N.R.S., Paris.
28. Nespoulous, J.-L., and Lecours, A. R. (1984): The clinical description of aphasia: Linguistic aspects. In: *Biological Perspectives on Language*, edited by D. Caplan, A. R. Lecours, and A. Smith. M.I.T. Press, Cambridge, Massachusetts.
29. Nespoulous, J.-L., Joanette, Y., Béland, R., Caplan, D., and Lecours, A. R. (1983): Is there a "markedness effect" in aphasics' production of consonantal clusters? Paper presented at the Academy of Aphasia Meeting, Minneapolis.
30. Shattuck-Hufnagel, S. (1979): Speech errors as evidence for a serial-ordering mechanism in sentence production. In: *Sentence Processing: Psycholinguistic Studies Presented to Merrill Garrett*, edited by W. E. Cooper and E. C. T. Walker. Lawrence Erlbaum Associates, Hillsdale, New Jersey.
31. Shattuck-Hufnagel, S., and Klatt, D. H. (1979): The limited use of distinctive features and markedness in speech production: Evidence from error data. *J. Verb. Learn. Verb. Behav.*, 18:41–55.
32. Stampe, D. (1979): *A Dissertation on Natural Phonology*. Garland, New York.
33. Trost, J. E., and Canter, G. (1974): Apraxia of speech in patients with Broca's aphasia: A study of phoneme production accuracy and error patterns. *Brain Lang.*, 1:63–80.
34. Troubetzkoy, N. S. (1970): *Principes de phonologie*. Editions Klincksieck, Paris.
35. Venneman, T. (1978): Universal syllabic phonology. *Theoret. Linguist.*, 5:175–215.

Advances in Neurology, Vol. 42: Progress in Aphasiology, edited by F. C. Rose.
Raven Press, New York © 1984.

Some Linguistic Components of Acalculia

Gérard Deloche and *Xavier Seron

*Unité INSERM U 84, Hôpital de la Salpêtrière, Paris, France; and *Cliniques Universitaires St. Luc, Unité NEXA, Université Catholique de Louvain, Brussels, Belgium*

Studies devoted to the acalculia syndromes have been classically centered on three interrelated topics: (a) description of the main varieties of calculation disorders, (b) analysis of the incidence on dyscalculia of some related impairments, such as spatial and linguistic defects, and (c) localization of lesions responsible for the different disorders. Such neuropsychologic approaches have developed from Henschen (16) to Hécaen et al. (15) and permit a gross delineation of the field into at least three classes of disorders: (a) alexia and agraphia for digits and numbers, (b) acalculia resulting from spatial defects, and (c) anarithmetia, or true acalculia, involving arithmetic operations per se (see ref. 4 for review).

Our own research into the numerical abilities of aphasics developed from a different perspective. Thus we first present and comment on our observations without direct reference to dyscalculia syndromes; at the end of this chapter, we return to the semiology of acalculia to indicate the level of pertinence of our observations.

The focus of our research is the study of transcoding, a complex linguistic activity, as performed by aphasic subjects in a restricted but complete domain, namely, the representation of quantities. It is hoped that the disruption provoked by the aphasic condition may highlight the processes used by normal subjects when handling such a task but which is difficult to perceive in normals because these processes are integrated into a whole that cannot be easily dissociated experimentally. Another expectation of this approach is that some notions developed to account for results obtained in the domain of quantities might apply to the analysis of language processing in general. Interest in linguistic transcoding processes is not new in neuropsychology, as has been recently exemplified in the neuropsychologic studies devoted to the disruption of reading and writing mechanisms (6).

One of the main reasons for analyzing how aphasic patients handle such tasks as converting an integrated digit string into the corresponding string of words, or the reverse, lies in the simplicity of the domain relative to other transcoding processes. The facets of this simplicity are manifold and can be summarized as follow: First, although the set of natural numbers is infinite, the lexicons of the two coding systems of quantities are finite; the digit lexicon is composed of 10 digits from 0 to 9 and a separator, the comma, while the alphabetic lexicon for integers from 0 to 1 million is composed of 25 elements in French, and is only slightly larger in English, with

31 elements. Not only are these lexicons small, they are also clearly distinct from other lexicons.

Second, and more important, is that the correspondence between the two notational systems is of a one-to-one nature in that, given an alphabetic form, there exists only one corresponding digit form; given a digit form, there exists only one corresponding alphabetic form. Such a one-to-one correspondence is virtually unique in linguistic transcoding processes. Consider, for example, what occurs in translating from one language into another, where ambiguity frequently occurs, or the complexity of grapheme to phoneme or phoneme to grapheme conversion rules, which intervene in reading aloud or in writing from dictation. The existence of such a one-to-one correspondence between the alphabetic and the digit codes does not mean that the transcoding processes are trivial and could be handled without syntactic knowledge by the simple transcoding of the individual words or digits by their corresponding lexical values. For example, the transcoding of the alphabetic string "one hundred forty-two" may not be done by transcoding "one" by the digit "1," "hundred" by the digit string "1 0 0," "forty" by the digit string "40," and so on. Similar remarks apply to reverse transcoding, in that the digit string "1 4 2" may not be transcoded by the alphabetic string composed of the lexical value of each digit element (one four two). The transcoding processes are complex; but here, too, they can be completely formalized by a set of rules containing few if any exceptions, as we have indicated in previous publications (9,21).

The third element of simplicity is that grammar can be easily written for both coding systems. For integers coded in digits, the only rule for acceptance of a digit string form is that it cannot begin with a "zero." For example, "0114" is not a legal digit string for integers. The grammar of the alphabetic notational system for integers is more complex, but it can be exhaustively described (19).

We studied two coding systems representing unambiguous quantities, with small and autonomous lexicons and two completely describable grammars that define one-to-one correspondence relationships. Such simplicity contributes to the success of the analysis and interpretation of disorders that occur in aphasic conditions and enables us to question the nature of the quantity transcoding difficulties we observe and their relationships to the impairments found in other linguistic tasks. First, we briefly present the alphabetic French lexicon for quantities, with emphasis on the concept of stacks that we use to structure it.

The French lexicon presented in Table 1 is sufficient for quantities less than 1 million. We subdivided the lexicon into three stacks: (a) the digit stack, containing the name of digits, (b) the tens stack, and (c) the particulars stack in French from 11 to 16, and in English from 11 to 19. A stack is a one-dimensional array of serially ordered elements. Each individual element of the lexicon is characterized by two elements of information: (a) the stack to which it belongs (units, tens, or particulars), and (b) its position in that stack. For example, "THREE" occupies the third position in the unit stack, "FIFTEEN" the fifth position in the particulars stack, and "TWO," "TWELVE," and "TWENTY" have the same position value but belong to different stacks. The other elements of the French lexicon are "MILLE" (thou-

TABLE 1. *Alphabetic coding system for quantities: lexical primitives and stacks*[a]

Position within stack	Three stacks		
	Units	Particulars	Tens
9	9 nine	19 nineteen	90 ninety
8	8 eight	18 eighteen	80 eighty
7	7 seven	17 seventeen	70 seventy
6	6 six	16 sixteen	60 sixty
5	5 five	15 fifteen	50 fifty
4	4 four	14 fourteen	40 forty
3	3 three	13 thirteen	30 thirty
2	2 two	12 twelve	20 twenty
1	1 one	11 eleven	10 ten

[a] One arithmetic operator: and; two syntactic ambiguities: thousand, hundred.

sand), "CENT" (hundred), "ZERO", and "ET" (and); "CENT" and "MILLE" play a special role and can be considered, at least in French, as syntactic ambiguities.

We now summarize some of the hypotheses proposed to account for the data we have gathered in transcoding tasks performed by relatively large groups of aphasic patients from the alphabetic system to the digital code, and vice versa (10,22). We have confirmed these hypotheses by recent studies designed for this purpose (11,12). All these tasks (transcoding, grammaticality judgments, and semantic grouping) were performed in writing in order to avoid memory problems and to involve as few different coding systems as possible. The difficulties experienced in the processing of number forms by aphasic subjects are analyzed by considering two levels in the material. Lexical errors concern single lexical primitives and are found in some paraphasic substitutions, such as 15 for 5 (20). Syntactic errors concern the syntactic structure of the serial ordering organization of alphabetic lexical primitives into well-formed numerals. These appear, for instance, in the omissions of syntactical functors such as "thousand" or "hundred" in "thirty nine seven forty two" for "39,742."

LEXICAL ERRORS

Since the two dimensions that characterize lexical primitives in a stack organization are by definition able to vary independently, two types of "pure" lexical confusions can be predicted (see Table 2). In stack position errors, such as the substitution of 8 for 7, 11 for 12, or 60 for 40, the confusion occurs between two elements that belong to the same stack but differ in their position in the stack. Conversely, stack errors, such as substitutions between 5, 15, and 50, preserve the position information but differ in the stack dimension.

Before discussing the relevance of the stack notion to the field of neuropsycholinguistic research, we first make a theoretical point. Our approach to the way the lexical primitives may be processed is in line with ideas developed by Warrington and Shallice (24), Deloche et al. (8), and others to account for data indicating that some semantic dimensions of words were preserved in patients presenting word

TABLE 2. *Alphabetic system: Two independent types of lexical primitive substitutions*

Stack position errors (stack information preserved)	
seven ↔ eight	units
eleven ↔ twelve	particulars
forty ↔ sixty	tens
Stack error (position information preserved)	
five ↙↗ ↖↘ fifteen ↔ fifty	5th

comprehension difficulties. Such data can be viewed as supporting the notion of a complex semantic preprocessing of lexical primitives (words) operating on several dimensions. Considered in this theoretical framework, our description of the alphabetic lexicon for numbers in terms of stack structures simply hypothesizes that the position-within-stack information and the stack-identity information are two candidates among the dimensions that specify lexical primitives for numbers.

In the particular field of the alphabetic coding system for quantities, our previous studies (9,10,21,22) provide converging evidence that supports interest in stack concepts for the analysis of aphasic impairments (see also Table 3). First, the vast majority of lexical primitive substitutions appear to result from one of the two predicted pure errors type, i.e., one dimension only was violated and the other was preserved, as in 50 for 40 or 13 for 30. Conversely, "mixed" errors that preserve neither of the two dimensions, such as 50 for 11, were rare. Such errors would be expected to occur in the case where the stack structure parameters do not affect the neuropsycholinguistic procedures at work in the transcoding tasks.

Second, in stack position errors, the absolute difference between the position of the correct lexical primitive and the error was not random. Cases such as 3 for 6 were the exception; most of the substitutions occurred with items adjacent in their stack.

Third, a double dissociation seems to exist between Wernicke's and Broca's aphasics with respect to their relative percentages of the two types of pure errors. The

TABLE 3. *Transcoding processes from/to alphabetic forms: two levels of impairments*

Lexical errors	Syntactic errors
Stack position errors	Thousand and hundred multiplicands
nine hundred and forty three → 953	thirty nine thousand seven hundred and forty two → 3917142
106,002 → one hundred three thousand and two	857 → eight fifty seven
Nondirectional stack errors	Directional (toward units) stack errors
one hundred and thirty → 113	sixteen thousands → 6,000
3 → thirteen	140 → one hundred and four

TABLE 4. *Nonnumbers stack-like structures*

Clue: Same position within stack		Clue: Same stack
(both 2nd)	February Monday March	(both months)
	similar to	
(both 2nd)	Two Twenty Three	(both unit names)

Wernicke's subjects were more likely to produce stack position errors than stack errors, whereas the reverse pattern was observed in the case of Broca's aphasics.

Fourth, stack errors seem to result from different sources of impairment in Broca's and Wernicke's aphasics. Whereas the few substitutions, such as 13 for 30 or 3, were equally distributed from and to the three stacks, thus indicating a nondirectional lexical difficulty in the Wernicke's subjects, the Broca's aphasics and, more particularly, the agrammatics, showed a marked tendency to produce unit names for tens and particulars names and encountered no evident difficulties with unit names. Those directional stack errors, such as 6 for 16 or 60, parallel the derivational errors reported in deep dyslexics and come under the heading of the syntactic errors discussed below.

The last two points suggest that, at least for some aphasic patients, the patterns of difficulties experienced with the limited domain of the alphabetic coding system for quantities and language in general are similar. If this is the case, the double dissociation stated in terms of stack notions is the particular application to quantities of a more general dissociation found with semantic versus syntactic dimensions of language. Consequently, there is no clear advantage in introducing stack concepts in neuropsycholinguistics.

In a subsequent experiment (see Table 4), we gathered evidence showing that the stack concept is in fact applicable to linguistic material other than numbers, since it allows the reconsideration of some so-called semantic confusions and the specification of the nature of the underlying disorder (11). In this study, a deep dyslexic and a Wernicke's aphasic with semantic paraphasias were asked to link two words out of three simultaneously presented words by means of a triadic technique. The material—ordinal adjectives, days in the week, and months in the year—was thought to be particularly suitable for processing by neuropsychologic procedures operating on stack-like structures. For instance, given the three words "February," "Monday," and "March," the link between February and Monday parallels the relationships between 20 and 12, 20 and 2, or 2 and 12; in each case, the elements grouped together refer to different stacks but have in common their within-stack position (here the second). Conversely, the association between February and March parallels the relationships between 2 and 3, 20 and 30, or 12 and 13; these groupings preserve the stack information but not the position dimension. If, because of brain damage, the system of neuropsycholinguistic procedures handling the two independent dimensions of the stack structure was selectively impaired, a unitary interpretation of the grouping strategy in the triadic paradigm and of lexical errors with the numeral lexicon could be proposed. The results actually indicate the double dissociation: the deep dyslexic grouping strategy preserved the position-within-stack information, whereas the Wernicke's aphasic preserved the stack dimension in the same way that these patients substitute 50 for 40 in the transcoding of nine hundred and forty-three by 9 5 3. Moreover, function word paralexias, such as "we" for "us" reported in deep dyslexics (6), are naturally and logically integrated into the position-within-stack procedure preserved in such cases.

SYNTACTIC ERRORS

As already noted, the directional stack errors (see Table 3), i.e., lexical primitive substitutions predominantly occurring on tens or particulars replaced by units, such as 4 for 40 or 6 for 16, paralleled derivational errors observed in deep dyslexics. This tendency to produce the root morpheme was preferentially found in Broca's aphasics with agrammatism, thus indicating, at least for the subjects in our studies, some similarity in the syntactic difficulties in the alphabetic notational system for numbers as well as in language.

Analysis of the grammatic structure of the strings of lexical primitives that constitute well-formed numerals, such as "CENT QUARANTE" (140) or "HUIT CENT CINQUANTE SEPT" (857) clearly indicates the two distinct functions of "CENT" (hundred) in French. In the first case, hundred appears in additive relationships and is marked in the corresponding digit string according to its lexical value by a 1 in the hundred position. In the second example, hundred is involved in a multiplicative relationship, and this functor receives no direct transcription in the digital forms. The results of the transcoding showed an impairment of handling complex syntactic structures with multiplicands that differentially affected Broca's aphasics (and more particularly agrammatics). The errors on the syntactically ambiguous words hundred and thousand occurred particularly with multiplicands: improper "1s" were inserted in digit strings such as "39*1*7*1*42" for "thirty-nine thousand seven hundred and forty-two"; in the reverse direction, the functors were frequently omitted, as in eight fifty-seven for 857. Such differential omission of a syntactic ambiguity parallels the selective omission by an agrammatic patient of the French word "car" (bus/because) when it was a conjunction, while it was uttered when it was a noun while reading aloud the sentence "*le car ralentit car le moteur chauffe*" (1).

So far, the dissociation of the performances by Broca's and Wernicke's aphasics according to the syntactic and semantic dimensions of the procedures engaged in the processing of alphabetic number forms, does not seem to be formally different from that observed with language at large. If this parallelism stands, insight into some syntactic disturbances might arise from the analysis of grammatic disorders in numeral systems, just as the notion of stacks introduced in the domain of quantities allowed the reconsideration of some kinds of unspecified semantic confusions. The results of a grammatic judgment experiment performed on numeral elements of lexicon strings, such as "three hundred and five hundred," are discussed in detail elsewhere (12). They indicate that the syntactic competence often reported in Wernicke's aphasics with sentences also exists with numbers. This finding strikingly parallels the interpretation of dyssyntaxia proposed by Lecours and Rouillon (17) in similar patients, whose sentences violate lexical restrictions (to hear over) but not abstract syntactic serial order constraints (a preposition can follow a verb).

CONCLUSIONS

After having discussed the incidence of some syntactic and semantic disorders in transcoding quantities and having emphasized the pertinence for language in general of the stack concept, we briefly indicate the relevance of our work to the acalculia syndromes and mention some of the major limits of our present investigations.

With some notable exceptions, until recently, investigations in the field (7,13,23) have been relatively insensitive to the code into which the operations (addition, multiplication, subtraction) are presented. The classic opposition investigated has been between written and oral calculation, with insufficient attention given to the fact that written exercises were either presented in advance in the digit script or dictated, which implies a transcoding process from the alphabetic to the digit form. Oral calculation always implies the alphabetic code as the source code with or without a transcoding process during mental calculation. Yet the code into which operations are presented and the existence of transcoding processes during calculation may be of crucial importance, a fact evidenced in the literature.

Gonzalez and Kolers (14), for example, have demonstrated that the time required for the identification of arithmetic operations is dependent on the code, Roman or Arabic, into which the elements of the operations are presented. Besner and Coltheart (3), in a stroop-like task in which normal subjects were required to decide which of two quantities was the larger, found a differential effect of the manipulation of the size of the symbols only for digit symbols. Finally, other data indicate that arithmetic skills in bilingual subjects may vary according to the language they use (18). In addition, there are also anecdotal clinical data. Some interesting observations made by Benson and Denkla (2) on single aphasic cases clearly indicate calculation difficulties due to transcoding disorders, and many of the errors presented by Cohn (5) under the general label of calculation developmental disorders observed in children are clearly of a transcoding nature. Such interference of transcoding difficulties in the performance of arithmetic operations may explain why, in their taxonomy of acalculia, Hécaen et al. (15) stressed the relationships frequently observed between difficulties in writing and reading numbers and anarithmetia or pure acalculia.

The present limits of our investigations are twofold. First, we have limited ourselves to the written code. With respect to tasks involving reading aloud or writing to dictation, we note that many errors observed seem closely parallel to examples observed in reading and writing tasks and reported in the neuropsychologic literature. Second, we have not presented any neuroanatomic correlations, a lack that is only temporary. Before searching for localization of function, we have focused on a fine-graded description of the disorders. Localization may, and must, follow.

REFERENCES

1. Andreewsky, E., and Seron, X. (1975): Implicit processing of grammatical rules in a classical case of agrammatism. *Cortex*, 11:379–390.
2. Benson, D. F., and Denkla, M. B. (1969): Verbal paraphasia as a cause of calculation disturbances. *Arch. Neurol.*, 21:96–102.
3. Besner, D., and Coltheart, M. (1979): Ideographic and alphabetic processing in skilled readers of English. *Neuropsychologia*, 17:467–472.
4. Boller, F., and Grafman, J. (1984): Acalculia. In: *Handbook of Clinical Neurology*, 2nd Ed., Vol. 1, edited by P. J. Vinken, G. W. Bruyn, and H. L. Klawans. North Holland, Amsterdam.
5. Cohn, R. (1971): Arithmetic and learning disabilities. In: *Progress in Learning Disabilities*, edited by H. R. Myklebust, pp. 322–389. Grune & Stratton, New York.
6. Coltheart, M., Patterson, K. E., and Marshall, J. C., editors (1980): *Deep Dyslexia*. Routledge and Keagan Paul, London.
7. Dahmen, W., Hartje, W., Büssing, A., and Sturm, W. (1982): Disorders of calculation in aphasic patients—spatial and verbal components. *Neuropsychologia*, 20:145–153.
8. Deloche, G., Andreewsky, E., and Desi, M. (1981): Lexical meaning: A case report, some striking phenomena, theoretical implications. *Cortex*, 17:147–152.
9. Deloche, G., and Seron, X. (1982): From one to 1: An analysis of a transcoding process by means of neuropsychological data. *Cognition*, 12:119–149.
10. Deloche, G., and Seron, X. (1982): From three to 3: A differential analysis of skills in transcoding quantities between patients with Broca's and Wernicke's aphasia. *Brain*, 105:719–733.
11. Deloche, G., and Seron, X. (1984): Semantic errors reconsidered in the procedural light of stack concepts. *Brain Lang.*, 21:59–71.
12. Deloche, G., and Seron, X. (1984): Grammaticality judgements in aphasics to alphabetically written numeral forms. (*In preparation.*)
13. Gardner, H., Strub, R., and Albert, M. L. (1975): A unimodal deficit in operational thinking. *Brain Lang.*, 2:333–344.
14. Gonzalez, E. G., and Kolers, P. A. (1982): Mental manipulations of arithmetic symbols. *J. Exp. Psychol. [Hum. Learning]*, 8:308–319.
15. Hécaen, H., Angelergues, R., and Houillier, S. (1961): Les variétés cliniques des acalculies au cours des lésions rétro-rolandiques: Approche statistique du problème. *Rev. Neurol. (Paris)*, 105:85–103.
16. Henschen, S. E. (1922): *Klinische und anatomische Beitrage zür Pathologie des Gehirns*. Nordiske Bofhandeln, Stockholm.
17. Lecours, A. R., and Rouillon, F. (1976): Neurolinguistic analysis of jargonaphasia. In: *Studies in Neurolinguistics 2*, edited by H. A. Whitaker and H. Whitaker, pp. 95–144. Academic Press, New York.
18. Marsh, L. G., and Makki, R. H. (1976): Efficiency of arithmetic operations in bilinguals as a function of language. *Memory Cognition*, 4:459–464.
19. Power, R. J. D., and Longuet-Higgins, F. R. S. (1978): Learning to count: A computational model of language acquisition. *Proc. R. Soc. Lond. [Biol.]*, 200:391–417.
20. Rinnert, C., and Whitaker, A. (1973): Semantic confusion by aphasic patients. *Cortex*, 9:56–81.
21. Seron, X., and Deloche, G. (1984): From 2 to two: An analysis of a transcoding process by means of neuropsychological evidence. *J. Psycholinguist. Res.*, 13:215–236.
22. Seron, X., and Deloche, G. (1983): From 4 to four: A supplement to "From three to 3." *Brain*, 106:735–744.
23. Warrington, E. K. (1982): The fractionation of arithmetical skills: A single case study. *Q. J. Exp. Psychol.*, 34A:31–51.
24. Warrington, E. K., and Shallice, T. (1979): Semantic access dyslexia. *Brain*, 102:43–63.

Advances in Neurology, Vol. 42: Progress in Aphasiology, edited by F. C. Rose.
Raven Press, New York © 1984.

New Approaches to the Developmental Dyslexias

Christine M. Temple

Neuropsychology Unit, Neuroscience Group, The Radcliffe Infirmary, Oxford, OX2 6HE, England

METHODS OF APPROACH

In any scientific discipline, a variety of different research designs and paradigms may be used to investigate similar phenomena. Fads, fashions, trends, and developments may mean that the approach of one decade is not the approach of the next.

When Hinshelwood (10–15) wrote about word blindness at the turn of the century, he was particularly concerned with the analysis of individuals. The investigation of individual case studies has been popular in both neuropsychology and neurology. Acquired dyslexia is just one of the cognitive disorders whose study has benefited from this approach. For much of this century, there have been individual case descriptions of alexia with agraphia and pure alexia. More recently, following the report of Marshall and Newcombe in 1966 (21), psycholinguistic analysis of individual cases of reading disorder has become popular. There have been case descriptions of the central dyslexias (deep, phonological, and surface dyslexias) and of the more peripheral dyslexias (letter-by-letter reading). These acquired dyslexias are taxonomized from the pattern of reading deficit exhibited. Concurrent neurologic or cognitive abnormalities do not form part of the diagnostic machinery. The theoretical interpretation of these psycholinguistic analyses is based on cognitive information processing models of the reading process.

It has already been noted that Hinshelwood investigated case studies of the developmental dyslexias. He was also concerned with the similarity between the developmental and the acquired cases, stating "without an adequate knowledge of [acquired word blindness] congenital word-blindness cannot be properly understood." Unfortunately, the work of Hinshelwood fell into disrepute. A new impetus to the study of dyslexia came from Orton in the 1920s and 1930s (24–26), who was also concerned with the analysis of individual case studies; his theoretical interpretation of these cases in terms of "competing" hemispheres is well known.

In contrast to these early case study approaches, the majority of research conducted into the developmental dyslexias has used a group study approach. These studies have been helpful in elucidating the general nature of the characteristics of dyslexic children in comparison to "normal" children. However, there is an obvious limitation to the amount of information that may be obtained, if the group involved is not homogeneous with respect to the factor under investigation. Group studies assume that developmental dyslexia is a single syndrome.

Since the early 1960s, a number of researchers have pointed out that developmental dyslexics do not all display similar patterns of disability (2–4,18–20,23) and have indicated the multiple syndrome nature. Despite this knowledge, few attempts have been made to pursue a detailed analysis of the different syndromes comprising the developmental dyslexias.

Recently, there have been new approaches to the developmental dyslexias, with a return to the investigation of individual case studies but now using a psycholinguistic approach and basing the theoretical interpretation on cognitive information processing models. The research is conducted in the light of the work done with the acquired dyslexias and the classification system used to differentiate them. In 1973, Holmes (16,17) indicated that there were striking parallels between the reading disorder of some developmental dyslexic children and some acquired surface dyslexics, a similarity recently substantiated by Coltheart et al. (7,9). I have been pursuing this approach, both with the type of children studied by Holmes, Coltheart, and Masterson (now referred to as developmental surface dyslexics) and also with the developmental phonological dyslexic (30,32,34). This approach is also helpful in the investigation of reading disorders in children who are not "pure" developmental dyslexics but may, for example, have mild hearing loss or chromosome abnormalities or suffer from seizures (33). To illustrate the new approaches, I compare and contrast three individual cases of "pure" developmental dyslexia; but it is first necessary to describe briefly two of the acquired dyslexic syndromes.

ACQUIRED SURFACE AND PHONOLOGICAL DYSLEXIAS

Acquired surface dyslexia was first described by Marshall and Newcombe (22) and acquired phonological dyslexia by Beauvois and Dérouesné (1). The two syndromes represent contrasting deficits in the reading process. Surface dyslexics are impaired in whole word recognition and frequently rely on "sounding out" words to obtain their pronunciation and meaning. Some theoretical interpretations suggest that this is done by utilizing an abstract set of grapheme-phoneme correspondence rules or rules based on larger orthographic units (5,28,29,31); these rules are viewed as part of a phonological reading route. As a result of this reading method, errors are prone to occur when reading words with irregular spelling to sound patterns. There are also homophone confusions.

In contrast, phonological dyslexics are good at whole word recognition but very poor at sounding out words, as exemplified by their poor reading of nonwords in comparison to their reading of words. They retain some phonological translation skills, but these are limited.

One interpretation of these two acquired dyslexic syndromes is in terms of the model in Fig. 1. Three reading routes are marked. The phonological route, c, is used by surface dyslexics but impaired in phonological dyslexia. The semantic route, a,

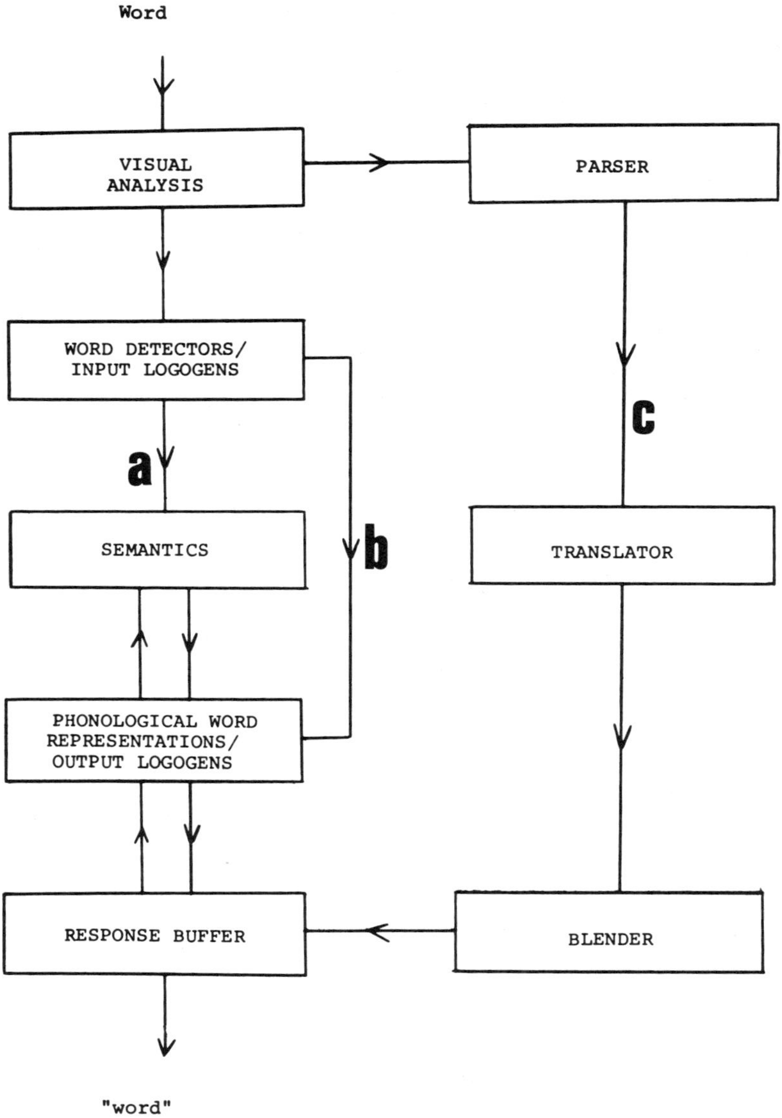

FIG. 1. A model of reading. (See text.)

is impaired in surface dyslexia but used in phonological dyslexia. The direct route, b, is impaired in both syndromes.

Since surface dyslexics use a phonological reading route, they should make more neologistic responses than phonological dyslexics. These neologistic responses may be valid or invalid. In surface dyslexia, many are valid. Valid errors may be regularizations where a more logical phonological translation of a word is given, e.g.,

TABLE 1. *Developmental dyslexics: Standardized results*

Parameter	A.H.	M.H.	R.B.
Age (years)	10.4	10.10	10.10
Sex	M	M	F
Handedness	Mixed, writes L	Mixed, writes R	Left
Verbal IQ	123	128	122
Performance IQ	117	118	104
Full IQ	123	126	115
Reading age (Neale Accuracy)	8.2	8.6	8.7
Reading age (Neale Comprehension)	10.8	10.11	10.11
Spelling age (Schonell)	7.8	7.7	7.6
Vocabulary (Peabody)	99th percentile	99th percentile	99th percentile

gnome → "/gɩnɔmeə/." Others, although not regularizations, are valid in the sense that the correspondences used would have been appropriate in some words, e.g., *four* → "/ʃɑɷ/" (cp s*our*). Invalid neologistic responses are interpreted as reflecting impairment of the phonologic route itself, e.g., *keep* → "/kit/". For in surface dyslexia, although this route is predominantly used, it is usually functioning imperfectly. Paralexic responses may also be regularizations, e.g., *sweat* → "sweet" or other valid errors, e.g., *hid* → "hide." The remaining paralexic responses are visual, e.g., *thigh* → "tight."

Phonological dyslexics, having a more severely impaired phonological reading route which they utilize less, should make fewer neologistic responses. Fewer neologistic and paralexic responses could be interpreted as valid. Phonological dyslexics, like surface dyslexics, make visual paralexias. In addition, they make derivational paralexias, e.g., *children* → "child," for which an adequate theoretical explanation has not yet been found. Phonological dyslexics also make visuosemantic errors, e.g., *satirical* → sarcastic, and what this author (32,34) has called pseudoderivational errors, e.g., *conscience* → "science," *organize* → "organ." Some phonological dyslexics make function word substitutions.

SURFACE DYSLEXIA AND PHONOLOGICAL DYSLEXIA: DEVELOPMENTAL CASES

Three developmental dyslexic children are described. Two, A.H. and M.H., are thought to be developmental phonological dyslexics and one, R.B., a developmental surface dyslexic. The three children are well matched for comparative purposes, since they have similar chronological, reading, and spelling ages. These and other standard background data are given in Table 1. All three children have above average intelligence and large receptive vocabularies. A.H. and R. B. have no neurologic abnormalities, although A.H. has poor imitation of gesture. M.H. has no significant neurologic abnormality, although there is mild dyspraxia in sequential finger movements.

TABLE 2. *Reading of nonwords in comparison to words*

Lists	A.H.	M.H.	R.B.
Three letter list ($N = 14$)	13 words 8 nonwords	14 words 5 nonwords	13 words 12 nonwords
Five or six letter list ($N = 15$)	13 words 4 nonwords	15 words 5 nonwords	12 words 11 nonwords
Coltheart list ($N = 25$)	25 words 6 nonwords	25 words 8 nonwords	23 words 20 nonwords
TOTAL	51 words[a] 18 nonwords	54 words[a] 18 nonwords	48 words 43 nonwords

[a] Statistically significant differences.

The most salient feature of phonological dyslexia is the impairment in nonword reading relative to word reading, an impairment not found in surface dyslexia.

Three lists were presented to the three children. The stimuli on the lists were presented individually to each child for reading aloud. Unless otherwise stated, all reading responses reported in this chapter result from individual presentation and reading aloud. On each list, half the stimuli were words and half were matched pronounceable nonwords made from the words by altering one letter. Two of the lists were constructed by the author. The first contained stimuli three letters in length, while the second contained stimuli five and six letters in length. The third list contained the shorter stimuli from a list by Coltheart (6). The results are reported in Table 2. Both A.H. and M.H. are significantly better at reading words than nonwords ($\chi^2 = 6.64$, $p < 0.001$). In contrast, R. B. is not significantly better at one or the other but is significantly better at reading nonwords than either A.H. or M. H.

The three children were also presented with a list of 40 nonwords used by Patterson (27) and a similar list of 48 nonwords constructed by the author. Once again, R.B. was significantly better than A.H. or M.H. at nonword reading ($\chi^2 = 21.2$, $p < 0.001$). On the Patterson list, A.H. read four of 40, M.H. read nine of 40, and R.B. read 24 of 40; on the Temple list, A.H. read nine of 48, M.H. read 11 of 48, and R.B. read 27 of 48.

Regularity Effects

A salient feature of surface dyslexia but not of phonological dyslexia is the presence of a regularity effect. Each child was presented with the 78 words on the Coltheart et al. (8) list. Half these words are regular, and half are irregular; they are matched for frequency, number of letters, number of syllables, and part of speech, but not for imageability. A.H. read 19 regular and 17 irregular words correctly; M.H. read 30 regular and 24 irregular words correctly. Neither of these differences is statistically significant. R.B. read 24 regular words correctly but only 10 irregular words. This is a significant regularity effect ($\chi^2 = 8.81$).

Error Patterns

Surface and phonological dyslexics also can be distinguished on the basis of their error patterns (see Table 3). Since surface dyslexics use a phonological reading strategy and phonological dyslexics do not, one would expect surface dyslexics to make more neologistic responses than paralexic responses. While 42% of A.H.'s errors and 31% of M.H.'s errors are neologistic, R. B. once more stands apart as 64% of her errors are neologistic. As a proportion of neologistic errors, one would expect a surface dyslexic to make more that are valid. Of their neologistic responses A. H. and M. H. make 13% and 11%, respectively, that are valid. R. B. makes 36% that are valid. Since R.B. made a higher proportion of neologistic errors in the first place, this percentage represents a sizeable number of errors. Since R.B. makes so many neologistic responses, she makes fewer paralexic responses than A.H. and M.H. However, a higher percentage of her paralexic responses are valid than those of A.H. and M.H. Given the neologistic results, it could be speculated that a number of R.B.'s errors are valid errors which happen by chance to be paralexias, whereas for A.H. and M.H., a number of their paralexic errors happen by chance to be valid. Some visual paralexic errors would be expected to be valid by chance, since both errors bear a strong orthographic resemblance to the target. Overall, 30% of R.B.'s errors are valid, whereas only 11% of M.H.'s and 10% of A.H.'s errors ae valid.

Phonological dyslexics also make derivational paralexias. These are also found in the corpora of A.H. and M.H. but only rarely in the corpus of R.B.:

A.H.			M.H.		
splendid	→	"splendor"	*weigh*	→	"weight"
children	→	"child"	*jewel*	→	"jewels"
grow	→	"grown"	*mechanic*	→	"machine"
image	→	"imagine"	*image*	→	"imagine"
refresh	→	"fresh"	*choir*	→	"chorus"
information	→	"inform"	*information*	→	"informant"
spend	→	"spent"	*high*	→	"height"
holder	→	"hold"	*reporter*	→	"report"
quick	→	"quickly"	*certain*	→	"certainty"
govern	→	"governor"	*management*	→	"manager"

A.H. and M.H. also make a number of pseudoderivational errors, an error type discussed elsewhere (32). It is to be observed in the error corpora of both acquired phonologic dyslexics and acquired deep dyslexics, who also make derivational errors:

A.H.			M.H.		
depth	→	"deepthness"	*entertainment*	→	"enter"
adjective	→	"adject"	*clear*	→	"cleaner"
sharpness	→	"shareness"	*government*	→	"glovement"
corner	→	"corn"	*refreshment*	→	"refusement"

TABLE 3. *Analysis of reading errors (%)*

Errors	A.H.	M.H.	R.B.
Paralexias	58	69	36
Neologisms	42	31	64
(Valid neologisms)	(13)	(11)	(36)
Paralexias			
Valid	6	11	19
Visual	60	61	74
Derivational	15	17	3
Visuosemantic	5	7	1
Pseudoderivational	5	3	0
(Neologistic pseudoderivational)	(7)	(6)	(0)

Finally, with respect to errors, A.H. and M.H. make some visuosemantic paralexias:

A.H.		M.H.	
click	→ "tick"	*bowl*	→ "barrel"
circuit	→ "circle"	*arrangement*	→ "agreement"
blast	→ "blase"	*truth*	→ "trust"
thinness	→ "thickness"	*argue*	→ "agree"

R.B. makes one visuosemantic error: *country* → "county"; M.H. and A.H. also make this error, as do a large number of dyslexic children tested by the author. It is probable that this is a visual error that by chance has a semantic component.

Stimulus Distortion

Beauvois and Dérouesné (1) reported that their patient with acquired phonological dyslexia was severely impaired when required to read words typed with the letters in reverse order, thereby prohibiting the use of global strategies. In contrast, handwritten stimuli were read easily. Temple and Marshall (34) noted that the developmental phonological dyslexic, H.M., performed slowly when required to read words typed with the letters in reverse order. The effect of stimulus distortion was further investigated with the three developmental dyslexics described here.

Four sets of stimuli were used: (a) normal typescript, e.g., hard, (b) reverse order lower case, e.g., drah; (c) reverse order upper case, e.g., DRAH; and (d) very poor handwriting. In each set, the same 25 words were used. Each set was presented on a different test occasion. The order of set presentation was normal, handwritten, reverse lower case, reverse upper case; thus, any effects of familiarity would be in the opposite direction to the effect found with acquired phonologic dyslexics. The results are shown in Table 4. There is a slight drop in performance of all three children with the handwritten stimuli. The handwriting was sufficiently poor to be ambiguous occasionally, so this drop was not surprising. However, whereas R.B.'s performance

TABLE 4. *Effects of stimulus manipulation*

Stimulus (*N* = 25)	A.H.	M.H.	R.B.
Lower case	16	19	10
Handwritten	10	15	6
Reverse lower case (e.g., tac)	2	8	12
Reverse upper case (e.g., TAC)	1	8	13

was at least as good with the stimuli presented in reverse order, M.H. and A.H. were significantly impaired with these presentations. (Smaller effect, that of M.H., $\chi^2 = 8.04$, $p < 0.001$.) Prohibiting the use of a global strategy for reading almost eliminates A.H.'s ability to read, significantly reduces M.H.'s ability to read, and leaves R.B.'s performance quite unimpaired.

Homophone Confusion

Surface dyslexics, but not phonological dyslexics, make homophone confusions. The three developmental dyslexics were presented with a list of 40 stimuli: 20 homophone pairs. All the words used were common, and none contained silent letters or features that were highly irregular, e.g., stair/stare, peace/piece. The words were randomized and presented individually for reading aloud. In addition, the children were requested to define the meaning of the words read. In three or four instances, A.H. and M.H. defined the words as their respective homophones, e.g., *thrown* → "What a king sits on." Given that both A.H. and M.H. make visual errors, confusing words with orthographic similarity, and that homophonic words resemble each other orthographically, the occurrence of some homophone confusion is not surprising. R.B.'s homophone confusion is much more marked. She defines half the words that she reads correctly as their respective homophones; i.e., when defining a word that has a homophone, she performs at chance level in selecting between it and its homophone.

CONCLUSIONS

All of the results are consistent with the notion that developmental surface dyslexics, like acquired surface dyslexics, are overreliant on a phonic route to reading. In contrast, developmental phonological dyslexics, like acquired phonological dyslexics, read by a whole word method and are severely deficient on tasks that require phonic segmentation and analysis. The existence of these two distinct groups of developmental dyslexics restresses the heterogeneity of the disorder. It also indicates that two independent systems of reading may develop in relative isolation from each other. In particular, developmental phonological dyslexia indicates that one may establish a substantial sight vocabulary without ever mastering the grapheme-to-phoneme correspondences of the language. Individual analysis of this sort reveals the specific type of difficulty that the dyslexic child encounters reading. The analysis may be important for constructing appropriate remedial schemes for each individual dyslexic child.

SUMMARY

Although Hinshelwood (10–15), at the turn of the century, was interested in both analysis of individual cases and comparisons between acquired and developmental dyslexia, the most widespread approach to the developmental dyslexias has been the investigation of large groups of dyslexics in comparison to normal readers on a variety of tests. These studies ignore the heterogeneity of the disorder. In contrast, progress has been made in the investigation of acquired disorders of reading by conducting individual psycholinguistic analyses of reading difficulties and utilizing input from cognitive psychology to construct explanatory models and theories. Two of the disorders described and elucidated by this approach are acquired surface dyslexia, in which there is an impairment in whole word recognition and overreliance on sounding out words to obtain their pronunciation and meaning, and acquired phonological dyslexia, in which whole word recognition is good but sounding out of words and nonwords is poor.

This approach has recently been used with cases of developmental dyslexia. This chapter compares and contrasts the pattern of performance of different dyslexic children when investigated in this way. Two of the children described are developmental phonological dyslexics; one is a developmental surface dyslexic.

The developmental phonological dyslexics are poorer at reading words than nonwords; the developmental surface dyslexic performs equally well on both. The developmental surface dyslexic is significantly influenced by spelling-to-sound regularity; the developmental phonological dyslexics are unaffected by this linguistic dimension. The developmental surface dyslexic makes more neologistic responses than the developmental phonological dyslexics, and also makes more valid errors. The developmental phonological dyslexics make derivational, pseudoderivational, and visuosemantic errors. Both groups make visual errors. The developmental phonological dyslexics are significantly impaired when stimuli are presented in a way that prohibits global analysis; the developmental surface dyslexic is unaffected by this manipulation. The developmental surface dyslexic makes homophone confusions, but these are not made by the developmental phonological dyslexics.

The developmental surface dyslexic has developed a system of reading predominantly based on phonological analysis or "sounding out"; the developmental phonological dyslexics have developed a system of reading predominantly based on whole word recognition. The development of these systems in relative isolation is of interest theoretically but may also have implications for the construction of individual remedial programs.

REFERENCES

1. Beauvois, M. F., and Dérouesné, J. (1979): Phonological processes in reading: Data from alexia. *J. Neurol. Neurosurg. Psychiatry,* 42:1125–1132.

2. Birch, H. G. (1982): Dyslexia and maturation of visual function. In: *Reading Disability: Progress and Research Needs in Dyslexia*, edited by J. Money. Johns Hopkins Press, Baltimore.
3. Boder, E. (1970): Developmental dyslexia: A new diagnostic approach based on the identification of three subtypes. *School Health*, 40:289–290.
4. Boder, E. (1971): Developmental dyslexia: A diagnostic screening procedure based on three characteristic patterns of reading and spelling. In: *Learning Disorders*, edited by B. Bateman. Special Child Publications, Seattle.
5. Coltheart, M. (1978): Lexical access in simple reading tasks. In: *Strategies of Information Processing*, edited by G. Underwood. Academic Press, London.
6. Coltheart, M. (1981): Analysing acquired disorders of reading. (*Unpublished.*)
7. Coltheart, M. (1982): Surface dyslexia and its implications for models of normal reading. In: *The Neuropsychology of Cognitive Function*, edited by D.E. Broadbent and L. Weiskrantz. The Royal Society, London.
8. Coltheart, M., Besner, D., Jonasson, J. T., and Davelaar, E. (1979): Phonological recoding in the lexical decision task. *Q. J. Exp. Psychol.*, 31:489–508.
9. Coltheart, M., Masterson, J., Byng, S., Prior, M., and Riddoch, J. (1984): Surface Dyslexia. *Q. J. Exp. Psychol.*, 35:469–496.
10. Hinshelwood, J. (1895): Word-blindness and visual memory. *Lancet*, 2:1564–1570.
11. Hinshelwood, J. (1900): *Letter-, Word- and Mind-Blindness*. H. K. Lewis, London.
12. Hinshelwood, J. (1900): *Congenital Word-Blindness. Lancet*, 1:1506–1508.
13. Hinshelwood, J. (1902): Congenital word-blindness, with reports of two cases. *Ophthalmol. Rev.*, 21:91–99.
14. Hinshelwood, J. (1904): A case of congenital word-blindness. *Br. Med. J.*, 2:1303–1307.
15. Hinshelwood, J. (1917): *Congenital Word-Blindness*. H. K. Lewis, London.
16. Holmes, J. M. (1973): Dyslexia: A neurolinguistic study of traumatic and developmental disorders of reading. Doctoral dissertation, University of Edinburgh.
17. Holmes, J. M. (1978): "Regression" and reading breakdown. In: *Language Acquisition and Language Breakdown*, edited by A. Caramazza and E. B. Zurif. The Johns Hopkins University Press, Baltimore.
18. Ingram, T. T. S., Mason, A. W., and Blackburn, I. (1970): A retrospective study of 82 children with reading disability. *Dev. Med. Child Neurol.*, 12:271–281.
19. Johnson, D., and Myklebust, H. (1967): *Learning Disabilities*. Grune & Stratton, New York.
20. Mattis, S., French, J. H., and Rapin, I. (1975): Dyslexia in children and young adults: Three independent neuropsychological syndromes. *Dev. Med. Child Neurol.*, 17:150–163.
21. Marshall, J. C., and Newcombe, F. (1966): Syntactic and semantic errors in paralexia. *Neuropsychologia*, 44:169–176.
22. Marshall, J. C., and Newcombe, F. (1973): Patterns of paralexia: A psycholinguistic approach. *J. Psycholinguist. Res.*, 2:175–199.
23. Myklebust, H. R., and Johnson, D. J. (1962): Dyslexia in children. *Except. Child.*, 29:14–25.
24. Orton, S. T. (1925): "Word-blindness" in school children. *Arch. Neurol. Psychiatry*, 14:581–615.
25. Orton, S. T. (1926): Reading disability. *Genet. Psychol. Monogr.* 14:335–453.
26. Orton, S. T. (1928): Specific reading disability—strephosymbolia. *JAMA*, 90:1095–1099.
27. Patterson, K. E. (1982): The relation between reading and phonological coding: Further neuropsychological observations. In: *Normality and Pathology in Cognitive Functions*, edited by A. W. Ellis. Academic Press, London.
28. Shallice, T., and Warrington, E. K. (1980): Single and multiple component central dyslexic syndromes. In: *Deep Dyslexia*, edited by M. Coltheart, K. Patterson, and J. C. Marshall. Routledge and Kegan Paul, London.
29. Shallice, T., Warrington, E. K., and McCarthy, R. (1983): Reading without semantics. *Q. J. Exp. Psychol.*, 35:111–138.
30. Temple, C. M. (1984): Developmental analogues to acquired phonological dyslexia. In: *Dyslexia: A Global Issue,* edited by R. N. Malatesha and H. A. Whitaker. Martinus Nijhoff, The Hague.
31. Temple, C. M. (1985): Surface dyslexia: Variation within a syndrome. In: *Surface Dyslexia in Adults and Children,* edited by J. C. Marshall, K. E. Patterson, and M. Coltheart. Lawrence Erlbaum, London.
32. Temple, C. M. (1984): Reading with partial phonology: Developmental phonological dyslexia. (*Submitted.*)
33. Temple, C. M. (1984): Surface dyslexia in a child with epilepsy. Neuropsychologia (*in press*).
34. Temple, C. M., and Marshall, J. C. (1983): A case study of developmental phonological dyslexia. *Br. J. Psychol.*, 74:517–533.

Advances in Neurology, Vol. 42: Progress in Aphasiology, edited by F. C. Rose.
Raven Press, New York © 1984.

A Physiologic Theory of Visual Dyslexia

J. F. Stein and Susan Fowler

University Laboratory of Physiology, University of Oxford, Oxford, England

Many workers in the field of developmental dyslexia would object to the title of this chapter, since it refers to two ideas thought to have been thoroughly discredited. It is now generally accepted that developmental dyslexia cannot be explained in terms of simple sensory or perceptual deficits, so the notion that there could be a simple physiologic explanation for dyslexia is unacceptable (28). For similar reasons, the proposition that there could be a type of dyslexia resulting from visual disorder is strenuously opposed. However, recent developments in sensory physiology make it necessary to reconsider the view that dyslexia is a purely cognitive disorder and, as such, not amenable to physiologic investigation. Not so long ago, few would have accepted the idea that physiology could ever offer any help with problems of perception; yet perceptual psychology and sensory physiology have now become totally interdependent.

We hope to show in this chapter that many of the difficulties faced by dyslexic children do relate to a classic perceptual problem: the optical space sense (20). How is it that we know where objects around us are located, despite the fact that our eyes move all the time? How are the transient pictures of the environment, offered to the mind's eye by the retina each time we fixate, converted to a stable view of the visual world with which we can operate confidently? This is the classic problem of how eye movement and position information are used to transform the changing retinal coordinates of the image of an object into stable mental coordinates representing its real position in the outside world. We suggest that a subtle disorder of this ability to reliably associate eye position signals, which indicate where the eyes are pointing, with retinal signals about which letter is being inspected may underly the difficulty many dyslexics have when learning to read.

Although the idea that dyslexia has anything to do with vision is contradicted, many dyslexic children are convinced that it is their eyes that are at fault; hence many appear at ophthalmology departments for check-ups. Many studies have established that there is nothing wrong with the visual acuity of these children (2), but the question of whether their eye movements are abnormal remains unresolved (1,21). Certainly the children's own complaints point to eye movement control problems. They report that letters appear to move around, flip and jump over each other, and reverse themselves; and they find that they are always losing their place on a page.

Conventional clinical testing of eye movements in dyslexics normally fails to show any obvious defects; ophthalmologists accustomed to looking for gross pareses or nystagmus are inclined to say there is nothing wrong with them, but closer examination of these children's eye movements reveals many subtle abnormalities. Careful measurements have demonstrated that a higher proportion of dyslexic children than normals have mild abnormalities of ocular motor control, such as esophoria, convergence inaccuracies, and a tendency to "cogwheel" during smooth pursuit. These abnormalities have not been considered significant, especially since major abnormalities of ocular motor control can usually be demonstrated only when such children try to read. Thus dysjunctive eye movements, failure to maintain stable fixation, mistimed, misdirected, and dysmetric saccades are often seen when dyslexic children attempt reading tasks (1). They are usually attributed to the cognitive load of reading and have been interpreted as being a result of the child's inability to understand what he is seeing rather than as an indication of the cause of his problems.

It is now clear that many dyslexic children may make these abnormal eye movements even when they are not trying to read, e.g., when they view simple targets, such as rows of light-emitting diodes (21) or moving spots of light (1). Such displays carry no cognitive load; thus the child's abnormal ocular motor control when inspecting them is probably a manifestation of a primary visuomotor disorder, which may underlie his reading difficulties.

Reading small print requires more accurate eye movement control than any task a 6-year-old child has hitherto been asked to perform. Small letters subtend only about ¼° of visual angle at the normal reading distance. Hence if each letter is inspected individually, as happens when a child first begins to learn to read, he must learn to control eye movements with better than ¼° precision in order to avoid confusing the shapes of letters and their order in a word.

The child learning to read must not only learn to control eye movements accurately, but he must also be able to record the position of his eyes at all times with this degree of precision. In order to determine where a letter is positioned on a page or within a word, it is necessary to correctly associate retinal signals about the nature of the letter, with extraretinal ocular motor signals about the precise position of the eyes with respect to the head. If this is not done properly, it is not possible to locate letters correctly. Hence children who cannot make reliable ocular motor/retinal associations when reading, mislocate and missequence letters and lose their place on the page.

A further problem resulting from inadequate retinal/ocular motor association when reading arises because eye position and retinal signals relating to the center of gaze are bilaterally represented. Both left and right visual cortical areas receive signals coming from the central portions of both halves of visual space. Some aberrant fibers project from up to 5° out in the temporal half of the retina, not to the ipsilateral lateral geniculate nucleus (LGN) but crossing over in the optic chiasm arrive at the contralateral LGN and hence project to contralateral visual cortex (6). Furthermore, the region of the visual cortex on one side representing the central 5° of contralateral visual space is linked, via the splenium of the corpus callosum and anterior commissure, to the homologous area in the other visual cortex representing the central 5° of the hemifield on the opposite side (7). Thus both left and right hemispheres receive signals relating to both sides of the maculae, the region of high retinal acuity used for reading. Similarly, both hemispheres receive signals relating to eye movements directed to both sides of the midline, although the pathways taken by these signals are not known with any certainty (18).

Duplication of retinal and eye position signals relating to the center of gaze in both hemispheres is essential for unification of the visual scene and for transferring information received first in one hemisphere over to the other. Hemispheric specialization would be impossible without it, but the cost is potential confusion. How does the observer know on which side of the midline a letter is situated if both sides are linked together in this way? What is needed to resolve the confusion is to know precisely where the eyes are pointing with respect to the head, using extraretinal, ocular motor cues. These provide evidence, independent of the retina, about where the letter is positioned in the outside world, enabling the subject to interpret the mixture of signals fed from both sides of the midline to the same hemisphere.

A further complication arises from the nature of the interconnections between the two hemispheres. These tend to be homotopic, i.e., homologous points on the two sides are linked together. Thus interhemispheric commissures connect together points equidistant from the midline on the retinotopic maps of each hemifield; 5° right projects to 5° left, and so on (24). The effect of transfer of information about an asymmetric object across such links is to cause it to be mirror reversed (e.g., a *b* is transformed to a *d*, and vice versa) (Fig. 1). Again the only way to compensate for this effect is to know in which hemifield the object appeared when it was first seen, i.e., to know precisely where the eyes were pointing at the time.

Accurate monitoring of eye position is vital, therefore, but it is made particularly difficult when reading small print, because the eyes are converged at the near point. The ocular motor signals that may be used to determine the direction in which the eyes are pointing consist of two types. The first are motor outflow signals, which report to sensory systems about the way in which ocular motor centers are moving the eyes; this enables them to discount retinal changes which are purely a consequence of the eyes moving, since these signals do not mean that anything in the outside world is moving (15). In addition, eye movements give rise to proprioceptive feedback from the ocular muscles and orbital tissues (8); this indicates whether the desired eye movement has been achieved. When the eyes are converged on a near object, feedback of proprioceptive ocular motor information may be highly confusing, because the two eyes are pointing in different directions; neither eye position can give reliable information about the direction of an object with respect to the egocenter, as this lies between the two eyes (4).

Thus precise eye movement control and accurate registration of eye position are particularly important when reading, but satisfactory achievement of this precision is made very difficult. First we consider how the problems may be overcome in normal subjects, then how they go wrong in certain dyslexic children.

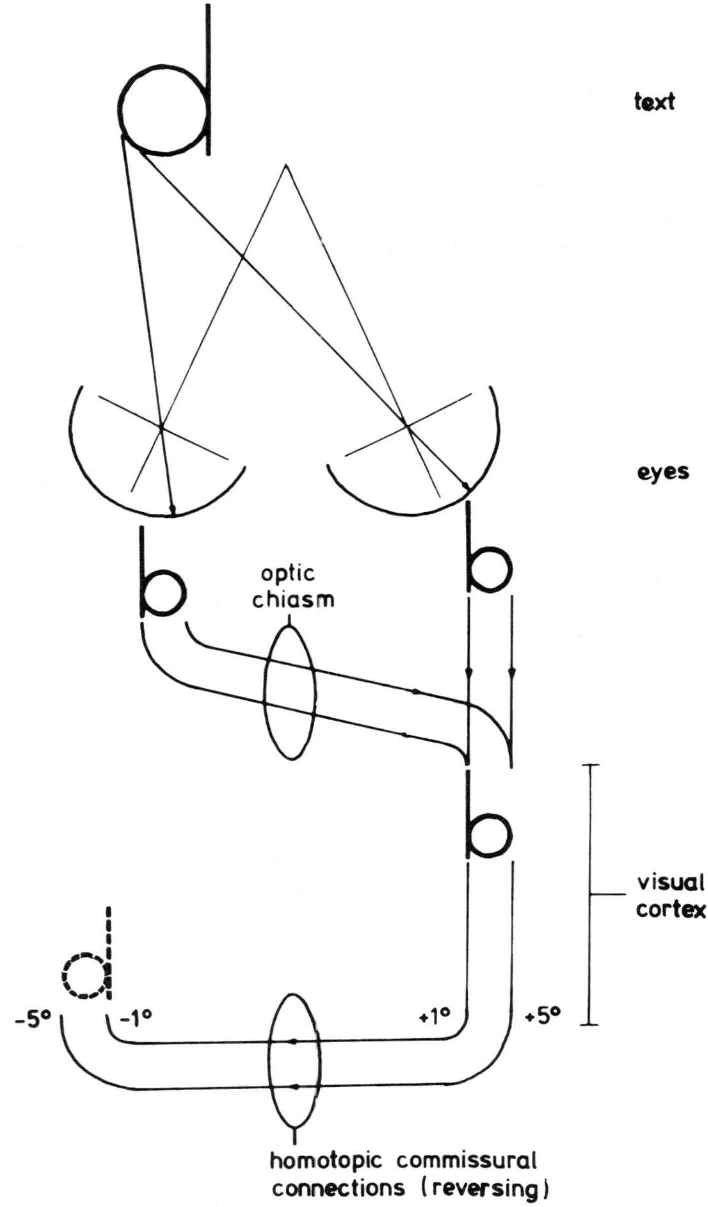

FIG. 1. The *d* is mirror reversed once by the optics of the eye when projected to the right hemisphere but is reversed again if transferred to the left hemisphere by homotopic commissural connections.

Recent evidence (9) has shifted attention away from the frontal eye field as the cortical center for eye movement control, back to where Ferrier (12) suspected it to lie: in the posterior part of the parietal lobe. Visually directed eye movements, together with accurate perception of visual direction (as opposed to spontaneous search movements) probably depend on visuomotor associations made in the posterior parietal lobe. Patients with lesions in the region of the inferior parietal lobule and angular gyrus make inaccurate eye movements in the contralateral hemifield; they mislocate objects in that half of extrapersonal space (14). If the inferior parietal lobule in monkeys is temporarily inactivated by cooling, the monkeys show similar symptoms (25); and neurons there have been shown by Mountcastle et al. (17) to receive both visual and eye position information and to discharge in advance of visually directed movements of hand or eye.

Of course monkeys cannot read. One should therefore, ask, what are the effects of hemispheric specialization for language on the organization of ocular motor control and visual direction sense? In humans, the left hemisphere contains semantic and lexical stores for language, whereas the right is specialized for spatial tasks and examining the environment. Thus gaze paresis and visual direction deficits are more common after right parietal lesions (11); and alexia, anomia, and sensory aphasia are more common with lesions of the left posterior parietal region (16). In humans, therefore, eye movement control, including vergence control, is probably dominated by the right hemisphere, whereas reading depends on the left inferior parietal lobule and angular gyrus. Hence eye movement signals, together with retinal information about letters viewed in the left hemifield, must always be transferred via the corpus callosum and anterior commissure from right to left hemisphere when reading, with all the dangers of confusion that this entails.

It is amazing that humans can learn to read at all. Accurate association of eye position signals with retinal information about the shape of letters or words is essential in order to locate, sequence, and recognise them, yet the eyes are converged when reading small print, so that position feedback from the two eyes differs and does not correspond to the direction of the object with respect to the egocenter. Furthermore, in many children, vergence is not always precise, so that temporarily, the foveae may not even be inspecting the same letter (3). Retinal and eye position signals, corresponding to objects seen with the central 5 to 10° of the visual field, are represented in both hemispheres; because of homotopic connections between these representations, however, information transferred from one side to the other is liable to be mirror reversed. Such transfer is essential for eye position signals that are organized primarily in the right hemisphere and for objects viewed in the left hemifield, since this information is required by the left hemisphere when reading.

The solution to many of these problems probably lies in the development of a "leading" eye (20,29). The word "leading" rather than "dominant" is chosen in order not to imply any relationship to the dominant left hemisphere. There is no reason to suppose that there are preferential optic or ocular motor connections between the left hemisphere and either eye. Development of a reliable leading eye may help in several ways to solve the problems of reliable retinal/ocular motor association outlined above. First, if a subject attends to the ocular motor signals of only one eye, confusion when those from the other eye disagree during vergence or dysjunctive movements is eliminated. Second, when inaccurate convergence is occurring, conflicting macular signals coming from the other eye may be suppressed. Third, since macular and ocular motor signals coming from one eye are identified as supplied by the leading eye, they are no longer confused with those coming from the other eye, whether they arrive directly in the left hemisphere or travel indirectly via the right hemisphere, and become mirror reversed.

Thus there are good reasons for supposing that the development of a stable leading eye is important for helping to resolve the confusions engendered by binocular convergence, bilateral representation of the maculae, and homotopic interhemispheric communication. Although the idea of eye dominance dates from as early as the sixteenth century (23), there has never been strong empirical evidence in its favor. Tests dependent on sighting dominance (the preferred eye for telescope or rifle sight) have proved unreliable and inconclusive (22). Most such tests are monocular and are highly affected by habit and handedness. A satisfactory test for the leading eye should determine whether the ocular motor and retinal signals relating to macular vision coming from one eye are successfully associated with each other, in preference to those coming from the other eye. Hence the test needs to employ the maculae, since these are bilaterally represented in both cortices, and to involve binocular vergence movements, so that conflicting eye position signals will be supplied to the two hemispheres. Such conditions are supplied in an orthoptic test introduced by Dunlop (10).

The two eyes view through a synoptophore macular sized pictures of a house with a central front door. In the slide viewed by the right eye, a large post is seen to the left of the front door; in the slide viewed by the left eye, a small post is placed to the right of the door. Thus the posts are positioned in the nasal field of each eye; initially, retinal signals about the post which each eye sees pass to the ipsilateral hemisphere. The child fixes the two images of the house and sees a large post to the left of the front door and a small post to the right. The synoptophore tubes are then diverged. Most children can preserve fusion for up to 5° during such divergence. The house may seem to move away from the observer but remains in the midline; one of the posts, however, usually appears to move toward the door of the house. Ocular motor signals relating to the divergence of each eye pass initially to the hemisphere contralateral to that eye, while the retinal signals about the post it views pass to the ipsilateral hemisphere. Hence retinal and ocular motor signals find themselves in opposite hemispheres; their successful association demands the use of the homotopic commissural links between the two sides (Fig. 2). Thus the ability to make reliable ocular motor/retinal associations is tested thoroughly. Most normal subjects report that one of the posts appears to move toward the door when the synoptophore tubes are diverged. If the test is repeated many times, it is always the post seen by this one eye that appears to move. The eye whose ocular motor signals are reliably associated with the post it views (in many cases the right eye) is termed the leading eye. Almost all normal readers are found to have a stable (or fixed) leading

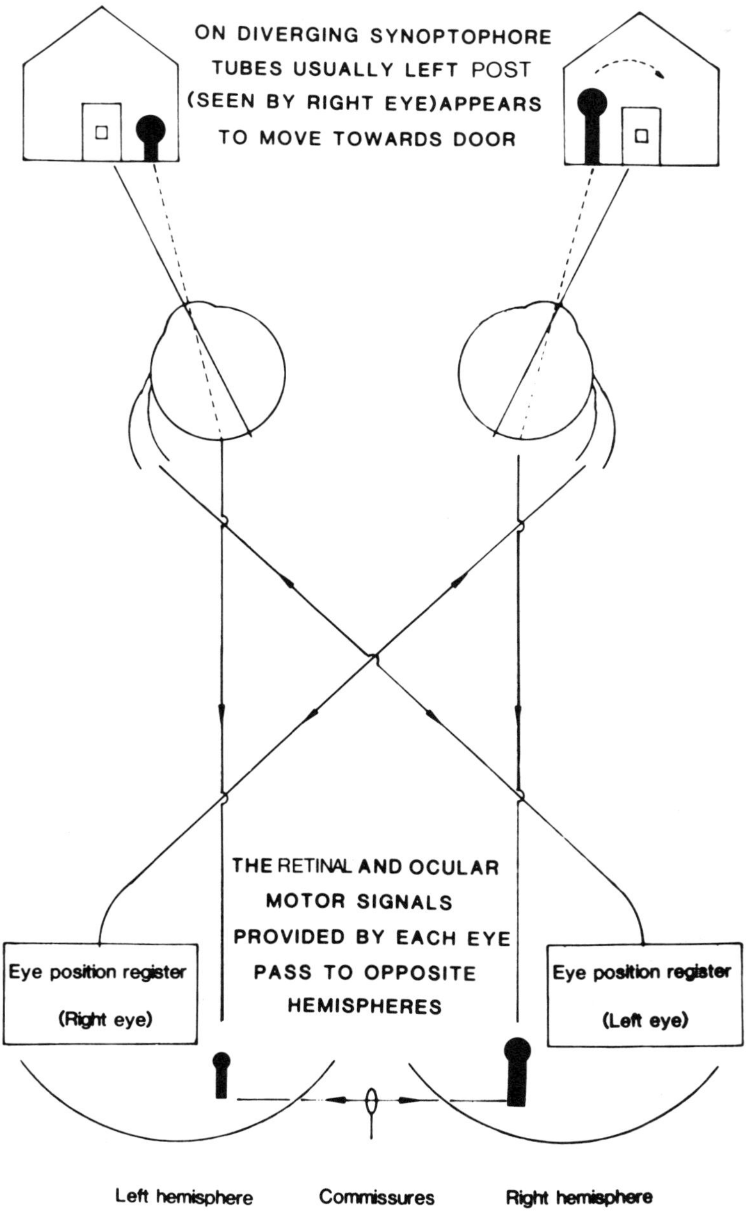

FIG. 2. The Dunlop test. (For details, see text.)

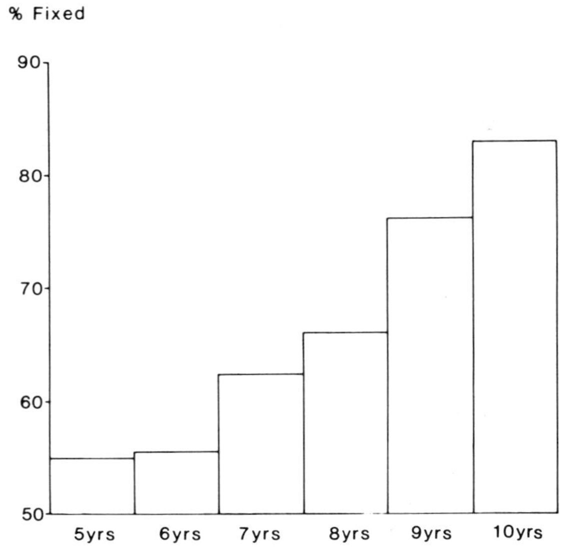

FIG. 3. Development of fixed leading eye in primary school children. $N = 632$.

eye on the Dunlop test, whereas many dyslexic children fail to develop such reliable ocular motor/retinal associations. When these children perform the Dunlop test repeatedly, either both posts appear to move or on one occasion the left and on the next the right post appears to move.

We performed the Dunlop test on more than 600 primary school children aged 6 to 10 years in order to see how stable ocular motor/retinal associations developed with age. We found that about 50% of children have achieved a stable leading eye by the age of 6 years, and about 7% more children achieve stability in each successive year; among 10 year olds, more than 80% have achieved a fixed leading eye (Fig. 3). We were also interested to find out if those children who had achieved a fixed leading eye were better readers. Figure 4 shows that this is the case and supports our hypothesis that development of a fixed leading eye helps to resolve the confusion of ocular motor and retinal signals encountered during reading.

We performed the Dunlop test in 80 dyslexic children and 80 normal readers matched for age and IQ (27). The orthoptist performing the test did not know which children were normal and which dyslexic. Two-thirds of the dyslexics were found to have unstable leading eyes, whereas only one normal child was unfixed (Fig. 5). We found that the dyslexic children with unfixed leading eyes made typically visual errors when attempting to read. These included missequencing, substitution, and reversal of letters when writing. To some extent, however, judgment of which errors are specifically visual is bound to be arbitrary.

Algernon Charles Swinburne was probably dyslexic: when reading poetry, he would stand in front of his audience with a hand clamped over one eye (19). We found that many dyslexics with unstable leading eyes had learned similar devices.

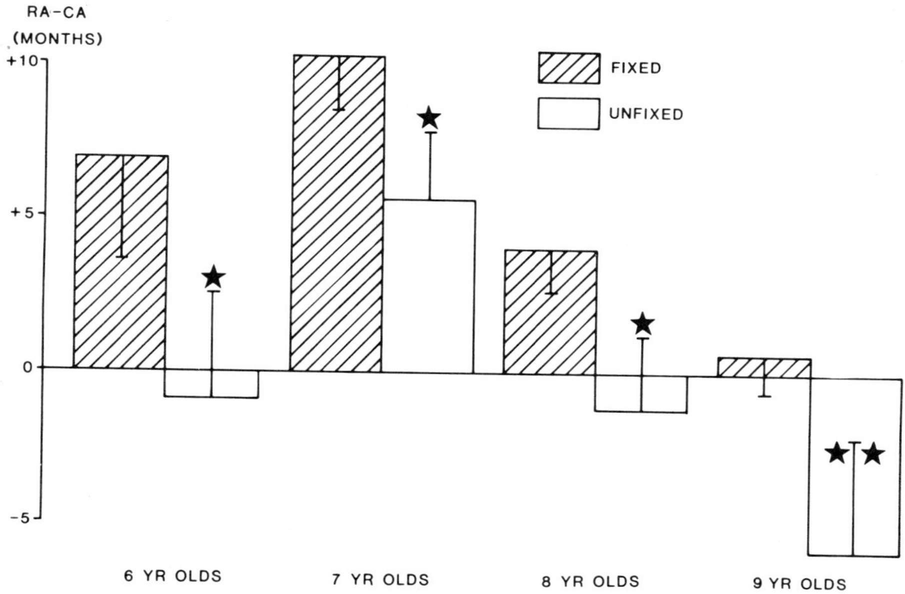

FIG. 4. Reading age (RA) of children with fixed leading eye is significantly higher than of those without. * $p < 0.05$; ** $p < 0.01$. CA, chronological age.

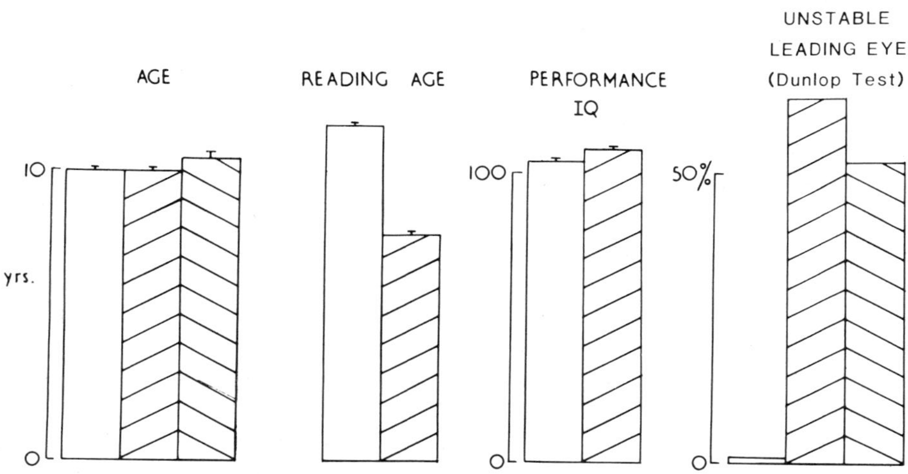

FIG. 5. More than 50% of dyslexics, matched with controls for age and performance IQ, have an unstable leading eye. □, Normal readers; ▨, 80 fully studied dyslexics; ▧, 274 other dyslexics.

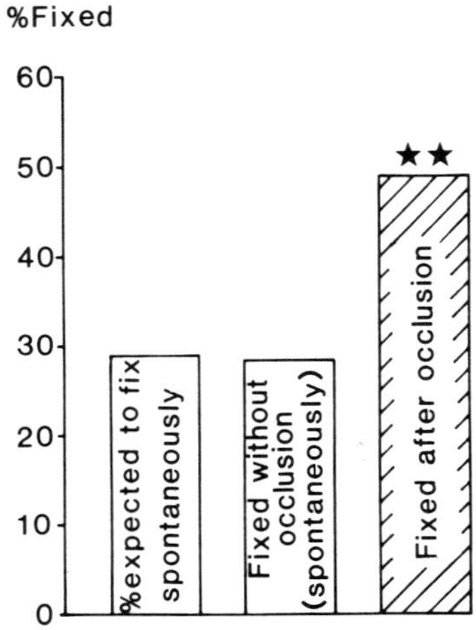

FIG. 6. Monocular occlusion helps children to develop a fixed leading eye.

Some would hold their hand over one eye; others got so close to the page that only one eye could see the print. Some developed a manifest squint when they first started to read, with visual suppression of the squinting eye (13). We have even seen a number of cases with the alarming symptom of sudden loss of vision in one eye presenting when they started to learn to read (13). All these maneuvers have the common effect of blanking out the retinal signals of one eye. This simplifies the retinal/ocular motor problems faced by the child by removing confusing retinal signals coming from the occluded eye and thereby encouraging the development of the other as the leading eye. We attempted similar treatment on our dyslexics with unstable leading eyes, by occluding their left eyes when reading, in order to encourage the seeing eye to form stable associations between its retinal and ocular motor signals and thus to become the fixed leading eye.

The results of our initial study were encouraging (26). A group of 15 dyslexics with unfixed leading eyes were given plain glasses with the left lens occluded with opaque material to wear when reading. Fifteen other dyslexics, matched for age and IQ, were not so treated. The treated dyslexics achieved a fixed leading eye, which persisted after the glasses were removed. At the same time, their average reading age improved by more than 12 months in the 6 months of observation. Those without treatment remained unfixed, and their average reading age barely improved by 6 months.

We have now almost completed a further double-blind study involving nearly 200 dyslexic children. All have been fully assessed by a reading specialist using the British Ability Scale tests together with writing and phonetic exercises of our own devising. All have been examined as well by an ophthalmologist and orthoptist who were not given the reading specialist's reports. A fourth person with no knowledge of the results of any of the tests then gave alternate children either plain spectacles or spectacles with the left lens occluded. Thus we have obtained four randomly selected groups of dyslexics: (a) children with unstable leading eyes who were given occluded spectacles, (b) those who were not, (c) children with fixed leading eyes

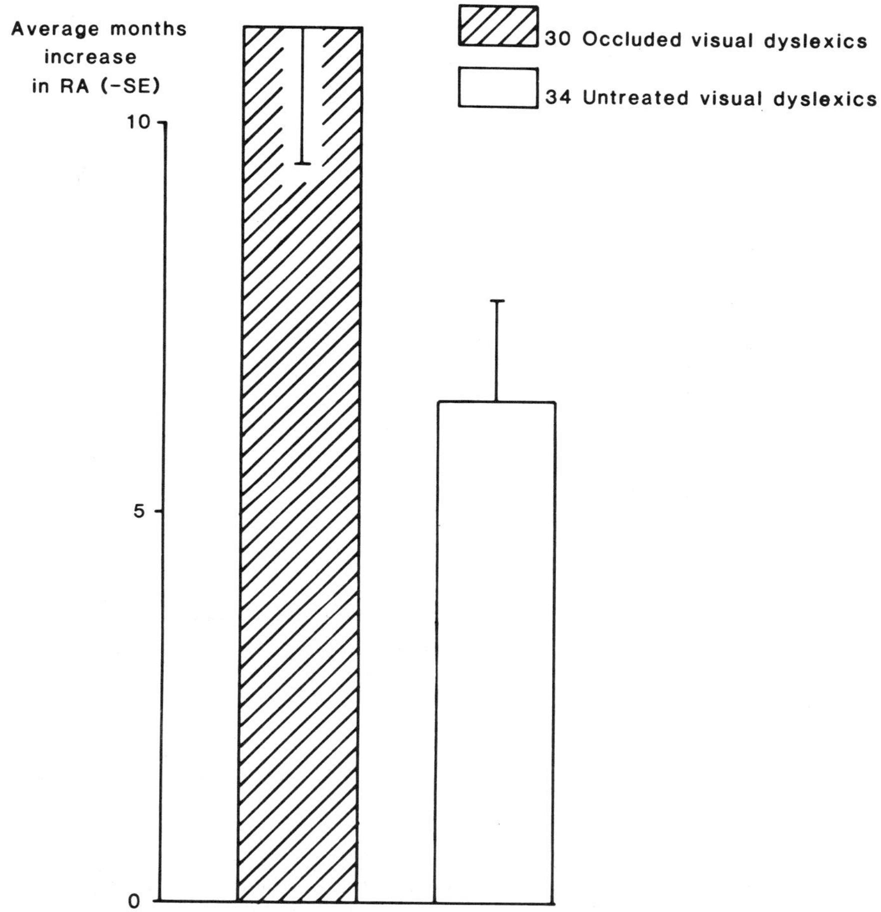

FIG. 7. Over 6 months of observation, occluded visual dyslexics who developed fixed leading eye improved their reading by almost 6 months more than those who were not occluded.

who were given occluded spectacles, and (d) those who were not. The children have been followed up by the orthoptist at intervals of 3 months. At 6 months, reading, writing, phonetic, and Dunlop tests were repeated. Those who had a stable leading eye then had their glasses removed, and those who were still unstable were given occluding spectacles. We will therefore have a group of more than 50 children with initially unfixed leading eyes who began with no treatment for a 6-month control period and then were changed to occlusion. The reading, writing, and Dunlop tests were repeated at the end of 1 year; in some children, they were repeated again 18 months after the children were first seen.

The results of this double-blind study fully support those of our preliminary trial of occlusion in dyslexics with unstable leading eyes. Nearly 50% of children who were initially unfixed on the Dunlop test become fixed after 6 months of occlusion,

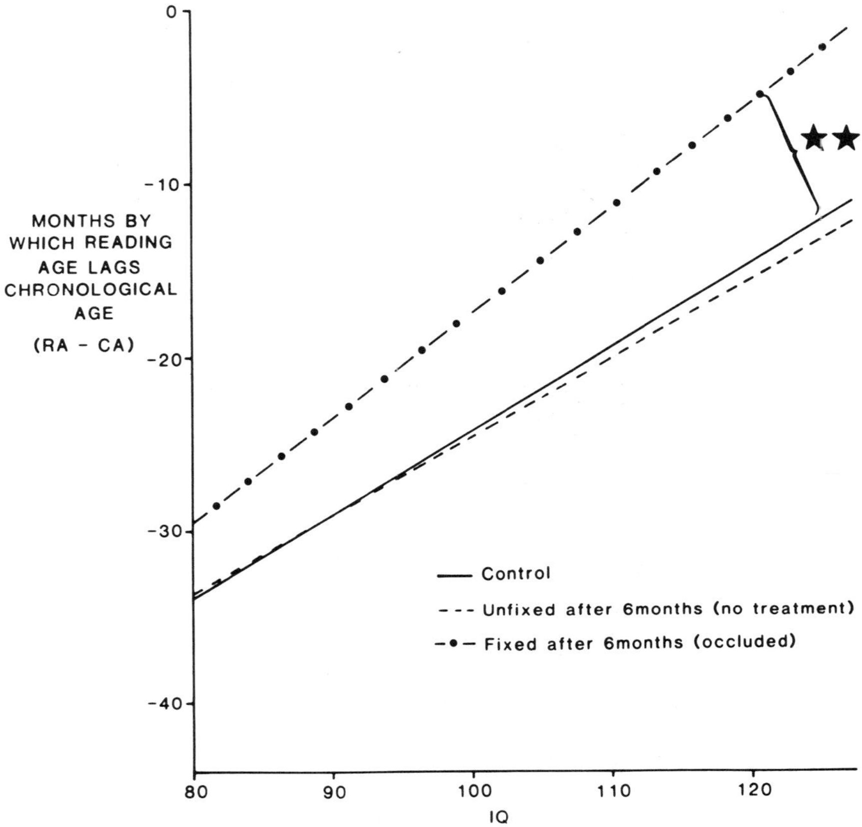

FIG. 8. Regression of reading retardation (reading age − chronologic age) on performance IQ for all children before treatment, 34 children who received no treatment, and 30 children who became fixed after 6 months occlusion. ** $p < 0.01$.

compared with approximately 25% who became fixed spontaneously wearing plain spectacles (Fig. 6). The percentage who achieved a fixed leading eye without occlusion is similar to the proportion of normal children still unfixed at this age whom one would expect to become fixed spontaneously (see Fig. 3). The average reading age of 30 dyslexic children who started with unfixed leading eyes but achieved stability after 6 months of monocular occlusion increased by 11.3 months, whereas that of 34 children not given occluding spectacles who remained unfixed increased by only 6.5 months (Fig. 7). The difference between these two groups is significant at the 1% level. When allowance is made for the IQ of each child by calculating the regression of their reading retardation (the difference between their chronologic and reading ages) against nonverbal IQ, for successfully treated and untreated children, the difference between the groups still remained highly significant (Fig. 8).

Thus monocular occlusion helps a substantial proportion of dyslexics with unfixed leading eyes to achieve stable ocular motor/retinal associations and thereby helps them to learn to read. This provides further evidence in favor of our basic hypothesis, namely, that many children are dyslexic because they fail to achieve reliable associations of ocular motor with retinal signals. We conclude, therefore, that visual dyslexia is indeed due to a child's failure to solve a classic problem of perception: they do not know properly where their eyes are pointing when they are trying to read.

REFERENCES

1. Adler Grinberg, D., and Stark, L. (1978): Eye movements, scan paths, and dyslexia. *Am. J. Optom.*, 55:557–570.
2. American Academy of Pediatrics, Ophthalmology and Otolaryngology (1973): The eye and learning disabilities. *J. Learn. Disabil.* 6:119.
3. Ashton, H., and Haines, J. (1982): Binocular coordination in severely disabled readers. Symposium on Visual Dyslexia, Worthing, England (*unpublished*).
4. Barbeito, R., and Ono, M. (1979): Four methods of locating the ego centre. *Behav. Res. Methods*, 11:31–36.
5. Bettman, J. W., Stern, E. L., Whitsell, L. J., and Gotman, H. F. (1967): Cerebral dominance in developmental dyslexia. *Arch. Ophthalmol.*, 78:722–729.
6. Bunt, A. H., Minckler, D. S., and Johanson, G. W. (1979): Bilateral projection of the central retina of the monkey. *J. Comp. Neurol.*, 171:619–630.
7. Choudhury, P. B., Whitteridge, D., and Wilson, M. E. (1965): The function of the callosal connections of the visual cortex. *Q. J. Exp. Physiol.*, 50:214.
8. Cooper, S., Daniel, P. M., and Whitteridge, D. (1955): Eye muscle spindles; their anatomy, physiology and connections in the brain stem. *Brain*, 78:564–583.
9. De Renzi, E. (1983): Gaze paresis and posterior parietal lobe. *Arch. Neurol.*, 39:482.
10. Dunlop, P. (1972): Dyslexia. The orthoptic approach. *Aust. Orthopt. J.* 12:16–20.
11. Ettlinger, G. (1977): Parietal cortex in visual orientation. In: *Physiological Aspects of Clinical Neurology*, edited by F. C. Rose. Blackwell, London.
12. Ferrier, D. (1876): *The Functions of the Brain*. Smith Elder, London.
13. Fowler, M. S., and Stein, J. F. (1983): Ocular motor dominance as a factor in some orthoptic problems. *Br. Orthopt. J.*, 40:433–445.
14. Hannay, H. J., Varney, N. R., and Benton, A. L. (1976): Visual localisation in patients with unilateral brain disease. *J. Neurol. Neurosurg. Psychiatry*, 39:307.
15. Helmholtz, H. von (1896): Treatise on physiological optics [in German]. *Physiol. Optik*, Hamburg. (Translated into English by J. P. C. Southall, Optical Society of America, New York, 1924.)
16. Kertesz, A., Lesk, D., and McCabe, P. (1977): Localisation of lesions causing aphasia. *Arch. Neurol.*, 34:590–601.
17. Mountcastle, V. B., Lynch, J. C., Georgopoulos, A., Sakata, H., and Acuna, C. (1975): Posterior parietal cortex of the monkey. *J. Neurophysiol.*, 38:871.
18. Mountcastle, V. B., and Motter, B. C. (1981): Light sensitive neurones in posterior parietal cortex. *J. Neurosci.*, 1:3–26.
19. Ober, W. B. (1979): *Boswell's Clap and Other Essays*. Southern Illinois University Press, Carbondale, Ill.
20. Ogle, K. N. (1962): Ocular dominance and binocular retinal rivalry. In: *The Eye, Vol. 4*, edited by H. Davson. Academic Press, New York.
21. Pavilidis, G. T. (1978): Dyslexics' erratic eye movements. *Dyslexia Rev.*, 1:1.
22. Porac, C., and Coren, S. (1976): The dominant eye. *Psychol. Bull.*, 83:880–897.
23. Porta, I. B. (1593): *De Refractione*. Carlinus, Naples.
24. Shatz, C., and Levay, S. (1979): Altered connections of visual cortex in siamese cat. *Science*, 204:328.
25. Stein, J. F. (1978): Effects of posterior parietal lobe cooling on reaching in the conscious monkey. In: *Active Touch*, edited by G. Gordon. Pergamon, New York.
26. Stein, J. F., and Fowler, M. S. (1981): Visual dyslexia. *Trends Neurosci.* 4:77–80.

27. Stein, J. F., and Fowler, M. S. (1982): Diagnosis of dyslexia by means of a new indicator of eye dominance. *Br. J. Ophthalmol.*, 66:332–336.
28. Vellutino, F. R. (1978): In: *Dyslexia*, edited by A. L. Benton and D. Pearl. Oxford University Press, Oxford.
29. Walls, G. L. (1951): A theory of ocular dominance. *Arch. Ophthalmol.*, 28:834–844.

Advances in Neurology, Vol. 42: Progress in Aphasiology, edited by F. C. Rose.
Raven Press, New York © 1984.

Involvement of Head Movement in Speech Production and Its Implications for Language Pathology

U. Hadar, T. J. Steiner, and F. Clifford Rose

Department of Neurology, Charing Cross Hospital, London W6 8RF, England

The relationship between speech and accompanying body movements is an important aspect of communication in general, and speech production in particular, bearing on many levels of linguistic performance (15). It offers a unique route for investigating cognitive processes underlying speech production (7,37), encoding and decoding processes (14), and the production of suprasegmental features, such as stress, intonation, rate, and rhythm (1,2,9).

The precise role of speech-related body movement and its relationship to linguistic and cognitive processes is a controversial issue. While some researchers view it as a highly structured system of communicative functions that are different from, independent of, and parallel to, speech (2,26), others claim that it reflects speech-related, prelinguistic processes at a motor level of cognition (29,36), and still others have conceived it as an independent part of the totality of communicative behavior, integrated with speech at a low level of general purpose control systems (1,10).

The latter approaches suggest the possibility that body movement is an integral part of speech production in both affecting and reflecting the motor processes of speech. Such interpretation does not exclude the possibility of independent cognitive functions, nor does it mean that body movements are part of the central programs for speech production, but it differs from cognitive and linguistic approaches in a number of implications.

While cognitive and linguistic approaches imply a correlation of movement with semantic and syntactic units of speech (7,25,43), the speech production thesis suggests a correlation with speech gestures (movement of articulators). This, in turn, implies that speaking as such may be accompanied by movement, irrespective of cognitive complexity or linguistic meaningfulness. Moreover, movement of certain body parts, such as the head or left hand (37), should correlate with the suprasegmental features of rate, duration, tone, and stress more significantly than with other speech features, as these are the most general products of speech gestures. Such body movement should possess differential physical properties analogous to or at least as rich and specific as those of the suprasegmental features. It was with this background that our study of head movement during speech was conducted.

METHODS

Although these introductory considerations appear theoretical, they offer clear methodologic indications. For instance, studies of the physical properties of kinesic behavior during speech (e.g., tempo, rhythm, intensity) have usually concentrated on head movement. Moreover, the hands and the head, moving during speech more than any other body part (14,40), are the best sources of kinesic information, but hand gestures are usually seen as dominated by symbolic rather than rhythmic functions (7,37); head movement is more relevant for our purposes. Similarly, the introductory framework for studying body movement with speech indicates, to a large extent, the monitoring techniques that can be employed: if physical richness of suprasegmental phenomena is to be found in movement, then measurement must be precise, with easy access to information regarding range, duration, speed, and intensity of movement.

For these reasons, the polarized light goniometer was employed. It operates by projecting strong light from a single source through a plane polarizer material and a rapidly rotating disk on to target and reference photosensors (38). Phase differences between the target and reference photosensors create a proportional voltage output, which can be processed, recorded, and then analyzed. In our studies, two photosensors were attached to the subject's head, one to the vertex directed upward, and one to the temple directed laterally (Fig. 1). Their output, rectified and summed, was proportional to the absolute, angular displacement of the head from an arbitrary external reference.

During conversation, movement of the head was recorded in synchrony with speech and a signal proportional to peak amplitude of sound waves (peak loudness). These signals were plotted on paper (Fig. 2) and analyzed both individually and in relation to each other.

While the head movement chart did not specify directions of movements, it offered an easy, almost immediate access to properties such as rate, duration, range, and speed of movement. Similarly, although the peak loudness chart could offer no information about segmental phonetic features of speech, it provided an easy access to suprasegmental features, e.g., pauses and their duration, prosodic phrases, their beginning and end, relative level of speech effort and, to some degree, stress. Most significantly, the technique made it simple to correlate speech with head movement features, allowing analysis of their covariation.

CHART ANALYSIS AND RESULTS

Initially, the head movement charts looked complex, suggesting that movements of the head are not all of one type. Thus we sought a classification to distinguish between qualitatively different movements. Preliminary experiments on the regulation of range and speed of head movement (20) suggested that frequency of move-

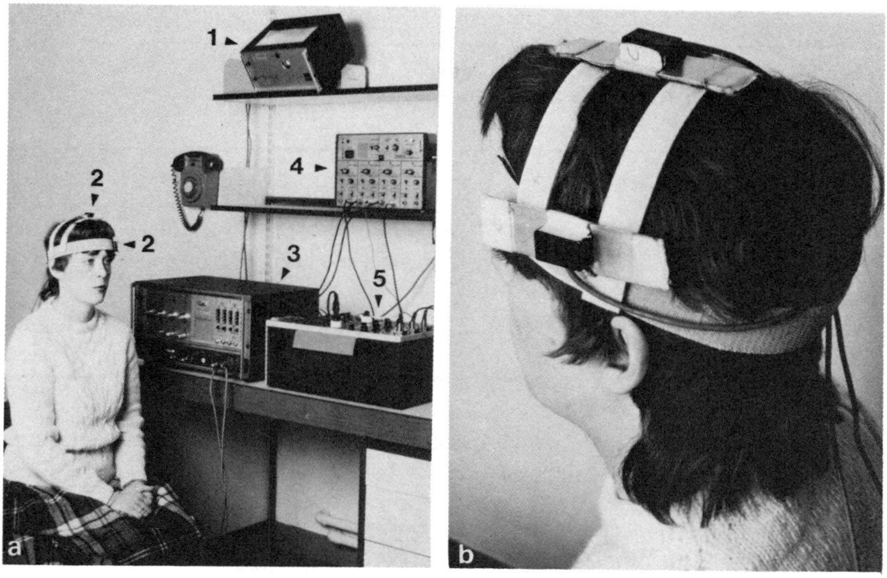

FIG. 1. The setting of instrumentation for recording head movement. **a.** General view. *1,* Projector unit; *2,* photosensors; *3,* processing unit; *4,* tape recorder; *5,* pen recorder. **b.** Arrangement of sensors on the head.

ment, in terms of cycles per unit time, is the most stable feature of a number of motor tasks and is essential to the motor regulation of speed, rhythm, intensity, and so forth. This indicated that a meaningful classification of movements might best refer to frequency features, an idea that was incorporated in our initial studies.

The first in a group of closely related studies recorded the frequencies and amplitudes of head movements at successive points in the chart 0.4 sec apart (21). Recorded frequencies were grouped into eight ranges, each spanning about 0.5 Hz

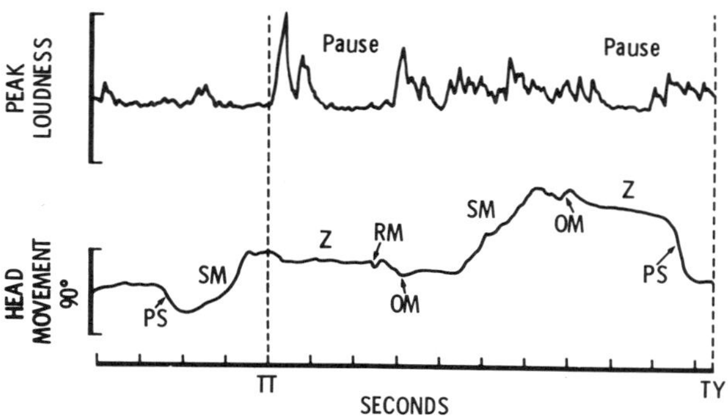

FIG. 2. Segment from an original recording featuring synchronous head movement and peak loudness. Movement types indicated are postural shifts (PS), slow movement (SM), stillness (Z), rapid movement (RM), and ordinary movement (OM). TT, turn taking; TY, turn yielding.

TABLE 1. *Distribution and amplitudes of points between various frequency ranges*

Frequency range (Hz)	No. of recorded points	Mean frequency (Hz)	Mean amplitude (deg)	SD amplitude
0.2–0.6	314	0.36	33.9	20.0
0.6–1.0	205	0.81	21.8	12.8
1.0–1.4	164	1.15	20.2	10.0
1.4–1.8	116	1.52	20.0	13.2
1.8–2.2	66	1.92	22.3	22.0
2.2–2.7	179	2.51	17.5	11.2
3.2–4.2	79	3.37	16.0	9.6
5.0–7.0	116	5.5	11.8	12.4

between 0 and 7 Hz. Table 1 shows the distribution of values between these ranges, revealing an inverse relationship between probability and frequency values. Most points recorded were of low frequency, with progressively fewer points as frequency increased, until a local minimum in the 1.8 to 2.2 Hz range. Probability then increased dramatically but fell again in the 3.7 to 4.2 Hz range, followed by a significant final increase near 5 Hz. These findings suggested a grouping of frequency values in three classes, with intermediate values being of low probability: a class of slow movements (SM) in the 0.2 to 1.8 Hz range; a class of ordinary movements (OM) in the 1.8 to 3.7 Hz range; and a class of rapid movements (RM) with frequencies higher than 3.7 Hz.

In the same study, amplitude of movement was found to be inversely related to frequency (Fig. 3). However, linear, nonrecurring movements at the higher ranges diverged from this rule, with wider amplitudes at higher frequencies. This suggested that wide linear movements of high frequencies belong to a separate kinematic class, referred to as postural shifts (PS). To the extent that these classes reflect a significant characteristic of head movement in the context of conversation and speech, they could be expected to correlate with differential aspects of speech, specifically with suprasegmental features. With this in mind, taking care not to exclude the possible

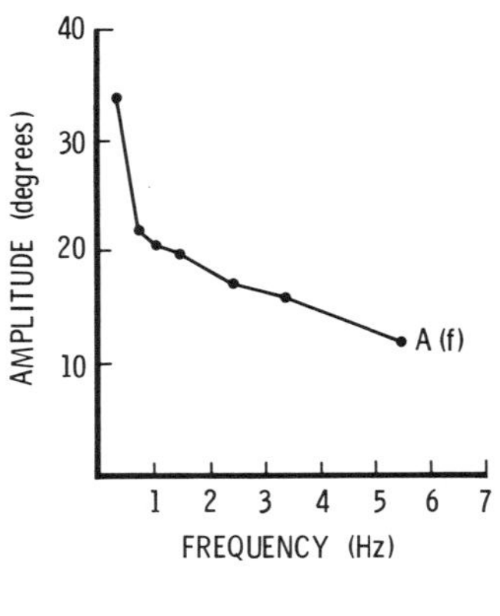

FIG. 3. Mean amplitude of each range plotted against mean frequency. The graph A(f) represents a rule by which amplitudes and frequencies are inversely related.

relevance of syntactic and semantic aspects, the timing of movements of various classes was investigated.

In the next study, PS were associated with progressively narrower speech categories: the wide domain of speaking was demarcated from listening and then subdivided into pause versus nonpause periods (22). As can be seen in Table 2, most PS occurred in association with speech, usually with pauses. Pause PS occurred roughly equally with pauses separating speaking turns (switching pauses) and with pauses inside speaking turns (inturn pauses); since the probability of occurrence of switching pauses was lower than that of inturn pauses, this indicated a greater tendency of PS to occur at turn taking (Table 2). Most inturn PS occurred between rather than inside syntactic boundaries (inter- and intrasentential, respectively). Furthermore, PS occurred primarily after half the duration of the pause had elapsed, in conjunction with the initiation of speech, and rarely either toward the termination of phonation (the beginning of the pause) or in the middle of pauses. Finally, PS occurred significantly prior to rather than after speech onset (prevocal).

These results suggested a general pattern of initiating speech with a PS, especially after long silences or with the transition from macro planning (6) to execution of speech. Although this could be interpreted as originating from cognitive processes, e.g., marking semantic boundaries (43), the recurring prevocal timing suggested a motor function. Specifically, PS seemed to be part of a complex of coordinated body movements, such as lateral eye and head movements (31) or eye blinking (45), that accompany speech onset. It was thought that the initiation of speech, being a highly complex task and involving many degrees of freedom (17), incorporated these movements to help regulate the initiation of speech by amplifying and scaling up the level of central, neural activity and by phasing the movements of the articulators. We thought that PS might serve to coordinate the onset of movement of the articulators, as an orchestra conductor coordinates the onset of play by raising his hands. The movement of a closely related organ may provide the articulators with an external reference against which their own movement can be phased. At the same time, inertic forces on the articulators, created by movement of the head, may elicit a basic level of tension necessary for onset of their movement (roughly analogous to the players positioning their instruments at the raising of the conductor's hands). Unlike the orchestra, in speech, the force for positioning gestures may be partly created by the "conducting" head movement itself.

The finding of a characteristic movement pattern at or around initial positions of speech suggested that terminal speech positions, i.e., those preceding pauses in speech, might also be of kinesic interest. Characteristic speech patterns toward pauses, referred to as terminal juncture, were thought of as establishing prosodic boundaries, thereby being of great linguistic importance. This, together with the basic affinity between movement and suprasegmentals, made terminal juncture an obvious target for kinesic studies (2), but the issue had not been investigated beyond Birdwhistell's observations.

Linguistically, terminal juncture is but one of a number of features that characterize speech across its segments (phonemes, morphemes) known as suprasegmental

TABLE 2. *Timing of PS in relation to speech, presented as their distribution between speech categories*[a]

<table>
<tr><th colspan="10">Location</th><th>Total</th><th>Significance ($df = 1$)[b]</th></tr>
<tr><td>Listening
10</td><td colspan="9">Speaking
89</td><td>99</td><td>$G = 94.5$
$p < 0.005$</td></tr>
<tr><td></td><td>Nonpause
11</td><td colspan="8">Pause
78</td><td>89</td><td>$G = 60.1$
$p < 0.005$</td></tr>
<tr><td></td><td></td><td colspan="5">Inturn
37</td><td colspan="3">Switching
41</td><td>78</td><td>$G = 4.1$
$p < 0.05$</td></tr>
<tr><td></td><td></td><td>Intrasen-
tential
10</td><td colspan="4">Intersentential
27</td><td colspan="3"></td><td>37</td><td>$G = 16.2$
$p < 0.005$</td></tr>
<tr><td></td><td></td><td></td><td colspan="2">Initiation
15</td><td>Midpause
8</td><td>Termination
4</td><td colspan="2">Initiation
30</td><td>Termination
11</td><td>68</td><td>$G = 14.5$
$p < 0.005$</td></tr>
<tr><td></td><td></td><td></td><td>Prevocal
13</td><td>Postvocal
2</td><td></td><td></td><td>Prevocal
17</td><td>Postvocal
9</td><td></td><td>41</td><td>$G = 8.2$
$p < 0.005$</td></tr>
</table>

[a] Levels of analysis consist of a pair of complementary categories, and each level is contained in all higher levels.
[b] Expected values for significance tests were derived from relative frequency of occurrence of each category. *G* values, corrected for continuity.

TABLE 3. *Distinct head movements and their relationship to stress*[a]

Movement	1 Share of movement classes in total of distinct movement (%)	2 Share of classes in head movement concurrent with primary peaks (%)	3 Percentage of movements in phase with peak loudness	4 Percentage of "on" movement with major peaks
RM	36.2	24.1	90.3	87.7
OM	40.2	35.5	42.5	75.0
PS	23.6	13.8	44.7	80.0

[a] RM implied a major peak in loudness.

features (34). These, comprising juncture, stress, speech rate, and duration of syllables, establish a unitary field of study; it was logical to investigate them together. In order to take advantage of the technical simplicity of our records, it was necessary to infer the suprasegmental features from the peak loudness charts. This virtually excluded both speech rate and duration of syllables from the investigation, while stress could be crudely associated with peak loudness. Terminal juncture was divided into patterns that preceded the last peak loudness prior to a long pause (terminal contour) and the pause itself (terminal pause).

A two-way analysis of the relationship between movement and peak loudness was conducted by establishing the position and amplitude of peaks with distinct head movements and the movement pattern coinciding with major peaks in loudness, with terminal contour and terminal pause (23). Although primary peaks of loudness were accompanied by distinct movements in 74.2% of cases, the probability of occurrence of each specific class of movement (Table 3) was roughly proportional to its overall probability of occurrence. However, RM occurred, most significantly, in phase with ("on") a peak in loudness, indicating a major peak, more than did other distinct movements. Movements with terminal contour (immediately prior to terminal pause) were OM in half the cases and SM in one-fourth; but only about 26% of all OM and 20% of all SM occurred at terminal positions.

In short, while major peaks in loudness did not necessarily imply a RM, RM implied a major peak. Conversely, while terminal contours correlated strongly with OM, the occurrence of an OM was only weakly indicative of terminal contour. These asymmetric rules suggested the primacy of head over articulatory movement in regulating high energies; the movement feature of intense sharpness was imposed on prosody, creating a major stress. At lower energies, such as in smooth variation of prosody toward boundaries, the prosodic position relative to the boundary invoked OM, but not vice versa. Furthermore, movements immediately following terminal contour were slow or still in 85.5% of cases, suggesting that boundaries are marked by the juxtaposition of distinct movement and stillness, which is an important factor in analyzing the relationship between motor and linguistic determinants (23).

We are currently conducting a study of head movement with speech dysfluencies, which further supports association of movement with suprasegmental features. Initial results indicate that a frequent pattern with speech onset following a grammatic pause (between syntactic boundaries) is intense movement prior to or with the first primary stress. Other than that, movement correlates with drastic prosodic transitions detectable in transitions of peak loudness rather than with grammatic categories. For instance, a head movement at the neighborhood of a dysfluency is more consistently indicated by a large increase in loudness than by semantic, syntactic, or phonologic characteristics, such as level of repetition (phoneme, word, clause), nongrammaticality of the related pause, semantic extent of self correction, and so on. In addition, where head movements occurred with sharp prosodic transitions, they seemed to start around 0.1 sec prior to the first major stress. This suggests that such movements may be involved in both the regulation of high energies, invoked for the transformation of current coordinative constants (determined by invariants of the ongoing performance), and the phasing of the articulators following breakdown of the set relationships between them prior to the dysfluency.

ROLE OF HEAD MOVEMENTS

Our results pointed to a clear and specific involvement of head movements with speaking, mainly with speech onset, stress, terminal juncture, and sharp prosodic transitions. We have offered a few specific suggestions as to their possible functions, with reference to two fundamental concepts in the theory of action: (a) the dissipation of energy, and (b) the phasing of movements of the articulators. While the first has been thought of as predominant in the regulation of stress, the latter is central in explaining speech onset. Both appear to combine in interpreting the role of head movements in speech dysfluencies. Indeed, it is most likely that the two concepts together explain complementary aspects of motor action, where the theoretical objective is reducing the computational load on the central programer, whatever that may be (33). Reduction in computational load suggests that actions are not actually programed; instead, the related organs and muscles may be constrained to operate as a group (coordinative structure) by fixing the relationships between them. In this case, the central system need specify only those constants that relate the operation of one muscle (or group of muscles) to another. Thus two groups of muscles, A and B, create a coordinative structure if the zero length, l^*, and tension level, t^*, of the one varies as a function, F, of these values in the other: $(l^*,t^*)\ (A) = F\ ((l^*,t^*)\ (B))$. Once these values are (centrally) set, a peripheral or external change in the values of one group is sufficient to bring about a coordinated change in the other without further central intervention. Such changes, referred to as perturbations, are limited in range, and changes outside this range require central resetting of F (see ref. 17).

These concepts are most suitable for explaining the role of head movements in speech production, as they allow for a functional integration into speech production of movements that are not articulatory. For instance, the set relationships between the variation of glottal closure, pharyngeal configurations, and movement of the larynx (4) mean that a sharp head movement, creating a sharp increase in air pressure followed by rapid release of the glottis, may be integrated into speech production as a stress-producing mechanism. It results in an acute increase in loudness, pitch, and syllable duration. In this manner, a single and simple command to muscles of the neck may bring about the complex movements required for stress, without involving detailed computations. Moreover, the concepts of constraint and immediate integration allow head movements to possess coordinative functions independent of their direct effects on the articulators.

Elastic properties of the musculoskeletal structures and external forces in the natural environment are such that moving organs tend to oscillate around their equilibrium states. Thus coordinative structures may be analyzed dynamically by analogy with mechanical mass-spring systems, approximated mathematically by second order differential equations (39). In the case of speech, an articulator can be thought of as an oscillator and speech gestures as a product space of oscillators (44), whose basic constituents are amplitudes, frequencies, and phases of the various articulators. In these terms, movements of the articulators may be characterized as having relatively high frequencies, narrow amplitudes, and variable articulatory phases (reflected in coarticulation, i.e., the simultaneous movement of the articulators toward different phonetic targets). Each of these characteristics may limit the articulatory system, which is compensated for, in part, by head movement.

Movements of the articulators are (inherently) of high natural frequencies because of their relatively low mass and the shortness of the muscles subserving them. Therefore, slowing down may impose an extra burden on the articulatory system, which may be alleviated by implementing externally some kind of slowing device. Indeed, terminal contour, which involves a characteristic lowering of speech rate (34), was most often accompanied by (ordinary) head movement. It may be that the regulation of slower articulatory movement is enhanced by coordinating it with head movement, which is of lower natural frequency. (Note that we use the term coordinating in the sense of fixing the relationships between variation of zero lengths and tensions.)

Since the dissipation of energy is dynamically correlated with amplitude, restriction of amplitude implies innate weakness of the articulatory system in regulating high energies. Moreover, the high frequencies required for speech may be disturbed by increasing amplitude. In continuous performances, an increase in amplitude involves the lowering of frequency (20,21). Dittman (14) recognized this weakness, claiming that the numerous movements associated with speech dysfluencies arise from a motor overflow or the spreading in the motor system of excessive energy. Unlike Dittman, we hold that body movements, especially head movements, serve consistently for the regulation of high energy: they occur when intense effort is required, either for reasserting coordinative constants following a dysfluency or for the production of stress. In addition, patients with motor dysphasia, who tend to speak with a highly redundant level of effort, also display the highest ratio of body movements to articulatory gestures (8). This thesis implies that excessive body movement should also occur with effort in other circumstances, such as when speaking loudly or with excitement. Such evidence would further support the functional as-

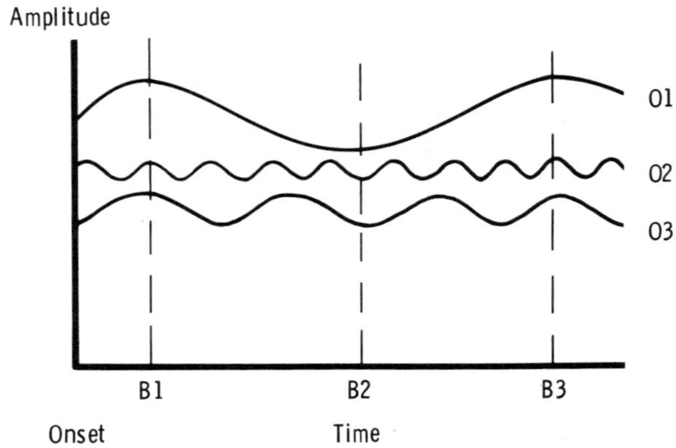

FIG. 4. Schematic illustration of the coincidence of phases in oscillators of different frequencies (01, 02, and 03). The conduction of such oscillators may be achieved economically if the reference beats are introduced where the phases coincide (B1, B2, and B3).

sociation of body movement with the regulation of high energy, developed in compensation for an inherent articulatory weakness.

Just as the restriction of amplitudes of the articulators could motivate the functional integration of head movement into speech for the regulation of high energies, the variable articulatory phases seem to motivate the integration of head movements for coordinative purposes. In terms of the orchestral metaphor, the conductor's role becomes more essential the more dissimilar the rhythms of different instruments; with complicated pieces of music, a coordinated performance may become impossible without an external pacemaker who himself has no playing part. Generally, this is the coordinating task we suggest for head movements. Coordination may be achieved more economically if the pacemaker's beats are given at the points where phases coincide (Fig. 4). These do not have to be at equal intervals, as they depend on the ratios of frequencies and phases of the related oscillators. Therefore, the beat of the pacemaker, in this case the head, does not need to be at equal intervals to be a useful conductor. Instead, the points in time at which beats (i.e., distinct head movements) are most likely to occur, in our model, should prove computable by a mechanical analysis of movements of the articulators. One obvious point is speech onset, which is self evident and does not require further discussion. Another point of crucial importance for this model is stress, where the characteristic impact on the articulators, reflected in the longer duration of the concurring syllable, may bring about the synchronization of phases. Other than at these points, coincidence of phases should depend on phonetic properties of the particular articulatory sequence.

Although head movements have hitherto been considered functional only in the motor sense, with sole reference to prosody and suprasegmental features, we think they bear on, and closely interact with, linguistic functions, i.e., the semantic, syntactic, and phonologic components of language performance. While the relationship between language and motor operations in speech is still largely unknown, some discussion of this issue is necessary to complete our argument.

The prime nature of motor operations was argued strongly by Kimura (30), who claimed that speech pathology may be accounted for, to a large extent, by motor impairment of skilled performance, with no independent language pathology. Others denied this, claiming that many clinical observations could not be explained purely in terms of motor operations (12,35). Another similar thesis, advanced by McNeill (36), stated that underlying linguistic performance, both phylogenetically and ontogenetically, was a whole level of gestural symbolism based on iconicity, i.e., on a morphologic similarity between the movement and its significance. This thesis is unsuitable for our model, for it refers to a mode of signification (iconicity) that is inapplicable to head movements; it does not possess the necessary morphologic sophistication. A third version of this concept, advanced by Kinsbourne (32), seems relevant—indeed, directly related—to the possible role of head movements in linguistic operations. Guided by evidence from head and eye movements during speech, Kinsbourne (32) stated that language has developed in the context of a semantic field created by orienting movements of the head and mediated by both auditory and visual perception. Such orienting responses do not signify in the usual sense of referring but rather in differentially synchronizing events in the environment (11). This synchronization, based on extended use of orienting responses, refers to an event by underlining or accenting its spatiotemporal constituents: the intensity of the response correlates, within limits, with intensity of the event, and their phases coincide. This mode of referring characterizes the semantic function of stress in language (3) and should prove the major route through which head movements affect linguistic operations. McNeill and Levy (37) recognized the importance of such movements, which they referred to as beats, but failed to note their semantic importance.

IMPLICATIONS FOR SPEECH PATHOLOGY

Suprasegmental impairment in aphasia has been studied since interest was first shown in speech pathology, with variable results regarding speech onset (13,19), speech rate (19,27), intonation (27,41), and stress (18). Although disturbances were often regarded as closely related to body movement, in the context of both speech production (8) and symbolic gesture (16), a number of important implications, highlighted by our studies, have escaped proper consideration. First, the extent to which the control of suprasegmentals relates to systems of general purpose motor control suggests that rehabilitation of faculties, such as speech onset, rate, intonation, and volume, may be enhanced by improvement of movement control in general. Second, head movements may be of unique importance in this respect because of their direct effects on both articulatory gestures and perceptual processing. Third, this association with head movements, together with Kinsbourne's (32) ideas, suggests that the linguistic functions of suprasegmentals, centered around the regulation of stress, may be both accounted for and rehabilitated by reference to head movements and orienting responses.

Although there is clear evidence that some of the prosodic impairment in aphasia originates directly from apraxia of one or more of the articulators (28), most of it has no organ-specific, but rather general motor, origin, closely related to the generation of rhythms by the nervous system (see also ref. 46). It is important to note that we do not refer here to general purpose, left hemisphere centers for skilled performances, but rather to the central mechanisms involved in the regulation of the dissipation of energy, with primary right hemisphere functions (30,47). Indeed, those hand movements that most closely correlate with suprasegmentals, i.e., beats, are notably movements of the left hand, unlike the iconic right hand movements (37).

Inasmuch as these central mechanisms apply to a wide range of motor operations, they depend heavily on the regulation of behavioral cyclicities (33); thus the rehabilitation of their normal function involves the reestablishment of behavioral cyclicities (see also Hadar et al., *this volume*). Even if the breakdown of speech-related cyclicities is not of cognitive consequence in itself, it may result in cognitive impairment, imposing an extra load on memory and retrieval systems (42). Furthermore, the possibility exists that various linguistic structures also involve the regulation of cycles (46) and may be restored, at least in part, by improving the related cyclic performances. The possibility of a linguistic gain from the reestablishment of behavioral cyclicities does not depend on a primary deficit in cyclic performance as such. A well-preserved general purpose capacity for cyclic performance could be used for restoring a linguistic function by approximating, step by step, the cyclic structure induced by the linguistic form. Although we are unable to specify the fine details of these approximations, they probably start at the low frequency end with the respiratory cycle, proceeding with the slow cycle of body movement and intonation (5) onto the various speech rhythms demonstrated in their pure form in poetic verse. The experimental use of these cycles for the rehabilitation of speech in aphasic patients is described in Hadar et al. (*this volume*).

We have not yet analyzed the patterns of head movements accompanying aphasic speech, but the results from normals suggest that these movements could play a major role in compensating for the loss of speech-related motor cyclicities. Cicone et al. (8) have reported a marked increase in body movements per speech gestures in Broca's aphasia, which should prove to be centered around and specific to speech onset, stress, maintenance of smooth contours, and sharp prosodic transitions. In this respect, it may be expected that head movements will play a role beyond their direct effects on the articulators, mediated by visual and vestibular processes. Some of these have already been reported (31,45), but much remains to be done.

Finally, the study of the linguistic deficits arising from impaired regulation of stress, even when of peripheral origin, is far from being exhausted. A firm basis has been laid by the work of Gleason and Goodglass and co-workers (18,19), which showed that some of the features of agrammatic speech may be accounted for by the distribution of stress at sentence level. For instance, unstressed grammatic words in initial positions were most likely to be omitted by agrammatic patients, whereas those that were stressed or in the middle position were preserved. More generally, agrammatic speech seems to be determined by the sentence level placement of stress and word level boundaries (open juncture) (24). It is possible that the creation of linguistic form in these patients has become heavily dependent on the linguistically prominent term, with the tendency to preserve words that contribute to the singularization of this term, i.e., to the placement of stress. Both cerebral hemispheres appear to be capable of producing this type of speech (5), and, in accord with Kinsbourne (32), it may be seen as a regressive type of linguistic formation based on the generative role of orienting responses. Although we feel that the generative function of stress in such linguistic formation is probably supported by the structuring function of smooth variation of contour, as in the differential establishment of declarative versus question versus commanding inflections, there is only indirect evidence from language pathology to that effect (11a).

SUMMARY

Analysis of head movement during speech, monitored by the polarized light goniometer, showed that head movement accompanies speech almost continuously in a manner specific to the concomitant, suprasegmental speech features. Thus initiation of speech after long pauses was accompanied by wide, linear movements (PS). The termination of speech in a pause (terminal juncture) was accompanied by movements of medium amplitudes and frequencies (OM). Sharp, intense movements (RM) were indicative of a peak in loudness, and often of a major phonetic stress. Finally, a speech disturbance was accompanied by movement if it involved a sharp prosodic transition.

We suggest that these correlations indicate that head movement may have a role in speech production, regulating the many degrees of freedom and the dissipation of energy in speech. Furthermore, head movements may play a role in linguistic processing through the generative functions of stress, prominence, and orienting responses. Implications for speech pathology, especially dysphasia, are discussed.

REFERENCES

1. Bennett, A. T. (1980): Rhythmic analysis of multiple levels of communicative behaviour in face to face interaction. In: *Aspects of Nonverbal Communication,* edited by W. van Raffler-Engel, pp. 237–251. Swets and Zeitlinger, Lisse, The Netherlands.
2. Birdwhistell, R. L. (1970): *Kinesics and Context.* University of Pennsylvania Press, Philadelphia.
3. Bolinger, D. (1980): Accents that determine stress. In: *The Relationship of Verbal and Nonverbal Communication,* edited by M. R. Key, pp. 37–48. Mouton, The Hague.
4. Broad, D. J. (1979): The new theories of vocal fold vibration. In: *Speech and Language: Advances in Basic Research and Practice, Vol. 2,* edited by N. J. Lass, pp. 203–255. Academic Press, New York.
5. Brown, J. W. (1982): Hierarchy and evolution in neurolinguistics. In: *Neural Models of Language Processes,* edited by M. Arbib, D. Caplan, and J. Marshall, pp. 447–467. Academic Press, New York.
6. Butterworth, B. L. (1980): Evidence from pauses in speech. In: *Language Production, Vol. 1,* edited by B. L. Butterworth, pp. 155–176. Academic Press, New York.
7. Butterworth, B. L., and Beattie, G. W. (1978): Gesture and silence as indicators of planning in speech. In: *Recent Advances in the Psychology of Language 4: Formal and Experimental Approaches,* edited by N. R. Campbell and P. T. Smith, pp. 347–360. Plenum Books, London.

8. Cicone, M., Wapner, W., Foldi, N., Zurif, E., and Gardner, H. (1979): The relation between gesture and language in aphasic communication. *Brain Lang.*, 8:324–349.
9. Condon, W. S. (1980): The relation of interactional synchrony to cognitive and emotional processes. In: *The Relation of Verbal and Nonverbal Communication*, edited by M. R. Key, pp. 49–66. Mouton, The Hague.
10. Condon, W. S., and Ogston, W. D. (1967): A segmentation of behavior. *J. Psychiatr. Res.*, 5:221–235.
11. Condon, W. S., and Sander, L. W. (1974): Synchrony demonstrated between movements of the neonate and adult speech. *Child Dev.*, 45:456–462.
11a. Danly, M., and Shapiro, B. (1982): Speech prosody in Broca's aphasia. *Brain Lang.*, 16:171–190.
12. Darley, F. L., Aronson, A. E., and Brown, J. R. (1975): *Motor Speech Disorders.* Saunders, Philadelphia.
13. Delis, D., Foldi, N., Hamby, S., Gardner, H., and Zurif, E. (1979): A note on the temporal relations between language and gesture. *Brain Lang.* 8:350–354.
14. Dittman, A. T. (1972): The body movement-speech rhythm relationship as a cue for speech encoding. In: *Studies in Dyadic Communication*, edited by A. W. Siegman and B. Pope, pp. 135–152. Academic Press, New York.
15. Dittman, A. T. (1978): The role of body movement in communication. In: *Nonverbal Behavior and Communication*, edited by A. W. Siegman and S. Feldstein, pp. 69–95. Lawrence Erlbaum, Hillsdale, New Jersey.
16. Feyereisen, P., and Seron, X. (1982): Nonverbal communication in aphasia—a review. 2: Expression. *Brain Lang.*, 16:213–236.
17. Fowler, C. A., Rubin, P., Remez, R. E., and Turvey, M. T. (1980): Implications for speech production of a general theory of action. In: *Language Production, Vol. 1*, edited by B. L. Butterworth, pp. 373–420. Academic Press, London.
18. Gleason, J. B., Goodglass, H., Green, E., Ackerman, N., and Hyde, M. R. (1975): The retrieval of syntax in Broca's aphasia. *Brain Lang.*, 2:451–471.
19. Goodglass, H. (1976): Agrammatism. In: *Studies in Neurolinguistics, Vol. 1*, edited by H. Whitaker and H. A. Whitaker, pp. 237–260. Academic Press, New York.
20. Hadar, U., and Steiner, T. J. (1982): Speed related motor behavior and its implications for motor control. *J. Physiol.*, 324:6.
21. Hadar, U., Steiner, T. J., Grant, E. C., and Rose, F. C. (1983): Kinematics of head movement accompanying speech during conversation. *Hum. Movement Sci.*, 2:35–46.
22. Hadar, U., Steiner, T. J., Grant, E. C., and Rose, F. C. (1984): The timing of shifts of head postures during conversation. *Hum. Movement Sci.* , 3 (*in press*).
23. Hadar, U., Steiner, T. J., Grant, E. C., and Rose, F. C. (1983): Head movement correlates of juncture and stress at sentence level. *Lang. Speech*, 26:117–129.
24. Kean, M-L. (1980): Grammatical representation and the description of processing. In: *Biological Studies of Mental Processes*, edited by D. Caplan, pp. 239–268. MIT Press, Cambridge, Massachusetts.
25. Kendon, A. (1972): Some relationship between body movement and speech. In: *Studies in Dyadic Communication*, edited by A. W. Siegman and B. Pope, pp. 177–210. Pergamon Press, New York.
26. Kendon, A. (1980): Gesticulation and speech: Two aspects of the process of utterance. In: *The Relation of Verbal and Nonverbal Communication*, edited by M. R. Key, pp. 207–228. Mouton, The Hague.
27. Kent, R. D., and Rosenbek, J. C. (1982): Prosodic disturbance and neurologic lesion. *Brain Lang.*, 15:259–291.
28. Kertesz, A., and Hooper, P. (1982): Praxis and language: The extent and variety of apraxia in aphasia. *Neuropsychologia*, 20:275–286.
29. Kimura, D. (1976): The neural basis of language qua gesture. In: *Studies in Neurolinguistics Vol. 2*, edited by H. Whitaker and A. H. Whitaker, pp. 145–156. Academic Press, New York.
30. Kimura, D. (1979): Neuromotor mechanisms in the evolution of human communication. In: *Neurobiology of Social Communication in Primates: An Evolutionary Perspective,* edited by H. D. Steklis and M. J. Raleigh, pp. 197–220. Academic Press, New York.
31. Kinsbourne, M. (1972): Eye and head turning indicates cerebral lateralization. *Science*, 176:539–541.
32. Kinsbourne, M. (1978): Evolution of language in relation to lateral action. In: *Asymmetrical Function of the Brain,* edited by M. Kinsbourne, pp. 553–565. Cambridge University Press, Cambridge.
33. Kugler, P. N., Kelso, J. A. S., and Turvey, M. T. (1980): On the concept of coordinative structures as dissipative structures, I: Theoretical line. In: *Tutorials in Motor Behavior*, edited by G. E. Stelmach and J. Requin, pp. 3–48. North Holland, Amsterdam.

34. Lieberman, P. (1974): A study of prosodic features. In: *Current Trends in Linguistics, Vol. 12, Part 10: Phonetics*, edited by T. A. Sebeok, pp. 2419–2451. Mouton, The Hague.
35. Marshall, J. C. (1980): Clues from neurological deficits. In: *Signed and Spoken Language: Biological Constraints on Linguistic Form*, edited by U. Bellugi and M. Studdert-Kennedy, pp. 275–290. Verlag Chemie, Weinheim.
36. McNeill, D. (1979): *The Conceptual Basis of Language*. Lawrence Erlbaum, Hillsdale, New Jersey.
37. McNeill, D., and Levy, E. (1982): Conceptual representations in language activity and gesture. In: *Speech, Place and Action*, edited by R. J. Jarvella and W. Klein, pp. 271–295. Wiley, New York.
38. Mitchelson, D. L. (1975): Recording of movement without photography. In: *Techniques for the Analysis of Human Movement*, edited by D. W. Grieve, D. I. Miller, D. L. Mitchelson, J. P. Paul, and A. J. Smith, pp. 33–69. Lepus Books, London.
39. Penev, G. D., and Tairov, O. P. (1979): Application of the principle of urgent identification in the control of complex motor systems (velocity control). *Biophysics*, 24:552–559.
40. Ragsdale, J. D., and Sylvia, C. R. (1981): Distribution of kinesic hesitation phenomena in spontaneous speech. *Lang. Speech*, 23:185–190.
41. Ryalls, J. H. (1982): Intonation in Broca's aphasia. *Neuropsychologia*, 20:355–360.
42. Saffran, E. M. (1982): Neuropsychological approaches to the study of language. *Br. J. Psychol.*, 73:317–337.
43. Scheflen, A. E. (1964): The significance of postures in communicative systems. *Psychiatry*, 27:316–333.
44. Sorokin, V. N. (1975): Analysis of the system of control of speech movements. *Biophysics*, 20:725–731.
45. Terzano, M. G., Parrino, L., Manzoni, G. C., and Mancia, D. (1983): Seizures triggered by blinking when beginning to speak. *Arch. Neurol.*, 40:103–106.
46. Turvey, M. T. (1980): Clues from the organization of motor systems. In: *Signed and Spoken Language: Biological Constraints on Linguistic Form*, edited by U. Bellugi and M. Studdert-Kennedy, pp. 41–56. Verlag Chemie, Weinheim.
47. Weintraub, S., Mesulam, M-M., and Kramer, L. (1982): Disturbances in prosody: A right hemisphere contribution to language. *Arch. Neurol.*, 38:742–744.

Advances in Neurology, Vol. 42: Progress in Aphasiology, edited by F. C. Rose.
Raven Press, New York © 1984.

Variability and Consistency in Picture Naming by Aphasic Patients

**David Howard, †Karalyn Patterson, ‡Susan Franklin, §John Morton, and *Virginia Orchard-Lisle

**Speech Therapy Department, Regional Neurological Unit, Eastern Hospital, London; **Psychology Department, University College, London; †MRC Applied Psychology Unit, Cambridge; ‡Speech Therapy Department, St. Mary Abbott's Hospital, London; and §MRC Cognitive Development Unit, London, England*

Head (10) was impressed by the variability of aphasic responses:

> It is not a sufficient test to hold up some object and ask the patient to name it; at one time he may be able to do so, at another he fails completely. No conclusion can be drawn from one or two questions put in this way; his power of responding must be tested by a series of observations in which the same task occurs on two or more occasions. (Vol. 1, p. 145)

Schuell et al. (14) argued that this variability concealed at least two types of consistency; while an individual item might elicit different responses on different days, aphasics were consistent in both the overall proportion of correct responses and the varieties of errors that they made.

The data reported in this chapter are based on the performance of 12 aphasics on three presentations of one set of 300 pictures and two presentations of a set of different pictures of the same objects. For each subject, we have a total of 1,500 naming responses, as well as the results of reading the 300 picture names. On this corpus, we conduct a number of different analyses in order to clarify a number of different claims that have been made about sources of variability in aphasic picture naming. Of particular concern is the question of whether effects reported for groups of aphasics are necessarily true for the individual patients of which the groups are composed. Group studies assume that their groups are homogeneous and combine data from different patients; is this procedure justified?

We examine the claim that aphasics may perform better in picture naming when they find neighboring items easy to name (2). We quantify the extent of the consistency of naming on different presentations of a particular picture and examine whether difficulty in naming is specific to individual pictures or whether there is a problem that is common to different pictures of the same name. Having quantified the internal consistency of individual patients' performance, we then consider the extent to which there is consistency between different patients. We examine the extent to which patients' difficulties in naming particular pictures can be accounted for by the length or frequency of its name. We then turn to the patients' naming errors and consider the extent to which they are consistent in the errors that they produce. Data are reported on how patients judge their own errors; do they believe them to be correct names for the pictures, or do they know them to be wrong?

SUBJECTS

The subjects were 12 aphasic patients aged between 44 and 76 years. One had been aphasic for only 9 months; the remainder were between 2 and 12 years post onset. On the basis of their performance on the Boston Diagnostic Aphasia Examination (BDAE) (8) six could be classified as Broca's, four as mild conduction, and two as anomic aphasics.

METHOD

Two sets of 300 pictures were prepared. Set A consisted of line drawings of objects whose names were agreed on by at least 90% of normal control subjects; set B consisted of different drawings of objects with the same names. So, where set A has a picture of a lion, set B has one too, but a different one.

The data comprise the naming performance of the 12 aphasics on the two sets of pictures and in oral reading of the picture names. The data were collected in two series. In the first, the patients named set A, then set B, and then set A again on three successive days. The second series followed approximately 3 months later; the subjects named set B, then set A, and on the third day read the written names of the pictures aloud. These six tests are referred to in this chapter as A1, B1, A2, B2, A3, and R, respectively.

Responses were scored as correct if they contained the target word; errors in plural marking were ignored. In addition, responses that had only one phonemic deviation from the target, that is, one phonemic deletion, metathesis, substitution, or addition, were counted correct. Pictures were presented for 5 sec or until the subject had produced a name with which s/he was satisfied.

Analysis 1: Effects of Success or Failure on the Previous Item

Brookshire (2) claimed that aphasics were less likely to name a picture presented in the middle of a series that they found difficult to name than when it occurred in a series of items that they could name with ease. This result could be attributable to either an effect on the subjects' "state of mind"—they get depressed by a long series of hard items and therefore are less likely to name the next item—or an inherent property of aphasic naming—that success on one picture increases the probability of success on the one that follows, and failure correspondingly lowers the probability of subsequent success, by, for instance, facilitating the links between semantic representations of pictures and verbal semantic representations of names.

If the second hypothesis is true, we would expect that successes and failures would show a tendency to occur in sequences. Therefore, we examined the data from all

TABLE 1. *Consistency between tests*

Patients	Contingencies between tests A1 & A2	A1 & B1	B1 & A2	A3 & R
Nonfluent				
T.M.	0.373	0.345	0.350	0.324
B.B.	0.329	0.361	0.382	0.091 (NS)[a]
R.B.	0.435	0.282	0.309	0.000 (NS)
J.B.	0.431	0.387	0.435	0.111 (NS)
C.R.	0.468	0.349	0.429	0.000 (NS)
P.W.	0.500	0.480	0.519	0.396
Fluent				
S.C.	0.442	0.361	0.368	0.239
M.R.	0.536	0.483	0.509	0.310
T.P.	0.468	0.453	0.405	0.000 (NS)
B.M.	0.309	0.203	0.320	0.074 (NS)
M.S.	0.525	0.506	0.490	0.205
G.G.	0.310	0.292	0.336	0.241
MEAN	0.427	0.375	0.404	0.166
Correlation by subjects	0.970	0.973	0.978	0.848
Correlation by items	0.810	0.726	0.769	0.485

[a] All contingencies and correlations are significant at $p < 0.001$, except where marked.

six tests with all patients with the "one sample runs test" (15). The results show no tendency for correct namings or failures to occur in sequences for any patient. The overall distribution of scores on the runs test does not differ from that expected by chance (Kolgorov-Smirnov test for rankable scores: $K = 1.10$; NS). We can, therefore, be confident that within a random ordering of pictures in which there are no deliberate sequences that are hard or easy to name, there is no effect of success or failure on one item on the one that follows. We can, in addition, conclude that our patients are not showing significant effects of fatigue in naming a series of 300 pictures; in that case, successes would tend to cluster toward the beginning of the test and failures toward the end.

Analysis 2: Consistency Between Different Presentations of the Same Set of Pictures

A perfectly consistent patient would invariably name a picture that s/he had successfully named on a previous occasion and always fail to name one that s/he had previously failed. A completely inconsistent patient would be equally likely to name a picture irrespective of whether or not it had been named on a previous occasion. The first patient would show a contingency coefficient (C) of 0.71, and the second of 0.00. (It is a peculiar property of contingency coefficients that, when derived from a 2 × 2 table, the maximum value is 0.71.) As can be seen from Table 1, none of our subjects was close to either extreme, but all were significantly more likely to name a picture on A2 that they had named correctly in A1 than one on which they had previously failed ($p < 0.001$). But, our aphasic subjects vary considerably in how consistent they are. At one extreme, the most consistent patient, M.R., names on A2 72% of pictures she had named on A1 but only 9% of those she had failed; the least consistent patient, B.M., names on A2 73% of his A1 successes and 38% of his failures. Success or failure on a particular item on A1 is not a reliable predictor of the patients' performance on the same item on A2. On the other hand, the correlation of 0.970 between the overall number of correct responses on A1 and A2 shows that, as Schuell et al. (14) claimed, the overall proportion of correct responses is highly predictable for each patient.

In Table 1 and all subsequent tables, the patients are assigned to the two groups—nonfluent and fluent—on the basis of their BDAE assessments. Within each group, the patients are ordered in terms of the severity of their naming impairment (mean score on tests 1–5), with the most impaired first. Inspection of Table 1 shows that consistency is not related to diagnostic group or severity of naming impairment.

Analysis 3: Consistency Between Presentations of Different Sets of Pictures

If aphasic patients are having problems only in the retrieval of picture names and not in recognition of the pictures, we would expect that they would be as likely to name a different picture of the same object as they are to name the same picture on a second attempt. For such patients, the contingencies between A1 and B1 and between B1 and A2 should be as high as the contingency between A1 and A2. If, on the other hand, subjects are having difficulty in recognizing the pictures, they should show substantially lower contingencies between different picture sets than between two presentations of the same set, because, to some extent, their difficulties will be specific to the particular pictures involved. Examination of the data in Table 1 shows that for 11 of the 12 patients, contingencies between sets A and B are as high as the contingency for the two presentations of set A; only R.B. shows substantially lower consistency between the two different picture sets than he does between the two presentations of set A. R.B.'s retrieval of a picture name appears to depend on the particular representation of the object concerned, suggesting that he alone of the subjects may have problems in the recognition of pictures as well as in retrieval of their names. Correlation of the scores by patients of 0.97 shows that the overall levels of performance on the two picture sets are closely related, and correlation by items shows that the pictures of the same name are causing problems in different tests, irrespective of the particular pictures involved. The problems of our aphasic patients, with one possible exception, are in the process of name retrieval rather than picture recognition. This result replicates, in an indirect fashion, for single subjects, the outcome of a number of group studies that show that patients' success in naming is independent of the representation of the object concerned, whether object, line drawing, or photograph (6,9).

All our patients, with the exception of T.M., are substantially better at reading picture names aloud than at naming the pictures. The contingencies between naming

TABLE 2. *Naming and reading for each patient correlated with the remaining patients as a group*

	Naming tests 1–5		Reading	
Patient	r	% var acc[a]	r	% var acc[a]
Nonfluent				
T.M.	0.452	20.5	0.147[c]	2.2
B.B.	0.573	32.8	0.144[c]	2.1
R.B.	0.552	30.5	0.158[c]	2.5
J.B.	0.453	20.5	0.209	4.4
C.R.	0.563	31.7	0.069 (NS)	0.5
P.W.	0.396	15.7	0.097[b]	0.9
Fluent				
S.C.	0.531	28.2	0.191	3.6
M.R.	0.648	42.0	0.289	8.3
T.P.	0.552	30.4	—	—
B.M.	0.460	21.2	0.159[c]	2.5
M.S.	0.559	31.3	0.216	4.6
G.G.	0.476	22.6	0.256	6.6

[a] Percentage of the variance accounted for by each correlation.
[b] $p < 0.05$; [c] $p < 0.01$; NS, not significant. Remainder are $p < 0.001$. T.P. made no errors in reading.

and reading (Table 1) suffer as a result from floor effects. Six of the 12 patients are significantly less likely to read a name where they cannot name a picture of the same name, showing that for these patients, difficulties with some words are independent of whether they are presented for reading or as pictures to name. The correlation of scores by items between A3 and R shows that the same words are causing difficulty in both tests.

(The scores of the patients on all five naming tests intercorrelate at between 0.916 and 0.983; the scores by items correlate between 0.665 and 0.805. As all the naming tests are so closely related, the analyses that follow are based on the combined scores on all five tests. Essentially identical patterns of results are found when the analyses are applied to each test individually.)

Analysis 4: Consistency Between Patients

Some pictures are consistently difficult for an individual aphasic to name; others are consistently easy. In this section, we address the question of whether different aphasic patients have difficulty with the same items.

For each patient, the naming and reading scores for each item were correlated with the scores of the remaining 11 patients combined. The results are shown in Table 2, together with the amount of variance accounted for by each correlation.

In naming, all the subjects show a highly significant degree of consistency with the remaining patients. Nevertheless, the correlations account for only 15 to 42% of the variance for each patient; for each subject, the majority of the variance must be accounted for by factors idiosyncratic to that patient. Of these, perhaps the most important is the day-to-day variability of performance with individual items. The correlations show that in reading, the patients are always less consistent with each other than they are in naming; this is not surprising when we consider that these patients show a variety of different and specific patterns of reading impairment. For example, P.W., B.B., and T.M. are deep dyslexics; R.B. and J.B. are phonological dyslexics; T.P. is a recovered letter-by-letter reader; and other patients, except for occasional slips, are able to read all isolated single words. Some pictures are hard for all the patients to name, and others are easy; in the next analysis, we examine two of the factors that may determine this.

Analysis 5: Effects of Word Frequency and Length

To what extent can the difficulty that patients have with particular words be attributed to word frequency or length? To examine this question, the frequencies of each word were taken from Kucera and Francis (11) [ranging from 867 words per million (wpm) to those that do not appear in the corpus], and the number of phonemes in each name were counted (range, 2–9). Log word frequency (WF, setting those with frequency 0 to 0.5) and phoneme length (WL) were correlated with mean probability of naming for the patients as a group; the effects of WF were significantly greater than those of WL. As these two measures correlate with each other, all WL effects reported are partial correlations.

The correlations between naming and reading and WF and WL are shown for the individual patients and the patients as a group in Table 3. For the patients as a group, there is a highly significant correlation with WF of 0.333 accounting for 11.1% of the variance; once this has been allowed for, there is a significant correlation with WL of −0.156, accounting for a further 3.2% of the variance. In reading, only WF affects the group scores, accounting for 10.0% of the variance.

Analysis 4 showed that there was much in common between the performance of individual patients. The high consistency between different picture sets (analysis 3) shows that this must be a property of particular names rather than particular pictures. Analysis 5 shows that word frequency and word length do account for a small proportion of the difficulties with names that the patients have in common; the remainder must be due to other properties of the names not related to their frequency or length.

With the individual patients, there is a remarkable degree of variation in the way they are affected by the variables of WF and WL in naming and reading. At one extreme, B.M. shows no effects of either variable in either task; at the other, B.B. is affected by both WF and WL in both tasks. There is a tendency for patients who show WF effects in reading to show them in naming too, but there is an exception (R.B.). Again, one could argue that there was a tendency for fluent patients to be less likely to be affected by word length than nonfluent aphasics; G.G. and J.B. are the exceptions. The only generalization these results allow is that aphasic patients may or may not show effects of word frequency and word length in either reading or naming. "Classical" diagnostic categories are no guide to whether they do or not;

TABLE 3. *Effects of word frequency and word length on naming and reading*[a]

Patient	Naming tests 1–5 correlation with		Reading correlation with	
	Word frequency	Word length	Word frequency	Word length
Nonfluent				
T.M.	0.166[c]	−0.099[d]	0.068 (NS)	0.046 (NS)
B.B.	0.313[b]	−0.161[c]	0.189[b]	−0.268[b]
R.B.	0.069 (NS)	−0.118[c]	0.152[b]	0.032 (NS)
J.B.	0.200[b]	−0.061 (NS)	0.071 (NS)	0.065 (NS)
C.R.	0.200[b]	−0.131[c]	0.124[b]	0.034 (NS)
P.W.	0.081 (NS)	−0.128[c]	0.041 (NS)	−0.136[b]
Fluent				
S.C.	0.332[b]	−0.032 (NS)	0.191[b]	−0.020 (NS)
M.R.	0.310[b]	−0.083 (NS)	0.334[b]	−0.024 (NS)
T.P.	0.340[b]	−0.050 (NS)	—	—
B.M.	0.007 (NS)	0.076 (NS)	−0.039 (NS)	0.046 (NS)
M.S.	0.266[b]	−0.093 (NS)	0.151[c]	0.013 (NS)
G.G.	0.135[c]	−0.227[b]	0.153[c]	−0.281[b]
Group	0.333[b]	−0.156[c]	0.316[b]	−0.093 (NS)

[a] Word length effects are partial correlations.
[b] $p < 0.001$; [c] $p < 0.01$; [d] $p < 0.05$; NS, $p > 0.05$: all one-tailed.

whether these variables affect a patient or not is surely related to the particular point(s) of breakdown in the processes of reading and naming, which are not captured by "classical" diagnoses.

The correlations with both word frequency and word length for the combined scores of all the patients are much higher than the mean correlations for the individual patients. Treating the patients as a group overestimates the influence of these variables and, of course, conceals the heterogeneity among the patients in whether word frequency and word length have any effect. In naming, word frequency accounts for 0.05 to 11.1% of the variance, and in reading 0.2 to 11.2%; while the effects of frequency on naming are significant for nine of the 12 patients, they are small, and much smaller than those reported previously, which are based on data from small numbers of items with large groups of patients (12).

A number of recent experiments have suggested that with normal subjects, in a variety of tasks, the effects of word frequency are due to particular difficulty with very low frequency words (1,7). Do aphasics, in the same way, show word frequency effects in picture naming that are attributable only to difficulty with pictures with very low frequency names? The correlation between mean probability of correct naming for the aphasics as a group and WF is 0.333; when only pictures with name frequencies greater than 8 wpm are considered, the correlation for the reduced set of 202 items is 0.216. This is significantly lower because of the restricted word frequency range; the relevant comparison is whether the fitted linear curve is flatter once low name frequency pictures have been eliminated. With the whole set, the gradient is 0.097 per log wpm; with words of frequencies greater than 8 wpm, it is 0.101 per log wpm. There is no evidence, then, that the effects of word frequency are attributable to specific difficulty in naming pictures with low frequency names.

Analysis 6: Consistency and Types of Errors

We showed in analyses 2 and 3 that patients were on average fairly likely to find the name for a picture that they had named correctly beforehand, and that they produced similar proportions of correct responses in different tests. Does the same apply to errors? That is: (a) Do patients produce similar proportions of errors of different categories in different tests? (b) Having made an error on one test, is the patient likely to produce an identical error, or another of the same sort, when the picture is presented for naming again?

For each of the patients, all responses in tests A1 and A2 were categorized as follows:

1. Correct responses (CORR)
2. Semantic errors (SEM): real word errors that bore a clear semantic resemblance to the correct response; these included semantically related circumlocutions
3. Word errors (WORD): real word responses that were not semantically related to the correct name
4. Phonological errors (PHON): nonwords that were phonologically related to the correct response
5. Neologisms (NEOL): all remaining nonword errors; these included phonologic errors made on semantic or word errors
6. No response (NR): where the patient made no response that was an attempt at retrieval of the name.

Where a subject produced a sequence of errors, the last of these was analyzed as the preferred response.

The proportions of errors that fell into each of these categories on A1 and A2 for each patient are presented in Table 4, together with the proportion of responses of all categories that were identical on A1 and A2 and the proportion of explicit errors (i.e., SEM + WORD + PHON + NEOL) that were identical. A number of conclusions are immediately apparent from Table 4. The different aphasics produce different patterns of errors; some (e.g., J.B. and S.C.) characteristically will not respond if they do not produce the correct name; others (e.g., P.W. and M.S.) nearly always produce some response. For all the patients, the overwhelming majority of explicit errors are semantically related to the target name. It is also apparent that the proportions of errors in each category are not in any systematic way related to the diagnostic categories or the severity of the naming impairment.

When the proportions of errors in each category for each patient on A1 and A2 are correlated, the results shown in Table 5 are obtained. It is clear that patients are consistent in the overall proportions of their errors that fall into each of these categories, with the exception of neologisms. In this case, the proportions of neologisms

TABLE 4. *Proportions of errors in each category for each patient, and the proportion of responses and explicit errors that were identical on A1 and A2*

	Proportions of incorrect Responses					Proportion identical	
Patient	SEM	WORD	NEOL	PHON	NR	Responses	Explicit errors
Nonfluent							
T.M.	0.602	0.120	0.007	0.000	0.271	0.35	0.23
B.B.	0.534	0.043	0.019	0.027	0.378	0.42	0.16
R.B.	0.673	0.057	0.014	0.000	0.253	0.54	0.24
J.B.	0.180	0.004	0.021	0.004	0.795	0.65	0.25
C.R.	0.410	0.057	0.017	0.000	0.516	0.67	0.30
P.W.	0.609	0.048	0.046	0.138	0.159	0.74	0.41
Fluent							
S.C.	0.285	0.020	0.023	0.022	0.651	0.54	0.16
M.R.	0.533	0.129	0.042	0.000	0.296	0.46	0.29
T.P.	0.367	0.012	0.008	0.012	0.600	0.66	0.23
B.M.	0.282	0.090	0.024	0.047	0.556	0.58	0.05
M.S.	0.509	0.127	0.098	0.015	0.252	0.69	0.30
G.G.	0.500	0.037	0.038	0.136	0.288	0.60	0.21

produced by all patients were low, which may misleadingly depress the correlation. In addition, it is clear from Table 4 that a substantial proportion of items produce identical responses on A1 and A2. This proportion varies considerably, from 35% for T.M. to 74% for P.W. When only the items that elicited explicit errors on A1 are considered, the proportion of identical errors falls to between 5 and 43%; a large proportion of the identical responses are attributable to omissions and correct names.

The differential probabilities of different classes of response on A1 being repeated or being replaced by an error in another category on A2 are analyzed in Table 6. It is apparent from the table that correct names are by far the most likely responses to be repeated on the second presentation. Otherwise, only semantic errors and no responses show any particular chance of being repeated. No class of error on A1 is more likely than another to be followed by a correct name on the second presentation; in this sense, no one error is any closer to success than any other. There is a slight tendency for WORD, NEOL, and PHON errors to change to a different error of the

TABLE 5. *Correlations of proportions of errors on A1 and A2 by patients*

Errors	*r*	*p*
SEM	0.917	<0.001
WORD	0.856	<0.001
NEOL	0.355	NS
PHON	0.933	<0.001
NR	0.957	<0.001

TABLE 6. *Mean proportion of responses in each category on A2 related to the responses on A1*

Response on A1	Mean proportion of responses on A2						
	Identical response	Different response					
		CORR	SEM	WORD	NEOL	PHON	NR
CORR	0.765	—	0.097	0.013	0.007	0.011	0.106
SEM	0.283	0.285	0.199	0.030	0.009	0.008	0.186
WORD	0.085	0.293	0.134	0.175	0.057	0.036	0.219
NEOL	0.037	0.407	0.257	0.030	0.146	0.000	0.123
PHON	0.152	0.265	0.041	0.000	0.000	0.105	0.438
NR	0.405	0.303	0.213	0.047	0.012	0.019	—

same category; the same does not apply to SEM errors; if the identical error is not produced, a different semantic error is not especially likely to occur.

The patients in this study show considerable consistency in producing correct responses; they show some consistency, albeit less, in naming errors. Patterns of errors vary from patient to patient but are consistent for each patient between tests. Semantic errors and omissions are more likely to be repeated in identical form than errors of other categories.

While the aphasics' naming errors can be categorized systematically, and in most cases unambiguously, into these four error types, each type of error includes a number of partly distinguishable varieties. Semantic errors include occasional responses which could be considered appropriate names; they just happen not to be the names produced by normal control subjects: e.g., SNAKE → "adder" (R.B.) and CLAW → "talons" (T.M.). The majority of semantic errors are "shared feature" errors (5a); these include many coordinates: e.g., FOX → "wolf" (T.M.), MAYOR → "judge" (S.C.), PYRAMID → "sphinx" (R.B.), LEEKS → "celery" (T.P.), CAMEL → "elephant" (C.R.), ARROW → "dart" (B.B.), MICE → "rats" (P.W.), GLOBE → "atlas" (M.S.), and SCREW → "nail" (G.G.). Much less frequent are superordinate errors: e.g., CASE → "luggage" (R.B.) and SHOULDER → "arm" (M.S.). Parts are sometimes named instead of the whole object: e.g., SINK → "tap" (M.R.) and BICYCLE → "wheels" (T.M.). Associative semantic errors are fairly common: THERMOMETER → "temperature" (P.W.), PYRAMID → "Carthaginian" (T.M.), NOOSE → "hangman" (R.B.), SPADE → "dig" (B.B.), and THIMBLE → "finger" (M.S.). Descriptions are, predictably enough, most common among the fluent aphasics: MASK → "a thing to put on your face" (M.R.), KENNEL → "a dog's box" (S.C.), RULER → "what you measure with" (M.S.), and COT → "a baby's bed" (T.P.).

Many word errors are probably a result of misrecognition of the picture; the aphasics, like normal subjects, do not invariably recognize the pictures for what they are intended to be: e.g., LIPSTICK → "candle" (T.M.), HAYSTACK → "house" (R.B.), and ANCHOR → "key" (M.R.). Entirely unrelated words are rare for all the subjects, apart from T.M., whose responses include TROWEL → "Spain", GARAGE → "dog", and INK → "doctor."

The majority of neologisms appear to result from the process described originally by Pick (13) and later by Brown (3); the patient makes a semantic error on which a phonological error is superimposed. In this corpus, these can be identified with some confidence, where on another test presentation, the patient produces the semantic error without phonological distortion. For example, on A1, M.R. named a CHICKEN as a /fɒld/ and on A2 as a "fowl." Other examples of this are WORM → "/keɪt/" (via snake, M.R.), WEB → "/spaɪdɪd/" (via spider, G.G.), BULL → "/hɒks/" (via ox, P.W.), and GLOBE → "/ætə/" (via atlas, M.S.). Examples of neologisms where an intermediary cannot be identified are rare but include FOX → "/mʌltz/" (M.R.) and SPAGHETTI → "/bɪdɪs/" (C.R.). The neologisms produced by jargon aphasics frequently have no identifiable intermediary (4,5); the patients in this study, none of whom produces many neologistic errors, may not be generating them in the same way as jargon aphasics.

The range of error subtypes produced by the patients in this study is large. The absolute numbers of errors of any one sort produced by different patients is not particularly meaningful, as many cannot be unambiguously categorized; for example, ZEBRA → "horse" (T.M.) could be either a coordinate or superordinate error; MOON → "balloon" (R.B.), could be either an associative error (via the title of one of David Niven's autobiographic books) or a result of misrecognition of the picture, and GRAVE → "coffin" (C.R.) could be counted as either a coordinate (in the category "dead body containers") or as an associate.

Analysis 7: Judgments of Naming Errors

The overwhelming majority of explicit errors are semantically related to the target; they also tend to be repeated. Is this because a patient thinks, for example, that "lion" is the correct name for a picture of a tiger? Or is it because "lion" is the most relevant name that s/he can find, even though s/he knows it is wrong?

In order to investigate this issue, we assembled for each patient all the explicit errors made in A3 together with the correct names and unrelated names randomly assigned to the pictures. Each subject was presented three times with the pictures that had elicited the errors with, in random order, either the correct name, his/her own error, or the unrelated name; each time, s/he was asked, "Is this the best name for the picture?" The results (Table 7) show that the patients consistently accept correct names and reject unrelated names; but they accept a substantial proportion (49–80%) of their errors as correct names (these are, of course, nearly all semantic errors). A patient, who named a picture of a tiger as "lion," will therefore tend to judge both "tiger" and "lion" to be correct picture names; this suggests that s/he is judging the appropriateness of these names on the basis of a semantic representation that is underspecified in a way that allows both names to fit the specification. If aphasic patients use the same semantic representation in the process of picture naming, they will not, typically, be making a semantic error as the best available

TABLE 7. *Judgments of errors*

Patient	Probability of "yes" response: Errors	Correct	Unrelated
Nonfluent			
T.M.	0.49	0.87	0.01
B.B.	0.64	0.99	0.00
R.B.	0.74	0.97	0.01
J.B.	0.58	0.98	0.00
C.R.	0.70	0.91	0.00
P.W.	0.63	0.88	0.00
Fluent			
S.C.	0.68	0.97	0.00
M.R.	0.69	0.77	0.02
T.P.	0.70	0.92	0.00
B.M.	0.53	0.97	0.00
M.S.	0.72	1.00	0.00
B.M.	0.80	1.00	0.00
MEAN	0.66	0.94	0.003

response, despite knowing it to be wrong; rather, they retrieve a name on the basis of a semantic representation that can specify a range of semantically related names, including, among others, the correct name.

CONCLUSION

Detailed analysis of the naming performance of 12 chronic aphasic patients shows that they are consistent in the overall proportions of correct names that they produce and in the proportions of errors that they make in different categories. This does not depend on the particular pictures involved. On the other hand, the response produced on any occasion is not, in general, an accurate guide to the response to that picture on another occasion. The responses most likely to be repeated are correct names and omissions, with some tendency for identical semantic errors to be produced.

In general, all the aphasic patients find the same items difficult; some of this variation can be accounted for by a tendency for the subjects, as a group, to have particular difficulty with lower frequency and longer words. It is interesting to note that treating the data from the patients as a group leads to much higher estimations of the importance of word frequency and length in determining the ease of name retrieval than is justified from their effects on individual subjects. For no patient does either of these variables account for more than 11% of the variance and in most cases much less. It appears that previous studies that have emphasized the importance of word frequency in aphasic word retrieval have overestimated the strength of these effects by combining the scores of individual patients.

Examination of the responses of individual patients shows that there are major qualitative differences that are not related to either diagnostic group or severity of naming impairment. Some patients consistently produce a correct response where they did before, or an error where there was an error; others are inconsistent. While the patients are internally consistent in the pattern of errors they produce across different tests, there is great variation between patients in the errors produced. Some patients nearly always produce a semantic error, while others rarely make any response if they cannot retrieve the correct name. Some patients are affected by the frequency of a word they are trying to find, others by its length; some patients are affected by both variables, and others by neither. Whether these variables affect a subject's performance in naming is no guide to whether it will in reading.

Thus while aphasic patients are consistent to a degree in their performance and show some consistency with each other in the items they find difficult, they show considerable qualitative variation in their naming impairments, which are not captured by assigning the patients to diagnostic categories. Detailed analysis of the performance of individual patients is necessary in order to determine the ways in which picture naming is breaking down.

ACKNOWLEDGMENTS

S. Franklin was supported by a grant from the Department of Health and Social Security to J. Morton and K. Patterson. D. Howard and V. Orchard-Lisle were supported by a grant from the North East Thames Regional Health Authority. We are grateful to the consultants of Addenbrooke's Hospital, Cambridge, for permission to study patients under their care, and to Dr. M. I. P. Wilkinson and Dr. N. E. Gilchrist of the Regional Neurological Unit, Eastern Hospital, Hackney, for permission to study their patients. We are particularly grateful to the 12 subjects of this study, who endured extensive testing with good humor and interest. During the preparation of this manuscript, D. Howard was supported by a grant from the Medical Research Council. A shortened version of this chapter was read at the 1983 Congress of the International Association for Logopaedics and Phoniatrics in Edinburgh.

REFERENCES

1. Bouwhuis, D. G. (1979): Word knowledge and letter recognition as determinants of word recognition. In: *Processing of Visible Language, Vol. 1*, edited by P. A. Kolers, M. E. Wrolstad, and H. Bouma. Plenum, New York.
2. Brookshire, R. H. (1972): Effects of task difficulty on naming performance of aphasic subjects. *J. Speech Hear. Res.* 15:515–518.
3. Brown, J. W. (1972): *Aphasia, Apraxia, Agnosia: Clinical and Theoretical Aspects*. Charles C. Thomas, Springfield, Ill.
4. Buckingham, H. W. (1981): Where do neologisms come from? In: *Jargonaphasia*, edited by J. W. Brown. Academic Press, New York.
5. Butterworth, B. (1979): Hesitation and the production of verbal paraphasias and neologisms in jargon aphasia. *Brain Lang.*, 8:133–161.

5a. Coltheart, M. (1980): The semantic error: types and theories. In: *Deep Dyslexia*, edited by M. Coltheart, K. E. Patterson, and J. C. Marshall. Routledge and Kegan Paul, London.

6. Corlew, M. M., and Nation, J. E. (1975): Characteristics of visual stimuli and naming performance in aphasic adults. *Cortex*, 11:186–191.

7. Erdelyi, M. H. (1974): A new look at the new look: Perceptual defence and vigilance. *Psychol. Rev.* 81:1–25.
8. Goodglass, H., and Kaplan, E. (1972): *The Assessment of Aphasia and Related Disorders.* Lea & Febiger, Philadelphia.
9. Hatfield, F. M., Howard, D., Barber, J., Jones, C., and Morton, J. (1977): Object naming in aphasics—the lack of effect of context or realism. *Neuropsychologia,* 15:717–727.
10. Head, H. (1926): *Aphasia and Kindred Disorders of Speech.* Cambridge University Press, Cambridge.
11. Kucera, H., and Francis, W. N. (1967): *A Computational Analysis of Present Day American English.* Brown University Press, Providence, R.I.
12. Newcombe, F., Oldfield, R. C., and Wingfield, A. R. (1965): Object naming by dysphasic patients. *Nature,* 207:1217.
13. Pick, A. (1931): *Aphasia.* Charles C. Thomas, Springfield, Ill. (Translated by J. W. Brown, 1973.)
14. Schuell, H. R., Jenkins, J. J., and Jimenez-Pabon, E. (1964): *Aphasia in Adults.* Harper & Row, New York.
15. Siegel, S. (1956): *Non Parametric Statistics for the Behavioural Sciences.* McGraw-Hill, Tokyo.

Advances in Neurology, Vol. 42: Progress in Aphasiology, edited by F. C. Rose.
Raven Press, New York © 1984.

Assessment of Understanding in Global Aphasia

Gill M. Edelman

The Hammersmith Hospital, London W12 OHS, England

Investigators of aphasia have always included in their classifications a group of patients who present with a pattern of profound impairment across all language modalities. Comprehension of spoken language, verbal expression, reading, and writing are severely affected. Such a pattern has been variously referred to as global aphasia, total aphasia, or irreversible aphasia syndrome (22), appellations that stress both the extent and persistence of these profound deficits.

Standardized assessments have allowed us to more closely define this group of patients according to the levels of performance reflected in test scores. On the Boston Diagnostic Aphasia Examination (BDAE) (11) for example, a score of more than 1.5 SD below the norm on each major subtest places the patient in the category of global aphasia. Similarly, on the Porch Index of Communicative Ability (PICA) (18), the critical measure is an overall performance score below the 20 percentile. Although these measures are frequently used in experimental studies as the criteria by which subjects are classified into different aphasia types, descriptions of their patterns of performance remain deficient. There is a commonality of both the extent and persistence of deficits, but patients with global aphasia may differ significantly in both these respects. For example, there are many language and nonlanguage skills that remain intact, and in some global aphasics, there is considerable improvement over time (20). Collins (7) states that: "An adequate definition of global aphasia should incorporate both strengths and deficits and somehow distinguish those patients, who within days or weeks move out of the global range." Thus Collins differentiates between those with acute, evolutional, or chronic global aphasia, pointing out that these subclassifications can often be made only in retrospect. Indeed, this will remain the case until assessment procedures are developed that are sensitive to these significant differences between global aphasics and the small but significant improvements that can occur over time.

The problems of assessing global aphasia are far greater with respect to measurement of comprehension than expressive skills. It is undisputed that global aphasics have sparse verbal output, which, in severe cases, is limited to perseverative utterance of a few meaningless syllables. In less severe cases, some isolated words may be used in appropriate but limited contexts. This performance is both observable and quantifiable, and improvements in verbal expression can be measured in terms of increase in amount of output and its meaningfulness. The ability of global aphasics to understand spoken language is a matter for greater speculation and enquiry, however, and the way in which comprehension is generally assessed in aphasia is an area of considerable controversy.

Traditionally, the methods of assessment have involved the presentation of verbal stimuli of graded difficulty, when the patient must demonstrate comprehension of these stimuli through nonverbal or limited verbal responses (e.g., require a patient to point to named objects). The difficulty of this task can be increased by increasing the demands on the auditory retention or linguistic complexity of the command by, for example, asking the patient to point to a series of objects or to one of the objects according to a description of its function. A typical test item requiring a limited verbal response might require a patient to answer yes or no to a simple question. The following example is from the Western Aphasia Battery (WAB) (14): "Is your name Brown?" The task would be made more difficult by increasing the linguistic complexity of the questions; for example: "Does March come before June?"

This method of assessing comprehension is based on a process of inference, since comprehension is not observable and measureable in the same way as verbal output. Furthermore, it is an underlying assumption of this approach that the patient is able to demonstrate his intact comprehension via response through a relatively intact motor system. Boller et al. (5) advise clinicians: "In reality when we obtain hardly any correct responses to most tests of comprehension, we may still entertain the possibility that the processes that patients use to respond are selectively impaired." According to Reidel (19): "It is difficult to know whether the adequacy/inadequacy of an aphasic person's response to controlled spoken units reflects actual comprehension."

This concern about whether test performance accurately reflects comprehension of spoken language is present for reasons other than the uncertainty about the relative preservation of the motor system; e.g., commands and questions are presented out of context in an attempt to measure comprehension of language structures. Many of the para- and extralinguistic variables that accompany normal spoken language are thus systematically eradicated. While normals can perform these acontextual language tasks with little difficulty, many aphasics may have considerable difficulty. The increased availability of contextual information, both verbal and nonverbal, increases the aphasics' understanding of spoken language. Although all the above statements are compatible, they do not lead us to any obvious conclusion about the role of contextual information in the process of normal language comprehension.

We are faced with the problem of designing an assessment tool for use with a brain-damaged population who may have associated deficits in nonlanguage behavior against a background of fragmentary knowledge about language comprehension in normals. This causes Reidel (19) to conclude: "The very nature of the comprehension dimension plus the fact that there is controversy about all aspects of comprehension deficits in aphasia, makes demands on test design that are almost impossible to meet."

Given this state of our present knowledge: "Abnormalities of language function should be described as accurately as possible in qualitative and quantitative terms. In the end a good rule to remember is that most aphasics comprehend more than testing indicates" (1). This applies not solely because of the above theoretical uncertainties but also because most aphasia tests are designed for use with the whole spectrum of aphasic patients, from the minimally to the severely impaired. These tests have a definite floor and ceiling effect, making them most sensitive to those with moderate deficits (4) and least sensitive to mild and severe deficits, an observation that holds for tests of both receptive and expressive skills. The need for a more sensitive measure of mild comprehension deficits has long been recognized and has led to the development of several tests to fulfill this need, e.g., the Token test (8), the Auditory Comprehension Test for Sentences (ACTS) (24), and the supplemental language test on the BDAE. The converse need for tests more sensitive to the comprehension skills that remain intact in severe aphasia has not been similarly recognized.

The need for such an assessment is evident. Many global aphasics score few correct responses on current tests and yet demonstrate some intact comprehension in the course of their everyday interactions. Clinical observation may convince us not only that some residual skills remain but also that there may be some significant signs of improvement. Unless this improvement is substantial, the patient continues to be unable to demonstrate those comprehension skills in formal tests, so that significant changes in performance remain undetected on standardized assessments. For those aphasics initially identified as global who do not remain global, a sensitive assessment would enable us to identify and monitor their improvement at an early stage. Furthermore, with the increased attention to the design of treatment programs for the global aphasic, such an assessment tool might enable us to better identify those patients for whom therapy might prove most effective. For those patients who are unlikely to make significant gains in performance, a fuller appreciation of even minimally intact skills would help the clinician in giving more appropriate management advice.

In part, the development of assessments that measure functional communication skills in natural settings has allowed us to bridge the gap between test and life situations. These assessments, however, such as the Communicative Activities of Daily Living (CADL) (13) and Functional Communication Profile (FCP) (21), are most sensitive to those with moderate aphasic deficits and tend to provide more extensive information on the patient's ability to send rather than to receive messages. Thus they are of limited value to this patient group. The remainder of this chapter discusses what remains intact in global aphasia and how comprehension may be facilitated, and offers some tentative suggestions about the way in which understanding might be assessed.

WHAT REMAINS INTACT

A number of investigators have addressed themselves to the question of what skills remain intact in global aphasia. The motivation and rationale are well expressed by Green and Boller (12):

> Our purpose . . . is to determine which features of rudimentary comprehension they may still retain. If comprehension consists of a sequence of processes, then the assumption is that severely impaired aphasics may still exercise some control over the initial steps in the sequence.

As has already been stated, it is extremely problematic to establish a hierarchy of difficulty for language comprehension tasks. Some speculation regarding the different processes and levels of decoding an utterance is necessary. It is rational that a fundamental step in comprehending would require the listener to distinguish between meaningful and nonmeaningful speech stimuli.

This hypothesis was tested by Boller and Green (6) in 15 aphasic subjects with severe deficits of oral comprehension (as measured on BDAE) who were presented with a test battery of 85 items of questions and commands. These were divided into meaningful (familiar English) and nonmeaningful (English semantic jargon, phonemic jargon, and French). Subjects' responses were recorded in four major categories: correct or incorrect, appropriate or inappropriate, refusal or quizzical behavior, and jargon. An analysis of the category of test item and the category of response was carried out in order to answer questions about the subject's ability to distinguish between stimuli. Thus it was possible to test several hypotheses.

The first hypothesis stated that aphasics would show some ability to distinguish between meaningful and nonmeaningful stimuli. Refusal to respond or quizzical behavior had been observed in a control group in response to nonmeaningful stimuli, and analysis of aphasic subjects' responses confirmed that they, too, selectively responded in this way. However, there was a greater reliability of response to phonemic jargon and French than to semantic English jargon, indicating, as anticipated, "some control over the *early steps* in the sequence of auditory processing" (author's italics).

The second hypothesis stated that aphasics would be able to distinguish between questions and commands, and measures of both correctness and appropriateness were used as indicators of subjects' ability to make this distinction. Test results indicated that "although aphasics were unable to carry out all commands and questions correctly, they responded appropriately to nearly half the meaningful test items." "Appropriately" means that subjects gave the correct type of response, although its content may have been incorrect. Furthermore, an analysis of jargon responses indicated that these occurred significantly more often in response to information questions than to commands, indicating "some retained appreciation of the difference between sentence structures." In other words, the aphasics recognized the sentence type and attempted to make the appropriate verbal response.

A follow-up study in 1974 (12) investigated further these areas of preserved function and looked in more detail at the aphasics' ability to recognize and respond appropriately to different sentence types. Subjects with severe comprehension loss again showed some ability to differentiate sentence types, even when commands and questions were phrased indirectly or were preceded by an introductory utterance. In this study, the authors also compared performance on axial and limb commands to simple questions and again confirmed the clinical and experimental expectation, with a marked superiority of the former over the latter.

Axial Commands

The response to axial commands has been regarded as an interesting anomaly in the study of aphasic behavior. Liepmann (15) first noted preserved ability in one of his subjects, who was able to carry out whole body movements in response to verbal commands but was totally unable to carry out commands of a similar or lesser linguistic complexity requiring individual limb or facial movements. Geschwind (10) later suggested that the neurophysiologic mechanisms underlying these behaviors are different and postulated that "the bundle of Türck may well represent the efferent pathway for whole body commands."

In 1982, Poeck et al. (17) investigated this contention that whole body movements are preserved in patients with ideomotor limb apraxia. Sixty aphasic subjects, subdivided into aphasia type (global, Wernicke's, Broca's, or amnesic), were required to execute whole body, limb, and oral movements to both imitation and verbal command. Results did not confirm Geschwind's theory that axial movements are generally preserved in patients with ideomotor apraxia, but global aphasics emerged as an interesting exception. In the verbal mode of testing, this group performed significantly better in response to whole body commands, but Poeck et al. (17) could not "offer an interpretation for this finding."

The anomaly lends support to the view that global aphasics may have more residual skills than are apparent on formal testing. Selective deficits in motor control may depress performance on simple comprehension tasks and lead to inferences about understanding that underestimate subjects' capabilities. More attention must be paid to assessment design, with respect to the motor responses required by different comprehension tasks. This is particularly pertinent to the assessment of global aphasia, where dependence on nonverbal response is essential due to extremely limited verbal output. A simple response, e.g., pointing, can be an area of considerable difficulty since, as Benson (1) points out: "Even the motor task of pointing can be failed by some patients with severe motor problems, and thus failure may inaccurately exaggerate the patient's problems in comprehension."

Wapner and Gardner (26) provided further evidence for the relative preservation of fundamental language skills in global aphasia. First, they hypothesized that certain lexical domains would be more readily comprehended by global aphasics because of the involvement of the nondominant hemisphere in processing. Testing required that patients identify by pointing to items named by the examiner in one of two picture conditions (the first, pieces of furniture in a room; the second, places named on a map of the United States). A number of nonsense words and associated words without visual counterparts were also included. It was hypothesized that subjects would do better with the map condition because of a greater reliance on visuospatial abilities mediated by the nondominant hemisphere and that they would readily reject the nonsense words as inappropriate, thereby confirming the findings of Boller and Green (6).

The second hypothesis stated that certain syntactic categories of words would be easier than others. Again, picture identification provided the format for the task. Words represented varied according to frequency and operativity (i.e., the extent to which an element is discrete and separable from its surroundings and lends itself to manipulation by an individual). Again, words were included for which there was no visual counterpart, those drawn from different grammatic categories, and nonsense words. High operativity words, high frequency words, and nonsense words were expected to elicit a greater percentage of appropriate responses.

Both hypotheses were upheld. The global aphasics were significantly better at the map condition than the room condition; they were better with operative than figurative words and had little difficulty in rejecting words drawn from different syntactic categories and nonsense words. Furthermore, on retesting, it was demonstrated that greater recovery had occurred on the tasks that had been performed previously with some degree of success than on those tasks that subjects had previously failed completely.

From these studies, the following conclusions can be drawn: Global aphasics do retain some ability to distinguish between meaningful and nonmeaningful stimuli and some ability to recognize and respond appropriately to the pragmatic function of utterances. Second, they may perform better on tasks in which there is greater reliance on the function of the right hemisphere, and it may be possible to speculate on the pattern or recovery following the early identification of these areas of spared function.

The aim of these early studies was to identify some basic skills in the complex process of auditory comprehension that may remain intact in global aphasia. The recording of responses according to the criteria of both correctness and appropriateness was fundamental to the achievement of this aim. Scores of correctness alone would not have revealed those intact areas of performance. Attention to the form and manner of patients' responses rather than to content alone encourages more sensitive appraisal of residual skills and "permits a study of comprehension, not as an all or nothing phenomenon, but as a process made up of distinguishable components" (12). The recent development of multidimensional scoring systems should allow even more sensitive recording of patients' responses, and could be usefully applied to the assessment of comprehension in global aphasia.

FACTORS INFLUENCING COMPREHENSION

Although the above studies attempted to identify residual language skills, a number of investigators have sought to identify those factors that might enhance these skills and facilitate comprehension in severely impaired aphasics. The emphasis has been to look more closely at the auditory message itself, its content and form, and the context in which it is uttered.

Content of the Message

Familiarity with material contained within a message would seem to have an effect on comprehension. Patients tend to respond more reliably to simple questions relating to themselves and their immediate environment than to simple questions that have no personal significance.

Boller et al. (5) studied this phenomenon, investigating the effect of emotional content on patients' responses. The authors compared subjects' responses to paired sentences with "high emotional" or "neutral" content, hypothesizing that "there would be a greater number of responses to sentences with emotional content than to neutral sentences, even if the responses might not be correct." Two judges were used to interpret responses. The actual test stimuli include some emotionally loaded items which, although the authors claim were selected not to offend, upset, or excite subjects, in some instances seem calculated to do just that; for example: "are you an alcoholic?" and "do you have a happy family?" Whatever the ethics of administering such a battery, the study convincingly demonstrated the greater responsiveness of subjects to questions/commands in which personal saliency and affective content were high.

These findings were borne out by clinical experience and are particularly pertinent to the issue of whether testing reflects real life communicative behaviors. Hierarchies are based on increasing linguistic complexity and ignore the effects of content, which may be a significant variable on which comprehension depends.

Context

The discrepancy between performance on factual tests of comprehension, through acontextual language tasks, has led several investigators to examine the facilitating effect of verbal and nonverbal context on comprehension. It is the author's impression that the predictability of an utterance occurring in a given context is a significant factor influencing comprehension. The severely aphasic patient is more likely to comprehend an utterance when it occurs in its expected context than when it occurs artificially as part of a test battery. For example, global aphasics are more likely to respond appropriately to the command "raise your arm" in the context of a physical examination than in the context of a miscellaneous selection of unrelated commands, such as, "pick up the pen, raise your arm, give me the comb" (27).

One way of investigating to what extent aphasics are able to derive meaning from context is to look at their ability to interpret the metaphoric use of language. In these instances, appropriate interpretation of the speaker's intent depends on the successful integration of the meaning of the message and the situation in which it is conveyed. Stachowiak et al. (25) examined aphasics' ability to interpret metaphor in a sentence comprehension task. The concluding statement of each of six short paragraphs contained idiomatic use of metaphor. For example, one paragraph describing a poker game concluded: "The others stripped him down to his shirt." Subjects were required to select, from a five-picture choice, the picture that most appropriately conveyed the intended meaning. Foils included pictures representing the literal meaning of the metaphor. The aphasic group demonstrated relatively intact ability in performing this task. Although high level aphasics performed more accurately than those with severe deficits, the overall pattern of error was similar.

In another study, Wilcox et al. (28) had 18 aphasics observe videotaped interactions between two participants, in which a speaker made requests of a listener. The requests were phrased indirectly: "Can you open the door?" The context in which the request occurred made it clear whether the intent of the speaker was to convey the literal or metaphoric meaning. Aphasic subjects were required to judge the appropriateness of the listener's response to such requests. Both high and low level aphasics, as measured on standard aphasia tests, were able to perform this judgment with a high level of success.

These studies indicate that aphasic individuals, who may demonstrate considerable deficits of language processing on formal tests, derive significant benefit from the natural context in which an utterance occurs. These studies confirm clinical observation.

To what extent aphasics benefit from an artificially augmented context is less clear. In normal communicative contexts, gesture and gesticulation frequently occur as the natural accompaniments of spoken language. In an attempt to facilitate comprehension, clinicians frequently use gesture paired with simple spoken commands, but studies have been less than conclusive concerning the aphasics' ability to derive meaning from gestured signs.

Duffy et al. (9) investigated the extent of impairment of pantomime recognition in aphasics and its relationship with severity of language impairment. They found a greater impairment in pantomime recognition in aphasics than in groups of right hemisphere-damaged subjects, subcortically damaged subjects, and normals. Furthermore, they found a high correlation between the levels of impairment in pantomime recognition and language skills. Similar findings emerged from a study by Schwartz (23), who looked specifically at sign comprehension in global aphasia. The author matched global aphasics and brain-damaged nonaphasics according to levels of residual intellectual functioning and compared performance on tests requiring comprehension of 30 visual and auditory signs. The performance of the global aphasics was significantly lower, leading to the conclusions that: "A severe sign comprehension disorder is demonstrated by left brain damaged adults with severe language impairment." However, both these studies investigated recognition of gestures and signs in isolation and not in combination with the spoken word. One study that looked at the combined presentation of verbal and gestural stimuli (2) found significantly improved comprehension under these conditions. The development of a number of specific treatment approaches using combined gesture and speech would indicate a general belief that gestural context facilitates the comprehension of spoken messages. Undoubtedly, this is an area that requires further experimental investigation.

Rate of Presentation

A number of studies have reported that aphasics' performance on auditory comprehension tasks varies considerably, according to the rate of presentation of auditory stimuli. In general, increased speed has an adverse effect on facility of decoding, with slowed presentation leading to improved performance. Liles and Brookshire (16) presented selected and modified sections of the Token test to aphasic subjects. Tapes were constructed in which the rate of delivery for each command was systematically manipulated with either standard or increased pause time. Increased pause time led to improved performance, but this was limited to the earlier sections of the test. The investigators concluded that increased pause time was beneficial only where the patient was failing due to deficits of auditory memory or retention and not due to the difficulty in processing units of language contained within the command.

Although other studies have not always replicated the above findings (3), the consensus is that some patients do benefit from additional time for decoding, usually created by inserting pauses in sentences, a procedure commonly advocated by clinicians to aid understanding in severely impaired patients.

Effects of Prosody

Little is known about the extent to which aphasic patients rely on stress and intonation to aid comprehension. The functions of prosody in clarifying both the meaning and form of utterances suggest that prosodic features might provide compensatory or facilitative cues, where verbal comprehension is deficient. Expectation has not been backed by experimental investigation, however, and studies in this area are scant. It is common clinical practice to emphasize stress and intonation to aid understanding, but experimental investigation might enable us not only to measure their effects but also to identify those features that are most facilitative.

AN ASSESSMENT FOR UNDERSTANDING IN GLOBAL APHASIA

The discussion so far has highlighted the lack of specific provision of an assessment capable of demonstrating the residual communicative assets of this group of patients and has explored the difficulties inherent in the assessment of comprehension in aphasia in general. The experimental evidence for greater residual function than is apparent on current assessments has been considered, along with an evaluation of some of the factors that might facilitate understanding. We now outline an assessment of understanding in global aphasia which takes into account these findings. It is based on the rationale that an evaluation should enable the clinician to identify both residual skills and deficits.

Tests of language function and communicative function in aphasia are generally based on two different kinds of assessment procedure. The former tends to be highly systematic, isolating different areas and levels of language processing acontextually. The latter examines behaviors in a natural communicative context and emphasizes the measurement of communicative outcome, i.e., it measures whether a patient understands a given message. It does not systematically analyze the significant variables affecting understanding. It is the author's intention to suggest a framework that would permit the systematic evaluation of understanding both contextually and acontextually, in the absence and presence of those variables that may be facilitative. The emphasis of such an assessment is on identifying those functions that can be performed by the global aphasic and on stating the conditions necessary to their performance.

The assessment of such severely impaired patients has always been problematic from the point of when to begin testing. Some patients may present following a severe stroke with such generalized cognitive deficits that any form of assessment is impractical; it would be helpful, therefore, to determine which patients are able to fulfill the requirements of the test situation. Such a screening procedure might precede the test proper, and comprise an evaluation of the following areas of function: levels of alertness, awareness, and attention. Behaviors observed might include response to sound/voice/greeting, establishment and maintenance of eye contact, and control and duration of attention. Levels of performance for each behavior might be established; these would form the criteria for proceeding to the actual test.

Given the fact that such an assessment might be carried out in the acute stages of recovery when the patient may still be confined to bed and traumatized by the sudden changes that have affected him, it would be both sensitive and practical for the clinician to have as few of the trappings of formal assessment as possible (e.g., test equipment, manuals, score sheets). Unfortunately, as one of the main aims of the assessment is to provide systematic analysis of behavior, it is not possible to do without a score sheet. The evaluation should be done with items readily available in a hospital; thus many of the commands and requests would be those that might reasonably occur in the context of a case history or physical examination.

The assessment would evaluate performance on a variety of tests, comprising both commands and questions at a relatively simple linguistic level, i.e., simple imperatives or interrogatives normally stressed and intonated using familiar vocabulary. All such instructions and requests should be reasonable and moderately predictable. Commands are divided into two sections: those relating to self and those relating to objects in the environment. Commands relating to self are further divided into three categories, according to the demands of the motor response: (i) whole body movements (e.g., "lean forward," "stand up"), (ii) limb movements (e.g., "raise your arm," "make a fist"), and (iii) orofacial movements (e.g., "open your mouth," "show me your teeth").

Commands relating to objects might be divided into tasks of object recognition and object manipulation. The former may be evaluated as follows: (a) recognition of an object in a natural verbal context (e.g., "Have you any water?" "Which is your bed?"); and (b) recognition of an object in an acontextual task, in other words, pointing to an object from an array of items in typical test format (e.g., "Show me the comb." "Show me the pen."). Commands relating to the manipulation of an object would also be carried out both contextually and acontextually. A natural command might be: "Can you pass the tissues?" A typical test command might be:

TABLE 1. *Test outline*[a]

Screening Procedure
Commands
Relating to self
Whole body movements
Limb movement
Orofacial movements
Relating to objects in environment
Recognition
In meaningful context
Acontextually
Manipulation
In meaningful context
Acontextually
Questions
Relating to self/high affective content
Relating to environment/low affective content

[a] Hierarchy of examiner cues and multidimensional scoring system applied to test.

"Pick up the comb." It is interesting to note the greater flexibility of use of syntactic structures when giving instructions and asking questions in the more natural condition.

Questions due to limited verbal output unavoidably require a patient to indicate affirmation or negation, but this need not be verbal, and the examiner might be directed to attend to nonverbal signs, such as facial expression or head nodding or shaking. Questions might be divided into two areas: (a) relating to self (e.g., "Are you married? Do you have any children?"); and (b) those of less personal saliency (e.g., "Are you wearing a watch?" "Is it lunchtime?"). See Table 1 for test outline.

Examiner Cueing and Scoring

As was pointed out by Boller et al. (5), greater attention to the appropriateness of behavior and partial performance of a task leads to a greater sensitivity to residual skills in testing. If an assessment for global aphasia can build into its framework the following dimensions, it will increase its sensitivity in this respect:

Hierarchy of cues:

1. Examiner states command/question
2. Repetition at slowed rate
3. Expansion of utterance
4. Addition of gesture.

An example of the application of such a hierarchy for the question "Are you married?" might be, for the expansion stage, "Are you married? Do you have a wife?" and for the gesture stage, repetition of the question pointing to a ring finger. This hierarchy of cues is intended to correspond to the identified facilitators of reduced speed, meaningful verbal context, and natural gesture context and perhaps reflect the order of the strategies adopted by the speaker to aid understanding.

Patients' responses accordingly would be scored not only with respect to success or failure, but with reference to the kind of cue necessary to elicit successful understanding. A modified PICA scoring system might be appropriate:

Scoring system:
10. Accurate, complete and prompt;
9. Accurate, complete but slow/delayed;
8. Accurate after self-correction of error;
7. Accurate after repetition of instruction;
6. Accurate after verbal expansion of instruction;
5. Accurate after gestural cue;
4. Inaccurate but related to correct response;
3. Inaccurate;
2. Attention to item, but no response;
1. No response—no awareness of test item.

Such an assessment currently is being developed by the author and to date has been applied to approximately 30 patients. So far it has only been possible to gain impressions of its potential value, but it seems to have some potential in providing clinicians with a new way of assessing this particular group of patients. It is not possible to eliminate entirely the problems of assessing comprehension, but this assessment aims to take more account of the variables that may affect performance.

Aside from the theoretical arguments that surround this form of assessment, one warning must be sounded. In our search for strengths as well as weaknesses, we must be careful not to overestimate performance that once we underestimated. It is hoped that this assessment might allow a more balanced appraisal of understanding in global aphasia.

REFERENCES

1. Benson, D. F. (1979): *Aphasia, Alexia and Agraphia*. Churchill Livingstone, New York.
2. Beukelman, D. R., Yorkston, K. M., and Waugh, P. F. (1980): Communication in severe aphasia: Effectiveness of three instructional modalities. *Arch. Phys. Med. Rehabil.*, 61:248–251.
3. Blanchard, S. L., and Prescott, T. E. (1980): The effects of temporal expansion upon auditory comprehension in aphasic adults. *Br. J. Disord. Commun.*, 15:115–128.
4. Brookshire, R. H. (1978): *An Introduction to Aphasia*. BRK Press, Minneapolis.
5. Boller, F., Cole, M., Vrtunski, P. B., Patterson, M., and Kim, Y. (1979): Paralinguistic aspects of auditory comprehension in aphasia. *Brain Lang.*, 7:164–174.
6. Boller, F., and Green, E. (1972): Comprehension in severe aphasics. *Cortex*, 8:382–394.
7. Collins, M. J. (1983): Global aphasia: Knowledge in search of understanding. *Communicative Disorders*, 8(9).
8. De Renzi, E., and Vignolo, L. A. (1962): The token test. A sensitive test to detect receptive disturbances in aphasics. *Brain*, 85:665–678.
9. Duffy, R. J., Duffy, J. R., and Pearson, K. L. (1975): Pantomimic recognition in aphasics. *J. Speech Hear. Res.*, 18:115–132.
10. Geschwind, N. (1965): Disconnexion syndromes in animals and man. Parts I and II. *Brain*, 88:237–294; 585–644.
11. Goodglass, H., and Kaplan, E. (1972): *The Assessment of Aphasia and Related Disorders*. Lea & Febiger, Philadelphia.
12. Green, E., and Boller, F. (1974): Features of auditory comprehension in severely impaired aphasics. *Cortex*, 10:133–145.

13. Holland, A. L. (1980): *Communicative Activities in Daily Living*. University Park Press, Baltimore.
14. Kertesz, A. (1979): *Aphasia and Associated Disorders. Taxonomy, Localisation and Recovery*. Grune & Stratton, New York.
15. Liepmann, H. (1900): *Das Krankheitsbild der Apraxie* (*Motorisdren Asymbole*), Berlin.
16. Liles, B. Z., and Brookshire, R. H. (1975): The effects of pause time on auditory comprehension of aphasic subjects. *J. Commun. Disord.*, 8:221–236.
17. Poeck, K., Lehmkuhl, G., and Willmes, K. (1982): Axial movements in ideomotor apraxia. *J. Neurol. Neurosurg. Psychiatry*, 45:1125–1129.
18. Porch, B. E. (1971): *Porch Index of Communicative Ability. Vol. II. Administration, Scoring & Interpretation*. Consulting Psychologists Press, California.
19. Reidel, K. (1981): Auditory comprehension in aphasia. In: *Acquired Aphasia*, edited by Martha Taylor Sarno. Academic Press, New York.
20. Samples, J. M., and Lane, V. W. (1980): Language gains in global aphasia over a three year period. A case study. *J. Commun. Disord.*, 13:49–57.
21. Sarno, M. T. (1969): *The Functional Communication Profile—Manual of Directions*. Rehabilitation Monograph 42. New York University Medical Center, New York.
22. Schuell, H. M., Jenkins, J. J., and Jimenez-Pabon, E. (1974): *Aphasia in Adults*. Harper & Row, New York.
23. Schwartz, L. (1978): Sign comprehension in global aphasia. *Cortex*, 14:112–118.
24. Shewan, C. M. (1979): *Auditory Comprehension Test for Sentences*. Biolinguistics Clinical Institutes, Chicago.
25. Stachowiak, F. J., Huber, W., Poeck, K., and Kerschensteiner, M. (1977): Text comprehension in aphasia. *Brain. Lang.*, 4:177–195.
26. Wapner, W., and Gardner, H. (1979): A note on patterns of comprehension and recovery in global aphasia. *J. Speech Hear. Res.*, 22:765–772.
27. Whurr, R. (1974): *Aphasia Screening Test* (*unpublished*).
28. Wilcox, M. J., Davis, G. A., and Leonard, L. L. (1978): Aphasics' comprehension of contextually conveyed meaning. *Brain Lang.*, 6:362–377.

Advances in Neurology, Vol. 42: Progress in Aphasiology, edited by F. C. Rose.
Raven Press, New York © 1984.

The Aachen Aphasia Test

Walter Huber, Klaus Poeck, and Klaus Willmes

Department of Neurology, RWTH Aachen, D-5100 Aachen, West Germany

During the last 5 years, the Aachen Aphasia Test (AAT) (4) was developed, validated, and standardized. It is designed according to well-defined linguistic criteria and fulfills modern psychometric requirements. It was set up for the German-speaking population rather than translating one of the more frequently used English aphasia tests for the following reasons:

1. The test should assess only language functions and should not embrace various neuropsychologic and neurologic functions. In our view, dysfunctions of memory, praxis, visual recognition, and spatial orientation should be assessed by specific test batteries.
2. A sufficiently large number of homogenous linguistic items should be selected for each task. Furthermore, the tasks should cover major linguistic modalities and levels of systematic linguistic processing. It should be empirically demonstrated that these requirements are met.
3. The variety and variability of aphasic symptoms call for a differentiated yet reliable scoring of individual items.
4. The test should accomplish selection of aphasic patients out of a brain-damaged population and probabilistic allocation to defined subgroups.
5. Furthermore, instead of an overall score, severity gradings should be provided with respect to each subtest.
6. The significance of differential impairment across subtests must be established for the individual patient, and its diagnostic relevance must be evaluated.
7. Repeated application should yield information on differences in level and shape of test profiles and should permit judgments on improvement or deterioration.

THEORETICAL BACKGROUND AND CONSTRUCTION OF THE TEST

Clinical Approach

If one observes the language behavior of a large number of aphasic patients, it becomes obvious that they can be divided into certain groups. These groups are not characterized by crude and linguistically irrelevant symptoms. On the contrary, patients within a given group share many features of language behavior that can be described on the basis of an experienced clinician's intuition or a detailed linguistic analysis. The coherence of symptoms within a group is strong enough to even permit predictions. Not every patient in a group displays the whole set of symptoms held to be characteristic for the group, but sufficiently many symptoms can be assessed in order to assign him to a specific group. The groups correspond to the aphasic syndromes (8).

Today, aphasiologists tend to distinguish standard from nonstandard syndromes. The distinction is based on both frequency of occurrence and agreement on profile characteristics of language performance. Even though there might be slight variation in the description and interpretation of certain symptoms, there is agreement that global, Wernicke's, Broca's, and amnesic aphasia are standard syndromes. Nonstandard syndromes are conduction aphasia and the transcortical aphasias. The status of modality-specific disturbances, such as optic aphasia and pure alexia, is still a matter of debate.

While these views are shared by many investigators who see a large number of aphasic patients, some important qualifications must be made. In a large collection of aphasic patients, the characteristic syndromes are found in only about 75% of cases. Most of these are the patients with cerebrovascular accidents (CVAs) in circumscribed territories of the middle cerebral artery, i.e., in neurologic terms, patients with a transient or permanent ischemic brain lesion.

A certain number of the vascular aphasias (approximately 15%) cannot be classified in terms of standard or nonstandard syndromes. In our experience, the main reason is that the examination is done too early, prior to the establishment of a well-defined syndrome, or at a late stage of recovery, with or without the effects of speech therapy. Some researchers claim to be able to unambiguously classify 60% of the aphasic population, while we give considerably higher figures. These differences probably are due to the psychometric properties of the tests applied and to a more or less generous allowance for intuitive judgment on the significance of test results (8).

Two of the classic standard syndromes are conspicuously dependent on ischemic lesions in the territory of well-defined arteries: Broca's aphasia occurs when the prerolandic branch of the middle cerebral artery is affected; in Wernicke's aphasia, the posterior temporal branch is affected. Global aphasia is often thought to indicate an occlusion of the main branch of the middle cerebral artery with total softening of its territory, but there are observations to the contrary showing that the lesions in global aphasia can be large or small, anterior or posterior, cortical or subcortical, single or multiple (9). Remarkably, the syndrome of amnesic aphasia does not have a distinct vascular correlate, and it is the most frequent aphasic syndrome when the etiology is not a CVA. These cases, roughly 20% of the aphasic population, are mostly patients with intracerebral hemorrhage, brain tumor, abscess, trauma, or diffuse inflammatory or degenerative brain disease. In the majority of patients with these diagnoses, the aphasic language disturbance does not fit in with the uniform picture of patients with CVAs in the left frontotemporoparietal area.

Psycholinguistic Approach

Analysis of aphasic language performance suggests that a distinction must be made between those components of language processing that are modality specific and those that are language dependent. The former are generally subdivided into primary ones, which are directly related to the sound structure of language (acoustic perception and articulatory performance), and secondary ones, which pertain to the grapheme structure of language (reading and writing). Among the linguistic components, phonologic, syntactic, lexical, and semantic-pragmatic levels of processing are distinguished. On each level, specific units (i.e., phonemes, morphemes, sentences, and texts) and regularities for their selection and combination are discerned.

The linguistic tasks included in an aphasia test battery can be characterized by three linguistic facets: modality, unit, and regularity. Regularity and unit are dependent, since the regularities of individual languages are always tied to particular units. For example, similarity relationships among phonetic features, classificatory relationships within semantic fields, and recursive hierarchical relationships among syntactic structures are descriptions for phonemes, lexemes (words), and sentences, respectively. On the other hand, regularities and units are modality independent. Words and sentences having the same regularities can be selected for all modalities. The three facets pointed out are found in all aphasia tests, although linguistic regularities are rarely given explicit attention.

Construction of the Test

The AAT consists of six parts: (a) spontaneous speech, (b) token test [revised German version by Orgass (7a)], (c) repetition, (d) written language, (e) naming on confrontation, and (f) comprehension. The six parts were designed to serve three diagnostic purposes: (a) classification of major aphasic syndromes, (b) assessment of overall severity of aphasia, and (c) description of aphasic impairment in various linguistic modalities. By means of the spontaneous speech sample, symptoms that characterize the four standard aphasic syndromes are observed and rated (5,7,10–12). Spontaneous speech is evaluated on the basis of six levels of observation, performance on each level being judged on a 6-point scale. The scores on each level are defined by the characteristic symptoms and their frequency of occurrence (see Table 1).

To assess the overall severity of the aphasic language disturbance, the token test has been included in the AAT. Subtests c to f check specific linguistic modalities. The nature of the stimulus material is such that it requires the processing of specific features of the German language. Highly automatized and imitatory tasks, such as serial speech, copying, and repetition in unison, are not included because they contribute little to the assessment of the creative use of language and hardly fulfill any communicative function. Tasks with great interindividual variability in normal performance also have been excluded, e.g., production of narratives elicited by pictorial or verbal material, interpretation of proverbs, and grammatic judgment tasks.

TABLE 1. *AAT criteria for spontaneous speech rating*

Criteria	0	1	2	3	4	5
1. Communicative behavior (COM)	No comprehensible language utterance; and very little language comprehension	Communication only by means of incomplete or mostly incomprehensible utterances; and the listener must deduce the meaning of the utterance by means of questioning, guessing, and interpretation	A conversation about familiar topics is possible with the assistance of the discussion partner; and frequently it is impossible to communicate the message he intends to convey	Patient can converse about almost any everyday topic with only a little assistance; and conversation is made difficult by obvious language disturbances	Fluency of language production reduced; and/or some language disturbances can be observed	No disturbance of verbal communication; and/or minimal difficulties in speech; and/or patient reports on language difficulties which the discussion partner does not notice
2. Articulation and prosody (ART)	No utterance	Very severe dysarthria; and/or very severe dysprosody	Severe dysarthria; and/or severe dysprosody	Mild dysarthria; and/or mild dysprosody; and/or slow speech rate	Minimal symptoms of dysarthria; and/or of dysprosody; and/or slightly slowed speech rate	No disturbance of articulation; and/or of prosody
3. Automatized language (AUT)	No utterance; or only recurring utterances; or cannot be evaluated because of very severe dysarthria	Almost exclusively automatic utterances	Many automatic utterances; and/or very frequent verbal stereotypes; and/or very severe echolalia	Frequent verbal stereotypes; and/or severe echolalia; and/or a few automatic utterances	A few verbal stereotypes; and/or mild echolalia	No automatic utterances; and no verbal stereotypes; and no echolalia
4. Semantic structure (SEM)	No utterance; or cannot be evaluated because of recurring or automatic utterances, very severe dysarthria, or phonemic neologisms	Almost exclusively meaningless fluent or nonfluent concatenation of words, set phrases, and verbal stereotypes	Very many semantic paraphasias; and/or semantic neologisms; and/or very many empty, often communicatively inadequate phrases	Many semantic paraphrases; and/or many empty phrases; and/or very severe word-finding difficulties	A few semantic paraphasias; and/or severe word-finding difficulties; and/or some empty phrases	No disturbance of word choice; and of the combination of words; and of word-finding
5. Phonologic structure (PHO)	No utterance; or cannot be evaluated because of recurring or automatic utterances or very severe dysarthria	Almost exclusively fluent or nonfluent concatenation or phonemic paraphasias or neologisms	Very many phonemic paraphasias; and/or many phonemic neologisms	Many phonemic paraphasias; and/or occasional phonemic neologisms	A few phonemic paraphasias; and/or phonemic uncertainties	No phonemic disturbances
6. Syntactic structure (SYN)	No utterance; or cannot be evaluated because of recurring or automatic utterances, very severe dysarthria, or phonemic neologisms	Mostly one- and two-word utterances; and almost no function words or inflected forms	Short, simple sentences which are syntactically mostly incomplete; and frequent absence of function words or inflected forms	Long, complex sentences with frequent phrase blendings or doubling of sentence parts; and/or with very many sentence interruptions; and/or with many incorrect function words or inflected forms	A few incorrect function words or inflected forms; and/or some phrase blendings; and/or many sentence interruptions or fragmentary sentences	No syntactic disturbances

In designing the linguistic subtests, three structural principles were observed. On the one hand, different linguistic modalities were considered: speech production with auditory input (subtest c), language production with graphemic-phonemic/phonemic-graphemic transcoding (subtest d), speech production on pictorial stimulation (subtest e), and matching of auditory and graphemic stimuli to multiple choice sets of pictures (subtest f). On the other hand, different linguistic units were distinguished: phonemes, words, and sentences. Four different types of words have been included: one- and two-syllable nouns functioning as labels, color terms, loan and foreign words, and compound nouns having a descriptive semantic structure which places them between words and sentences. Finally, the subtests were designed in such a way that different linguistic regularities are focused on in the various subtests.

The stimuli used for repetition were such that typical combinations of German on the phonologic, morphologic, and syntactic level are tested. In the Written Language subtest, characteristic correspondence rules between phonemes and graphemes on the word and sentence level are checked. In naming, the availability of semantically simple and complex labels from various semantic fields as well as from a single one (namely, color terms) is assessed. In addition, pictures of everyday events that can be described in one sentence have been included. The syntactic form of these sentences, as well as their propositional content, have been standardized. In the comprehension subtest, discrimination is required between semantically similar words. The similarity is either one of function between the objects depicted in the multiple choice set or one based on the semantic ambiguity of homonymous words. Comprehension of sentences is not possible by a keyword strategy but requires the matching of either nondescriptive sentences or highly pronominalized sentences with pictures.

The linguistic parameters of the four linguistic subtests are summarized in Table 2. The items in each subtest are grouped together in linguistically well-defined sets of 10 items. In all subtests, items are scored on a 4-point scale, roughly according to the following scheme: 3, correct response; 2, close similarity to the target; 1, remote similarity to the target; and 0, no similarity to the target. These scorings are specified in the manual by detailed neurolinguistic descriptions of possible aphasic responses. For repetition and written language, the scoring criteria focus on phonemic, morphologic, and syntactic errors; for naming and comprehension, on semantic errors. Thus phonemic paraphasias are disregarded in all naming responses.

VALIDITY, RELIABILITY, AND OBJECTIVITY

The validation study was based on 30 patients of each standard syndrome and on 30 right brain-damaged patients and normal controls. Classification of the aphasic syndrome was unanimously reached by neurologists, speech pathologists, and neurolinguists who were familiar with the patient. Etiology was mainly vascular. Mean age of groups varied between 49 and 59 years; mean duration of brain-damage was between 1 and 7 months.

TABLE 2. *Linguistic structure of AAT subtests*

Item group (10 items each)	
	Repetition
1	Single phonemes; increasing articulatory difficulty
2	Monosyllabic nouns: increasing number of initial/final consonants
3	Loan and foreign words: increasing number of consonant-vowel syllables
4	Compound nouns: increasing number of free/bound morphemes
5	Sentences: increasing length and syntactic complexity
	Written language
1	Reading aloud: nouns, compound nouns, and sentences with increasing length and complexity
2	Selecting/combining on dictation (multiple choice set of letters/words) stimuli parallel to 1 and 3
3	Writing on dictation: stimuli parallel to 1 and 2
	Confrontation naming
1	Nouns: different semantic fields, functioning as labels
2	Color terms
3	Compound nouns: different semantic fields, descriptive semantic structure
4	Sentences: varying length and propositional complexity
	Comprehension
1	Auditory for words: multiple choice set with semantic similarity among pictures
2	Auditory for sentences: multiple choice set with situational similarity among pictures
3	Reading for words: stimuli parallel to 1
4	Reading for sentences: stimuli parallel to 2

The grouping of item sets according to the modalities repetition, processing of written language, naming and description on confrontation, and comprehension is confirmed by a complete linkage hierarchical cluster analysis. This method implies that a set of items is combined with an existing cluster only if similarity (correlation) to all sets within this cluster is greater than that to all sets lying outside. The results are illustrated in the tree diagram in Figure 1 (6). Although a cluster analysis only permits recognition of unspecified similarities, the results of this analysis can easily be interpreted in terms of the linguistic modalities that are common to AAT subtests.

By means of nonmetric multidimensional scaling procedures, we could demonstrate that the combined facets of linguistic units/regularities also have an impact on the performance in the written language and comprehension subtests (16).

Studying the differential validity of the AAT, we (15) found that spontaneous speech reclassifies 81.7% of the aphasic patients correctly, the entire test 85.8%, and the subtests 65%. The medians of spontaneous speech ratings and of subtest scores are shown in Table 3. All differences in level of performance were statistically assessed by distribution-free tests. The results are illustrated in Table 4.

For spontaneous speech ratings, differences in both gradation and grouping of the four standard syndromes were found for all levels of observation. With respect to

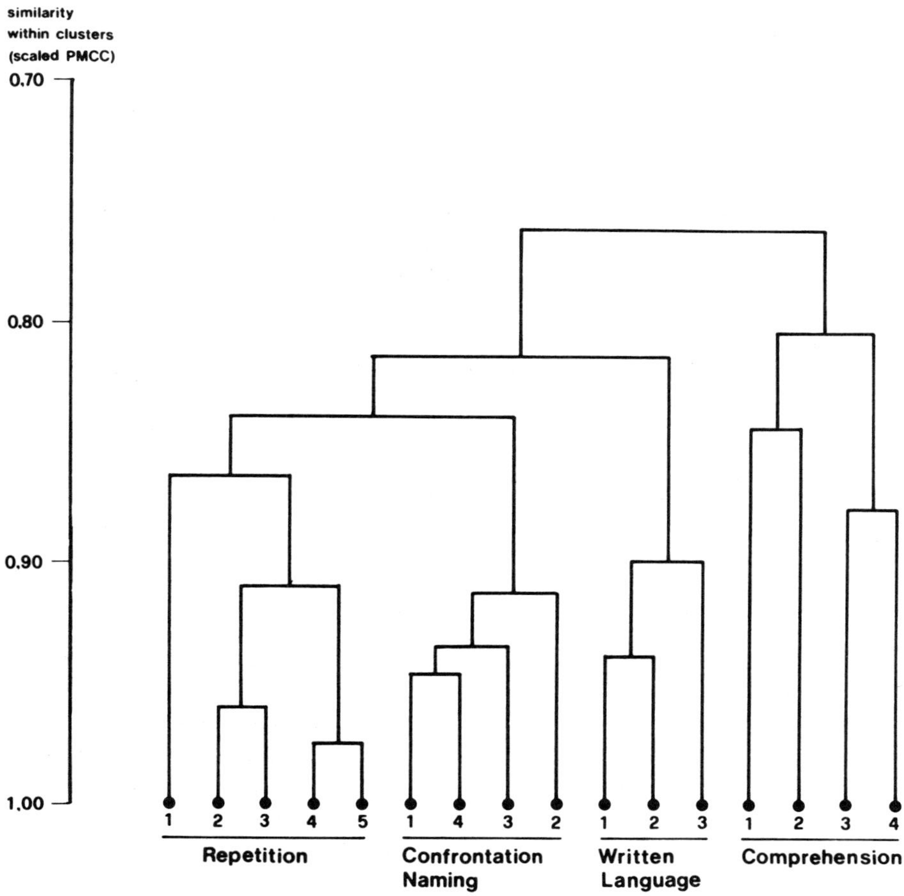

FIG. 1. Grouping of AAT item sets according to a complete linkage hierarchical cluster analysis. $N = 120$ aphasic patients of the validation sample; PMCC, product moment correlation coefficient.

subtests, the same gradation was present, but there were characteristic groupings among aphasic syndromes and the two control groups.

As can be expected, the AAT has good selection properties: 91% of the aphasic and 95% of the nonaphasic patients are correctly classified. It is worth noting that this result was already achieved when we considered performance on the written language and token test subtests taken together.

Reliability was demonstrated as follows:

1. High internal consistency of subtests could be shown by using both consistency and generalizability coefficients.
2. Test-retest reliability was studied in 40 patients (10 of each standard syndrome) over an interval of 2 days. High intercorrelations and no significant changes in

TABLE 3. *Descriptive statistics for AAT spontaneous speech ratings and subtests*[a]

		Global		Wernicke's		Broca's		Amnesic	
		Median	Range	Median	Range	Median	Range	Median	Range
Spontaneous speech[b]									
COM	(0–5)	0.59	0–3	2.50	1–4	2.50	1–4	4.13	3–5
ART	(0–5)	2.05	0–5	4.67	3–5	2.24	1–4	4.28	3–5
AUT	(0–5)	1.17	0–4	3.50	2–5	4.21	3–5	4.50	3–5
SEM	(0–5)	0.75	0–4	2.83	1–4	3.64	3–4	3.85	3–4
PHO	(0–5)	1.50	0–4	3.74	1–5	3.33	2–5	4.00	3–5
SYN	(0–5)	0.44	0–2	3.09	0–5	2.05	1–4	4.08	3–5
Subtests									
Token test[c]	(0–50)	42.0	20–50	31.0	5–50	16.0	3–32	5.5	0–28
Repetition	(0–150)	48.5	0–130	107.5	17–149	122.0	73–148	144.5	103–150
Written language	(0–90)	3.5	0–55	51.5	2–87	68.0	12–84	82.5	39–90
Naming	(0–120)	11.5	0–86	58.5	16–96	96.0	70–115	105.5	64–112
Comprehension	(0–120)	54.0	0–78	76.0	21–93	91.0	62–114	102.5	78–114

AAT median raw scores (after linear interpolation) and ranges from the validation samples.
[a] $N = 30$ for each subgroup.
[b] For abbreviations, see first column of Table 1.
[c] Error score.

level of performance were found for patients with duration of aphasia more or less than 3 months (13).

3. Interrater agreement studies were conducted for spontaneous speech and each expressive linguistic subtest separately. Subjects were students of speech pathology ($N = 29$ and $N = 18$) and test users in other departments of neurology ($N = 20$). For the six observational levels of spontaneous speech, coefficients between 75 and 86% were found for the clinical users. For the subtests, there was almost perfect agreement of about 99%.

TABLE 4. *Differences in AAT performance among aphasic subgroups*

Spontaneous speech[a]					Subtests						
COM	G	W[b]	B	A	Token test	G	W	B	A	R	N
ART	G	B	A	W	Repetition	G	W	B	A	R	N
AUT	G	W	B	A	Written language	G	W	B	A	R	N
SEM	G	W	B	A	Naming	G	W	B	A	R	N
PHO	G	B	W	A	Comprehension	G	W	B	A	R	N
SYN	G	B	W	A							

[a] Nonaphasic control groups were not considered for statistical analysis because of too small variability of scores. For abbreviations, see first column of Table 1.
[b] Underlining indictes nonsignificant differences obtained by nonparametric tests.

TABLE 5. *AAT standardization sample*

		Sex		Age (years)		Duration (months)	
Subgroup	*N*	M	F	Median	Range	Median	Range
Global	90	60	30	52.8	22–70	2.5	1–70
Wernicke's	74	44	30	58.5	36–70	1.5	1–124
Broca's	79	50	29	51.2	22–68	7.1	1–102
Amnesic	71	49	22	50.8	21–68	3.4	1–132
Nonclassified	62	38	24	53.8	22–70	4.0	1–43
Controls	100	63	37	50.8	23.70	—	—

Standardization

Norm data are based on 376 aphasic and 100 nonaphasic patients. Sample characteristics are given in Table 5.

Syndrome assignment was done by means of a nonparametric discriminant analysis using as a learning sample the subjects of the validation study. In addition to patients with a standard syndrome, there was a group of nonclassifiable aphasic patients. Their probability of allocation to one of the standard syndromes was below 70%. In this stage of test standardization, the nonstandard syndromes could not yet be established; we did not have a sufficiently large number of patients to yield learning samples.

Norms were derived from both the total sample and each standard syndrome group. Because of the highly skewed distributions of raw scores, only percentile ranks and stanine scales are given for the whole aphasic group and tercile norms for the syndrome groups.

PROCEDURE OF AAT DIAGNOSIS

The diagnostic procedure is illustrated in a flow chart in Fig. 2. Basically, there are three lines of evaluation. Selection and classification are done by a nonparametric discriminant analysis procedure (ALLOC) (2). An example of the (translated) computer output for patient N.N. is shown in Fig. 3. Based on the six spontaneous speech ratings and the five subtest raw scores, the patient was 100% aphasic; he was allocated to the Broca's subgroup with a posterior probability of 92.6%.

The program recognizes patients as aphasic when the probability for aphasia is at least 80% and gives a syndrome classification if one probability exceeds 70%. Probabilities between 50 and 80% for aphasia are considered as indicating a borderline situation, which can be present in case of recovery from aphasia or, e.g., in case of dysarthria or nonlocalized brain damage to either hemisphere.

Next, percentile ranks (PR) and stanine scores (SN) for each case are read from the norm tables; they are available for subtests and item groups per subtest. Stanine information is used to distinguish four clinical levels of severity: SN 1–3, severe; SN 4–5, medium; SN 6–7, mild; SN 8–9, minimal/no aphasic impairment. It is under-

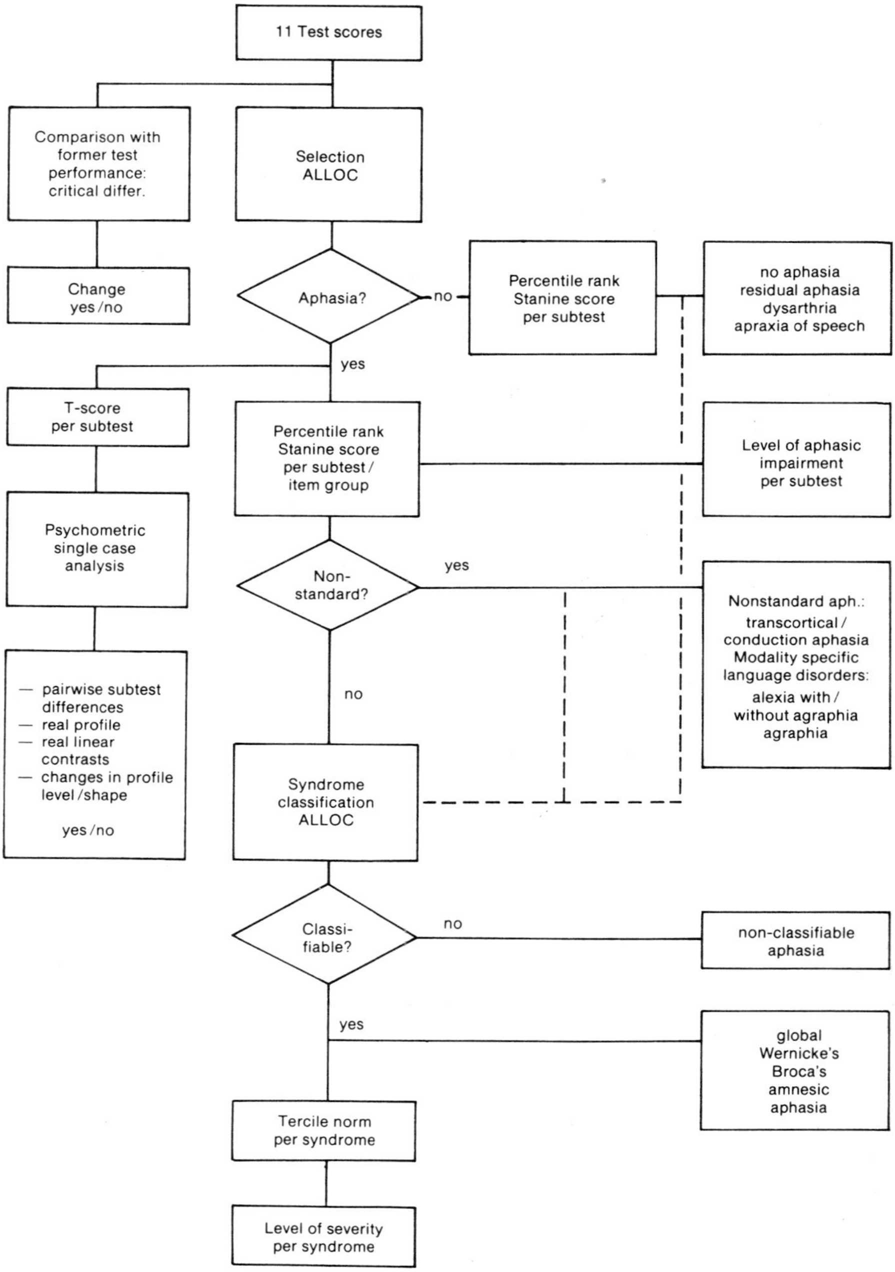

FIG. 2. Flow chart for procedure of AAT diagnosis. ALLOC, nonparametric discriminant analysis program.

```
****************************************************************************
*           AACHEN APHASIA TEST / A L L O C - D I A G N O S I S           *
*(LEARNING SAMPLE: 314 APHAS., 100 CONTR. / 90 GL,74 WE,79 BR,71 AM) *
*--------------------------------------------------------------------------*
* FAMILY NAME,FIRST NAME    :N.N.                                          *
* DATE OF BIRTH             :03.02.1927                                    *
* DATE OF EXAMINATION       :10.05.1982                                    *
* PATIENT IDENTIFICATION    :0507              1-ST EXAMINATION            *
*-------------------- A A T - P R O F I L E ------------------------------*
*    SPONTANEOUS SPEECH (1-6)         TT   REP WRIT NAME COMP              *
*      2  3  2  3  4  1               25   110   29   54   71              *
*--------------------------------------------------------------------------*
************************* CLASSIFICATION **********************************
*--------------------------------------------------------------------------*
*** DIAGNOSIS ***           POSTERIOR PROBABILITIES ( % )                  *
* 1.APHASIA      *          APHASIA   :100.0 %  NO APH.   :  0.0 %         *
* 2. SYNDROME ***                                                          *
*   BROCA        *          GL:  7.4%  WE:  0.0%  BR: 92.6%  AM:  0.0  %*
****************************************************************************
```

FIG. 3. Computer output of the ALLOC classification program for patient N.N. TT, token test; REP, repetition subtest; WRIT, written language subtest; NAME, naming on confrontation subtest; COMP, comprehension subtest. GL, global; WE, Wernicke's; BR, Broca's; AM, amnesic aphasia.

stood that 90% confidence intervals for raw scores are taken into account when the decision on degree of severity is made. In order to diagnose nonstandard syndromes and modality-specific impairment, we follow operational definitions that are based on percentile differences between subtest scores (1). For example, for the diagnosis of stable conduction aphasia, we require repetition to be below PR 50 and all other subtest scores to be at least 20 PR higher; these patients should have no severe dysarthria. If the criteria for nonstandard aphasias and modality-specific disturbances are met, this overrides, at present, the ALLOC classification.

In the case of a standard syndrome, tercile norms allow a differentiation between severe, medium, or mild impairment with respect to the syndrome. Again, confidence intervals must be considered.

Detailed analyses of the subtest profiles can be done by psychometric single case analysis procedures (3,14). The application of these methods is illustrated using the test results of patient H.C. with Wernicke's aphasia tested twice, during the first month postonset and 3 months later. In Fig. 4, both profiles are depicted based on *T*-standardized scores. (The statistical procedures require that PR are transformed into standard norms, such as *T*-scores.) Both profiles were found to be "real" profiles; i.e., there were reliable differences between subtest scores beyond measurement error. Pairwise comparisons yielded the following patterns of significant subtest differences:

First testing: <u>COMP TT NAME</u> REP WRIT
Second testing: <u>COMP NAME REP TT</u> WRIT

Subtests are ordered with respect to increased performance; underlinings indicate nonsignificant subtest differences.

In addition, the test procedures allow the computation of the diagnostic validity of reliable (pairwise) subtest score differences; i.e., one computes the probability of

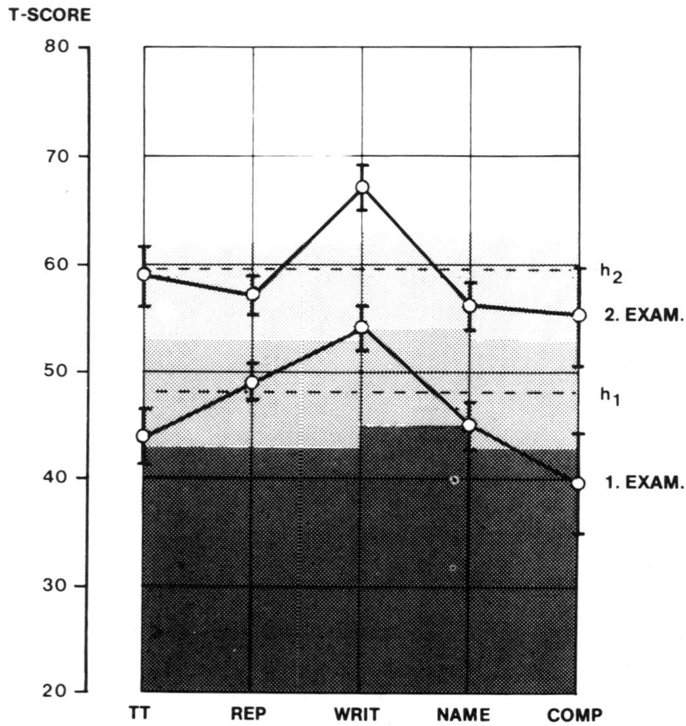

FIG. 4. *T*-score profiles of patient H.C., first and second examination. h_1, h_2, Estimated profile level for first and second examination. TT, token test; REP, repetition subtest; WRIT, written language subtest; NAME, naming on confrontation subtest; COMP, comprehension subtest.

obtaining still larger differences in *T*-scores among the aphasic reference population. Only if this probability is sufficiently small, e.g., less than 20%, is the score difference considered diagnostically valid. In the example given, performance on the written language subtest was reliably better than on all other subtests. Only the difference on the repetition subtest was not diagnostically valid for the first examination.

Single case analysis procedures also permit comparison of two *T*-score profiles of one patient. Profiles can be tested for overall differences in level and/or shape. If differences in shape are present, changes in pairwise differences among pairs of subtests can be evaluated with respect to both reliability and diagnostic validity. In the case of H.C., there was a significant increase in profile level and a significant difference in shape. Only the relationship between token test and repetition performance changed reliably, and this change was diagnostically valid.

A less detailed comparison of both test profiles is also possible. The test manual gives critical raw score differences for individual subtests or item groups within subtests.

CONCLUSION

The linguistic and psychometric properties make the AAT a useful, reliable, and valid tool for the clinical diagnosis of the aphasias. The test is also suited for follow-up studies, e.g., the efficacy of speech therapy in groups and single cases. Furthermore, baseline data for research purposes can be obtained.

ACKNOWLEDGMENT

The development and standardization of the Aachen Aphasia Test was supported by grants from the Deutsche Forschungsgemeinschaft.

REFERENCES

1. De Bleser, R. (1985): Localization of aphasia: Science or fiction? In: *Proceedings of the First European Workshop on Cognitive Neuropsychology*, edited by F. Denes. Erlbaum, Hillsdale, N.J. (*in press*).
2. Habbema, J. D. F., Hermanns, J., and van den Broek, K. (1974): A stepwise discriminant analysis program using density estimation. In: *Compstat 1974, Proceedings in Computational Statistics*, edited by G. Bruckmann, pp. 101–110. Physica Verlag, Wien.
3. Huber, H. P. (1973): *Psychometrische Einzelfalldiagnostik*. Beltz Verlag, Weinheim.
4. Huber, W., Poeck, K., Weniger, D., and Willmes, K. (1983): *Der Aachener Aphasie Test (AAT)*. Hogrefe Verlag, Göttingen.
5. Huber, W., Stachowiak, F.-J., Poeck, K., and Kerschensteiner, M. (1975): Die Wernicke-Aphasie. *J. Neurol.*, 210:77–97.
6. Huber, W., Weniger, D., Poeck, K., and Willmes, K. (1980): Der Aachener Aphasie Test: Aufbau and Überprüfung der Konstruktion. *Nervenarzt*, 51:475–482.
7. Kerschensteiner, M., Poeck, K., Huber, W., Stachowiak, F.-J., and Weniger, D. (1978): Die Broca-Aphasie. *J. Neurol.*, 217:223–242.
7a. Orgass, B. (1976): Eine Revision des Token Tests, Teil I und II. *Diagnostica*, 22:70–87,141–156.
8. Poeck, K. (1983): What do we mean by "aphasic syndromes"? A neurologist's view. *Brain Lang.*, 18:79–89.
9. Poeck, K., De Bleser, R., and Keyserlingk, Graf von, D. (1984): Neurolinguistic status and localization of lesion in aphasic patients with exclusively consonant-vowel recurring utterances. *Brain*, 107:199–217.
10. Poeck, K., Kerschensteiner, M., Stachowiak, F.-J., and Huber, W. (1974): Die amnestische Aphasie. *J. Neurol.*, 207:1–17.
11. Poeck, K., Kerschensteiner, M., Stachowiak, F.-J., and Huber, W. (1975): Die Aphasien. *Aktuel. Neurol.*, 2:159–169.
12. Stachowiak, F.-J., Huber, W., Kerschensteiner, M., Poeck, K., and Weniger, D. (1977): Die globale Aphasie. *J. Neurol.*, 214:75–87.
13. Weniger, D., Willmes, K., Huber, W., and Poeck, K. (1981): Der Aachener Aphasie Test; Reliabilität und Auswertungsobjektivität. *Nervenarzt*, 52:209–277.
14. Willmes, K. (1984): An approach to analyzing a single subject's scores obtained in a standardized test with application to the Aachen Aphasia Test (AAT) (*Submitted for publication*).
15. Willmes, K., Poeck, K., Weniger, D., and Huber, W. (1980): Der Aachener Aphasie Test: Differentielle Validität. *Nervenarzt*, 51:553–560.
16. Willmes, K., Poeck, K., Weniger, D., and Huber, W. (1983): Facet theory applied to the construction and validation of the Aachen Aphasia Test. *Brain Lang.*, 18:259–276.

Advances in Neurology, Vol. 42: Progress in Aphasiology, edited by F. C. Rose.
Raven Press, New York © 1984.

Approaches to Aphasia Treatment

*Leonard L. LaPointe

Veterans Administration Medical Center, Gainesville, Florida 32602

It is indeed appropriate to interweave opinions and data to advance aphasiology—a singular cause—bypassing the differences of culture and boundary and nation to the common purpose of discussion, perhaps even of discovery, as a noted bard once said (30): ". . . [of] some sweet oblivious antidote . . . [to] raze out the written troubles of the brain." This volume is a reflection of an ongoing concert of research and thought that continues to explore variations on a relevant theme: that of the restoration of communication to those people whose lives and identities have been wrenched by aphasia.

HISTORIC APPROACHES

The charge of this chapter is to review strategies and approaches to aphasia treatment from antiquity to the present. Since shortly after the discovery of the tongue, humans have been taken aback and fascinated by the peculiar and convoluted utterances that fell from the mouths of their brain-injured companions. The confusing disorder that came to be known as aphasia has proved to be fertile ground for scholars who seemed to develop an evolving obsession to record it, label it, rename it, sort it, resort it, categorize it, argue about it, and generally regard it as a weird and wonderful subject to study. However, the idea that shattered language can and should be mended, and that research should be done on these mending strategies and particularly on their outcomes, is all too recent.

Early interest attributed diseases to demons, the disfavor of celestial gods, or evil spirits who roamed the earth creating havoc. Therapies, even in the time of the Greek philosophers Socrates, Pericles, and Hippocrates, consisted of attempts to influence the balance of the various humors of blood, phlegm, black bile, and yellow bile. Without attempting to trace in too much detail these early efforts, we do know the treatment of aphasia had to pass through the eras of cautery and cupping, a process in which small suction cups were attached to offending levels of the nervous system (2). Most of these medieval treatments were applied to the neck to stimulate what was thought to be a sluggish tongue. As our eminent colleague Macdonald Critchley (7) has pointed out, it is difficult to explain how most of the healers of the 17th and

**Present address:* Department of Speech and Hearing Science, Arizona State University, Tempe, Arizona 85287.

18th centuries could have overlooked or misinterpreted such dramatic features as use of the wrong words, recurrent utterances, and the inability to read or even comprehend words; particularly, as Critchley stated (7): "The striking phenomenon of a prolix torrent of gibberish" (p. 54). Further tracing of the early days of the rise of rehabilitation are cataloged in considerable detail elsewhere (19) and need not be considered here.

CASE STUDIES

The 1860s witnessed a confluence of clinical and scholarly energy devoted to aphasia. The principal tools were careful observation and the detailed study of single cases. Little attention was paid to treatment, though, and much less to measuring treatment outcomes. Nevertheless, the early case studies did much to define the peculiar symptomatology of this condition that seemed to exist in a vast spectrum of varieties. Of course the classic case studies by Pierre Paul Broca, Bouillaud, Bastian, Wernicke, and others set the stage not only for the delineation of distinctive syndromes (some of which are argued to this day), but also to the formulation of the theoretical foundations of brain and language behavior.

A few of the early case studies provided sketchy plots of the recovery process. A short case study by Trousseau in 1864 has been called "perhaps the first description of the reeducation of speech in amnesic aphasia" (27):

> A very intelligent and cultivated woman became affected with complete aphasia. . . . She lost the memory of all words, but regained them in the following way: First, she repeated every question after the person who made the question, thus reviving the memory of spoken words. Then a friend recalled to her memory with utmost patience the most usual terms, word by word. . . . She now asked for a notebook in which she put down for six weeks and with admirable regularity not only the words pronounced in her presence, but also those she could evoke herself. . . . She wrote down in her notebook: "inkstand." This evoked "pen"; the latter evoked "bird". . . bird led to "fowl" and fowl to "stuffed goose liver". . . . In this way the patient re-constituted her language.

Observation and recording of special cases continued to dominate the research approach to aphasia for nearly 100 years. It was popular after World War II and continues as a viable research tool today. There is nothing as useful as careful observation and description filtered through the deductive and analytic mind of a clinician-researcher. From these observations, and from testing clinical hunches, particularly with the emerging technology of single case experimental design, come strategies that can alleviate some of the devastating effects of aphasia.

CONTEMPORARY APPROACHES

Most contemporary approaches to aphasia treatment are not atheoretic. A set of assumptions usually forms the foundation of a clinician's *modus operandi*, although the clinician may not be fully aware of what these assumptions are. Assumptions are made that consider the nature of language, the nature and definition of aphasia, beliefs about the recovery process, and ideas on the effects of neuropathology on the language system. Questions of competence versus performance, loss versus interference, access and retrieval impairment, and processing disruption all guide the clinician in deciding exactly what to treat, how to treat it, and why it should be treated. Without a model or a theoretic framework, the clinician is not unlike a sailor without navigational charts, wind, or even an anchor; both can drift aimlessly and with a good deal of randomness.

Fortunately or unfortunately in aphasia treatment, no singular model or approach has proved to be unequivocally better than the others. There is no doubt, however, that we urgently need an accumulation of clinical research designed to test hypotheses on the relative effectiveness of various approaches to treatment. Single case research, such as alternating treatment designs, and the ingenuity of clinical researchers will provide relevant answers in the ensuing years. What follows here is a synthesis of some of the major models and approaches to aphasia treatment. These approaches have been reviewed by others (8,14,18), who have used a variety of terms and labels for similar concepts.

One review (14) suggests that four distinct model-specific approaches to aphasia treatment can be distinguished: (a) linguistic, (b) cybernetic, (c) modality or input-output, and (d) multi- or cross-theoretic approaches. Those who take a primarily linguistic orientation to aphasia work from the premise that communication is generally "rule bound", that the essence of the problem is a "loss" of linguistic rules or competencies, and that language content and rules must be relearned during the therapeutic process. The focus of attack is directly on the deviant systems of language, be they lexical-semantic, morphosyntactic, phonologic, or orthographic. Readily manipulable by the clinician are such psycholinguistic properties of language as form class, word frequency, and abstractness.

Those who subscribe to the cybernetic model view language as being strongly influenced by cognitive processes and by the cybernetic factors of attention, fatigue, arousal, and the other effects of brain damage in general. The problem, according to the subscribers to this model, is one of "interference"; the rules and components of language are not obliterated, but they are not always accessible or retrievable. Reorganization and strategy learning are needed to stimulate or facilitate access to language. This is accomplished by the clinician's selection and manipulation of such things as the physical characteristics, order, or temporal aspect of the language stimuli.

Another orientation emphasizes the importance of communication being "modality bound." Performance across modalities of expression and comprehension are carefully evaluated, and both intra- and intermodality compromises and strategies are devised for treatment. Transcoding, deblocking, and intersystemic reorganization are concepts that are the basis of modality intervention strategies.

Much overlap can be seen across some of these approaches, but the multi- or cross-theoretical model is the most eclectic of all. This is the particular approach to aphasia treatment that I find most comfortable, since I believe that the state of the art of our appreciation of the precise nature of aphasic breakdown is not complete enough to allow one to subscribe to a singular view of the disorder. Therefore, some

TABLE 1. *Characteristics of the stimulation-facilitation approach*

1. Intensive auditory stimulation
2. Varied, abundant, and meaningful clinical material
3. Repetitive sensory stimulation
4. High patient response rates
5. Avoidance of struggle or forced responses
6. Avoidance of defective response correction
7. Manipulation of stimuli to make them adequate

aspects of all the previous models seem attractive to an explanation of the problem of aphasia as it occurs in all its wonderous and variegated forms, across individuals, and within individuals across time. Linguistic content, form, and use are affected by a host of modality and cybernetic factors, and although aphasia appears to be primarily a problem of interference and access, in some patients, the argument of a complete loss of certain aspects of language competence is compelling. Therefore, the treatment approaches for those who embrace a cross-theoretic model include relearning, facilitation, and compensation, since the linguistic, cybernetic, and modality deficits interact in a highly individualized way from patient to patient due to differences in lesion site, depth, extent, etiology, and other subject variables.

PRINCIPAL APPROACHES

Contemporary approaches to aphasia treatment are an outgrowth and amalgamation of models perpetuated by education, psychology, linguistics, and medicine. Approaches that reflect these models have been refined, blended, and pruned by the relatively new profession of speech and language pathology, and a few new twists have been added.

Perhaps the most prevalent form of aphasia treatment, at least in the United States and perhaps more extensively as well, is that called stimulation-facilitation, an outgrowth of concepts, some of which were fathered by Joseph Wepman and then nurtured and refined by Hildred Schuell. This approach is widespread and can be observed in clinics from Pretoria to Hammersmith and from Melrose, Florida to Oak Creek, Arizona.

Intensive and repeated sensory stimulation with focus on the auditory channel is characteristic of this approach. In fact, this emphasis on input has been termed auditory bombardment, since Schuell et al. (29) believed that disrupted auditory retention and comprehension skills were the underlying culprits in most aphasic deficits. Table 1 lists specific treatment characteristics of this approach. Finally, Schuell et al. (29) abhored rigidity in treatment and suggested that if the method leaves the patient behind or if the patient progressed faster than the method, the method must be changed. The authors recognized and advocated often that there is no room for rigidity in clinical practice. Perhaps that is one of the reasons why those concepts persist in being relevant and defy the quaintness that make some approaches appear somewhat dated.

TABLE 2. *Characteristics of programed-operant approaches*

1. Measurement of baseline behaviors
2. Definition of terminal behaviors
3. Stimulus control
4. Progress plotting, frequent evaluation
5. Reinforcement

PROGRAMED-OPERANT

Behavioristic, or programed-operant, approaches to intervention view language rehabilitation more as an educative or reteaching process. The experimental analysis of behavior and principles of operant conditioning provide the theoretic basis for this approach. The chronology of the major steps can be found in many sources (e.g., 3,13). Table 2 presents some of the characteristics of programed approaches to treatment.

Programed-operant methods were at their peak of fashion in the 1960s and 1970s and for some reason appeared to be strangely correlated with the crest of popularity of the Beatles. At any rate, both have left their legacy, and in fact behaviorists have not disbanded but have left us principles and strategies that permeate language intervention.

BASE-10 PROGRAMED STIMULATION

In recent years, an amalgamation of principles from both the programed-operant and stimulation-facilitation schools has been incorporated into a system of therapy called programed-stimulation (18). Table 3 shows features of this approach. As can be seen, this strategy of organizing intervention features clearly defined tasks, baseline performance measurement, session-by-session progress plotting, and the flexibility to incorporate a rich array of stimulation procedures designed to facilitate many responses from aphasic patients. With our particular variety of the programed-stimulation approach, speech and language performance can be converted to a graphic display of progress (or lack of it) in percentage over 10 treatment sessions

TABLE 3. *Base-10 Programed stimulation characteristics*[a,b]

1. Clearly defined treatment tasks
2. Baseline performance measurement
3. Adaptable to wide variety of treatment approaches, tasks
4. Session-by-session progress plotted
5. Graphic display of change in percentage
6. When used with single subject research designs, provides means for documenting treatment effectiveness

[a] From LaPointe (16).
[b] Blends principles of stimulation-facilitation and programed-operant approaches.

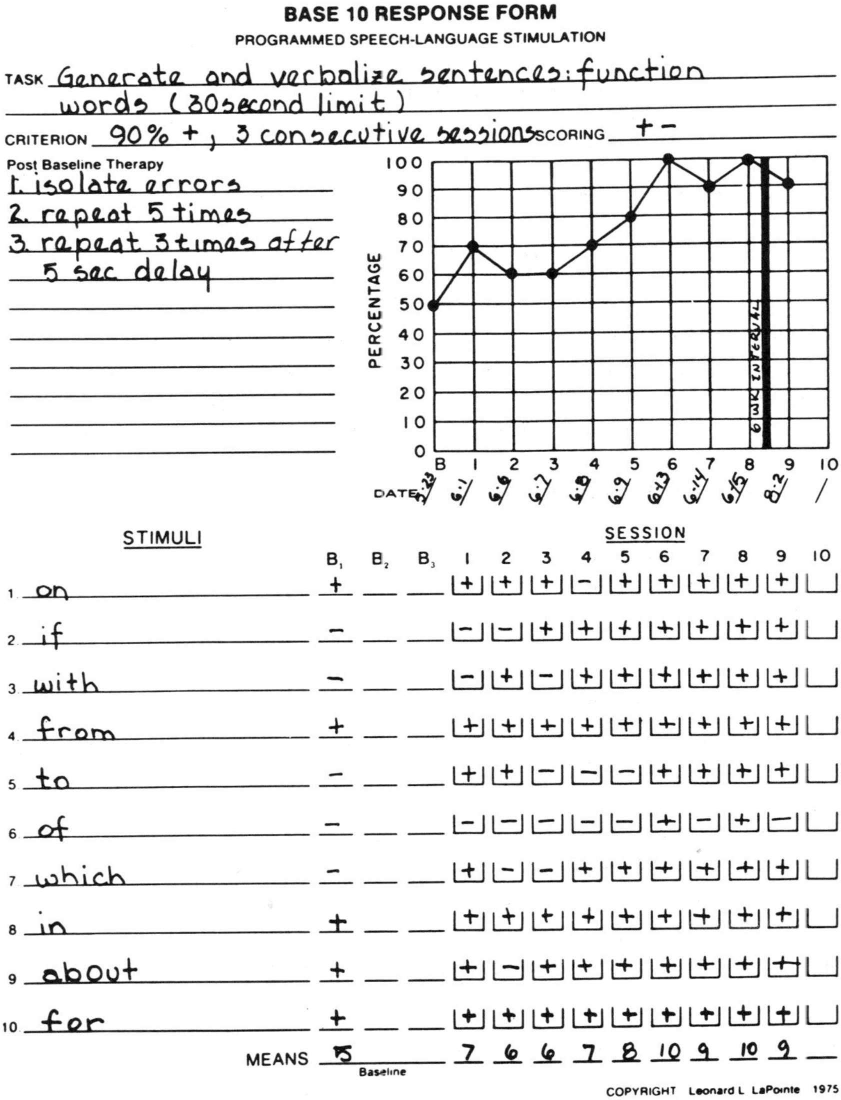

BASE 10 RESPONSE FORM

PROGRAMMED SPEECH-LANGUAGE STIMULATION

TASK Generate and verbalize sentences: function words (30 second limit)

CRITERION 90% +, 3 consecutive sessions SCORING + −

Post Baseline Therapy
1. isolate errors
2. repeat 5 times
3. repeat 3 times after 5 sec delay

STIMULI	B_1	B_2	B_3	1	2	3	4	5	6	7	8	9	10
1. on	+			+	+	+	−	+	+	+	+	+	
2. if	−			−	−	+	+	+	+	+	+	+	
3. with	−			−	+	−	+	+	+	+	+	+	
4. from	+			+	+	+	+	+	+	+	+	+	
5. to	−			+	+	−	−	−	+	+	+	+	
6. of	−			−	−	−	−	−	+	−	+	−	
7. which	−			+	−	−	+	+	+	+	+	+	
8. in	+			+	+	+	+	+	+	+	+	+	
9. about	+			+	−	+	+	+	+	+	+	+	
10. for	+			+	+	+	+	+	+	+	+	+	
MEANS	5 (Baseline)			7	6	6	7	8	10	9	10	9	

FIG. 1. Example of base 10 response form.

(Fig. 1). This approach has been adequately addressed in other sources (8,16) and need be mentioned only briefly here.

This approach, and other attempts to add a degree of organization and quantification to the therapeutic process, does not obviate the need for counseling, providing realistic hope, being a source of information and emotional support, communicating with related professionals, or all the other details that constitute the sum of efficient and compassionate patient management. In the past, much aphasia management has been long on rapport, warmth, support, and coffee and tea consumption, but not too long on the planning and drudgery necessary to document the removal of specific language barriers. Some might argue that in the past few years, we have seen more "trends away from structured treatment," but certainly this cannot mean abandonment of systems that aid us in getting a firm grasp of our goals, enhancing therapeutic planning, organizing what transpires in a therapy session, and documenting change in a person's communication performance.

THEME VARIATIONS

A rich array of contemporary variations on the theme of aphasia intervention is evident in recent literature. We read about and are influenced by such concepts as PACE therapy, pragmatics, and incorporation of parameters of natural discourse in treatment; thought-centered therapy; strategies related to divergent semantic therapy that attempt to more firmly resist the separation of cognition from language; self-adjusting therapy and systems of self-cueing; psychosociolinguistic and environmental systems of intervention; Melodic Intonation Therapy; and many other innovative and inherently sensible strategies of refinement of our treatment form, content, and medium. Many of these approaches are reviewed in greater detail by Sarno (28), Chapey (4), Darley (8), and Davis (9). A recent addition to our appreciation of approaches to aphasia treatment has come from Britain (5) and provides a summary of aphasia treatment that ranges from the ubiquitous issue of the efficacy of aphasia intervention to a treatise on single case research.

THE FUTURE OF APHASIA TREATMENT

It is doubtful that we can predict with any degree of accuracy what the future holds for aphasia treatment. Certainly the area of neurodiagnostics is undergoing a technologic revolution. Positron emission computed tomography, xenon and regional blood flow studies, nuclear magnetic resonance, and the remarkable contributions of computerized axial tomography scan technology have contributed mightily to answering the riddles of "Lesion, lesion, where is the lesion?" and to an even greater understanding of brain and behavior correlates.

With a few exceptions, however, the technology of aphasia treatment is still a Model A Ford in a space shuttle world. The materials that a present-day aphasia clinician takes into the clinic room for treatment are not that much unlike those that were set before the aphasic patient by the starch-collared French physicians in the 1880s. We absolutely must explore (and some aphasiologists do) the vast potential of the creative application of existing computer hardware and software science and the contributions of other breakthroughs in instrumental assistance to our traditional behavior treatment approaches. Table 4 displays some of the areas of computer use in aphasia treatment.

Microcomputers are being used and introduced into at least four areas of clinical management. First, they are used for direct word retrieval and communication aids, as in the California project by Colby et al. (6) and the SPLINK project in Britain

TABLE 4. *Areas of computer use in aphasia treatment*

Direct word retrieval aids: Communication aids
California project (15)
SPLINK project (12)
Software
Adaptable
Designed for aphasia treatment
Records: Number crunching
Clinical administration
Data retrieval on demographics
Prediction
Prognosis, counseling
Treatment duration, levels of achievement

(12). Second, a variety of software is being adapted as well as developed specifically for aphasia treatment. Most notable in this area is some of the work by Deloche and colleagues (10), who reported on 8 years of experience in developing computer-based training programs. In the United States, the work of Richard Katz (15) and some of his co-workers has focused on programs for reading activities that imitate actual treatment activities and on a project that represents computerized adaptation of tachistoscopic "flash card" drills that utilize features unique to the computer and cannot be duplicated by a clinician alone. Third, clinical administrative chores and data retrieval are giving us a better appreciation of the demographics of our case loads. Finally, the problems of prediction, prognosis, estimation of treatment duration, and the plotting of celeration rates and slopes of performance are adaptable to computer analysis. Some of this latter work has been elaborated upon by Matthews and LaPointe (23,24).

PREDICTION

We have been concerned with the concepts of trend analysis, reacquisition slopes, and celeration rates in our clinic and in our clinical research. Questions we are currently addressing include: "Can reacquisition rates be measured? How fast do skills change? How can we measure celeration rates or slope of change? Is change curvilinear? Can we plot or predict trends of performance or perhaps outcome levels?"

We have been experimenting with a simple 4-step method called the quarter-intersect method of determining degree or slope of change on communication tasks. This method has allowed us to determine such features of performance as the trend envelope (the upper and lower limits of performance variability) and the prediction envelope (the probable range of performance if progress continues at a predictable rate). These concepts are listed in Table 5.

Much more research is needed in this area, but it is vital to begin to address these crucial questions related to rate of reacquisition of language skills and prediction of eventual performance outcomes. Perhaps some day we can be less than vague when

TABLE 5. *Celeration rates and trend analysis in aphasia treatment*[a]

Concepts for study, research, and clinical application
Quarter intersect method: Means of determining degree of slope of change (4-step method)
Trend envelope: Upper and lower limits of performance variability
Prediction envelope: Probable range of performance if progress continues at same rate

[a] From Matthews and LaPointe (23,24).

families and patients ask us: "How long must this go on?" We owe them data-based answers rather than gossamer promises and guesses.

SELF-CUEING

Another area that is gaining much long-neglected interest is that of teaching strategies of self-cueing or self-correction to our patients. Somehow, we must free our patients from the tether of dependence on the clinician's cues and prompts. We are currently working on this problem; in clinical aphasiology, we have underutilized the material that has been established in studies of normal verbal learning and verbal behavior.

Table 6 shows some results of studies on aids to cued recall in normal subjects that may have some application to aphasic word retrieval problems. The relative effectiveness of these types of cues must be thoroughly investigated in aphasia, including studies of strategies for altering depth of processing as we attempt to retrain retrieval of words that are not consistently accessible (25,26,31). Perhaps some of these strategies that have proved successful in normal verbal learning can be adapted to the development of self-cueing strategies useful when aphasic persons get stuck and are out of the range of our influence.

Self-cueing deserves much more attention. Even a small degree of freedom and self-reliance can be a breath of fresh air in the smothering communicative environment of aphasia.

TABLE 6. *Aids to cued recall from studies of normal verbal learning and verbal behavior*

1. Recall improves when cued with category names, other list items (20)
2. Recall improves when cued with restrictive attributes (22) ("animal . . . small . . . begins with M")
3. Cue is effective if it formed part of initial encoding of items (31)
4. Recall improves with synonym, homonym cue (21)
5. Recall improves with subset cues (11) (cities . . . "eastern, western"; sports . . . "indoor, outdoor")

In terms of what to expect in the future, we welcome any contributions from neuropharmacology, biochemistry, and basic neuroscience. It is unlikely that breakthroughs in these areas will eradicate neuropathology or make our services unnecessary in the near future, but we encourage anything that would augment or enhance our efforts.

Of course, the approaches reviewed in this chapter are not the only attempts that have been made in aphasia rehabilitation. Many have gone unmentioned, and this chapter is simply one person's view of what has been done by some to try to unravel this enigma so that we can help these people to more efficiently get on with learning and living.

No doubt we will continue to learn slowly and build on the past, as we have done. The impressive contemporary thinker from the University of Colorado, Kenneth Boulding (1), has expressed optimism about the potential of human discovery. He states that estimates have been made that only 10% of the brain is used, even by academics, and that the information potential of the human brain, with 10 billion neurons capable of being on or off and assuming difference states, would be $2^{10,000,000,000}$ (two to the 10-trillionth). This is a very large number; if we could write it at one digit per second, it would take 90 years to complete it. It seems hard not to believe, therefore, that the potential for structure of this extraordinary organization, and for solving some of our enigmatic problems in aphasia, is great, and that it is extremely improbable that we have even approached its boundary.

Many of us feel that the field of clinical aphasiology is poised on the threshold of tangible advancements in knowledge. The recent past justifies this optimism. We are finally moving from a clinical art to a fledgling clinical science. The thunderous effect of the loss of speech is such that, without it, life can become lonely, frustrating, morbid, and barren. Our profession is dedicated to support the beauty and efficiency of communication and more than ever to advance our knowledge of strategies of restoration when language becomes shattered (17).

REFERENCES

1. Boulding, K. (1981): Human knowledge as a special system. *Behav. Sci.*, 26:93–105.
2. Brookbank, W. (1954): *Ancient Therapeutic Arts*. W. Heinemann, London.
3. Brookshire, R. H. (1967): Speech pathology and the experimental analysis of behavior. *J. Speech Hear. Disord.*, 32:215.
4. Chapey, R. (1981): *Language Intervention Strategies in Adult Aphasia*. Williams & Wilkins, Baltimore.
5. Code, C., and Muller, D. J. (1983): *Aphasia Therapy*. Arnold, London.
6. Colby, K. M., Christinaz, D., Parkison, R. C., Graham, S., and Karpf, C. (1981): A word-finding computer program with a dynamic lexical-semantic memory for patients with anomia using an intelligent speech prosthesis. *Brain Lang.*, 14:272–281.
7. Critchley, M. (1970): *Aphasiology and Other Aspects of Language*. Arnold, London.
8. Darley, F. L. (1982): *Aphasia*. Saunders, Philadelphia.
9. Davis, G. A. (1983): *A Survey of Adult Aphasia*. Prentice-Hall, Englewood Cliffs, N.J.
10. Deloche, G., Seron, X., Coyette, F., Wendling, I., Hirsbrunner, T., and Van Eekhout, F. (1983): Microcomputer-assisted rehabilitation programs for patients with aphasia or visual neglect. Presented at International Neuropsychology Society Meeting, Lisbon.
11. Dillon, R. F., and Bitter, L. A. (1975): Analysis of retrieval cues and release from proactive inhibition. *J. Verb. Learn. Verb. Behav.*, 14:616–622.

12. Enderby, P., and Hamilton, G. (1983): Communication aid and therapeutic tool: A report on the clinical trial using SPLINK with aphasic patients. In: *Aphasia Therapy*, edited by C. Code and D. J. Muller, pp. 187–192. Arnold, London.
13. Holland, A. (1970): Case studies in aphasia rehabilitation. *J. Speech Hear. Disord.*, 35:377–390.
14. Horner, J., and Rothi, L. (1979): Recovery processes and treatment of aphasia. Presented to Annual Convention of the American Speech-Language-Hearing Association, Atlanta.
15. Katz, R. C. (1984): Using microcomputers in the diagnosis and treatment of chronic aphasic adults. *Semin. Speech Lang.*, 5:11–22.
16. LaPointe, L. L. (1977): Base-10 programmed-stimulation: Task specification scoring and plotting performance in aphasia therapy. *J. Speech. Hear. Disord.*, 42:90–105.
17. LaPointe, L. L. (1977): What the speech pathologist expects from the neurologist. In: *Clinical Aphasiology Conference Proceedings*, edited by R. Brookshire, pp. 5–9. BRK Press, Minneapolis.
18. LaPointe, L. L. (1978): Aphasia therapy: Some principles and strategies for treatment. In: *Clinical Management of Neurogenic Communication Disorders*, edited by D. F. Johns, pp. 129–190. Little, Brown, Boston.
19. LaPointe, L. L. (1983): Aphasia intervention with adults: Historical, present, and future approaches. In: *Contemporary Issues in Language Intervention*, edited by J. Miller, D. E. Yoder, and R. Schiefelbush, pp. 127–136. ASHA Reports 12, Rockville, Md.
20. Lewis, M. Q. (1971): Categorized lists and cued recall. *J. Exp. Psychol.*, 87:129–131.
21. Light, L. L. (1972): Homonyms and synonyms as retrieval cues. *J. Exp. Psychol.*, 96:255–262.
22. Loftus, E. F., and Cole, W. (1974): Retrieving attribute and name information from semantic memory. *J. Exp. Psychol.*, 102:1116–1122.
23. Matthews, B. J., and LaPointe, L. L. (1981): Determining rate of change and predicting performance levels in aphasia therapy. In: *Clinical Aphasiology Conference Proceedings*, edited by R. Brookshire, pp. 17–25. BRK Publishers, Minneapolis.
24. Matthews, B. J., and LaPointe, L. L. (1983): Slope and variability of performance on selected aphasia treatment tasks. Presented at 1983 Clinical Aphasiology Conference, Phoenix.
25. Nelson, D. L., Wheeler, J. W., Borden, R. C., and Brooks, D. H. (1974): Levels of processing and cueing sensory vs. meaning features. *J. Exp. Psychol.*, 103:971–977.
26. Nelson, T. O. (1977): Repetition and depth of processing. *J. Verb. Learn. Verb. Behav.*, 16:151–171.
27. Riese, W. (1947): The early history of aphasia. *Bull. Hist. Med.*, 23:322.
28. Sarno, M. T. (1981): *Acquired Aphasia*. Academic Press, New York.
29. Schuell, H., Jenkins, J., and Jiminez-Pabon, E. (1964): *Aphasia in Adults*. Harper & Row, New York.
30. Shakespeare, W. *Macbeth*, Scene V, iii, 40.
31. Tulving, E., and Pearlstone, M. (1966): Availability vs. accessibility of information in memory of words. *J. Verb. Learn. Verb. Behav.*, 5:381–391.

Advances in Neurology, Vol. 42: Progress in Aphasiology, edited by F. C. Rose.
Raven Press, New York © 1984.

Reeducation Strategies in Neuropsychology: Cognitive and Pragmatic Approaches

Xavier Seron

Neuropsychologie Expérimentale de l'Adulte (NEXA), Cliniques Universitaires St. Luc, Neurology, B-1200 Brussels, Belgium

Important developments in neuropsychologic reeducation in the United States and in a number of European countries involve theoretical, methodologic, and pragmatic matters. This chapter examines reeducational practice from the point of view of the theoretical concepts at their origins. As Martin (26), Sarno (29), and Albert et al. (1) have stressed, the theoretical underpinnings largely determine the methods employed in therapy. Such critical examination is of particular utility today, because false unifiers can give the illusion that there is incipient homogeneity developing among the different therapeutic practices. For example, every neuropsychologic therapy has recently become "cognitive," but it is not clear if this new label indicates the nature of the disturbances involved, if it qualifies the logic of reeducational strategies, or if it is merely a passing fad.

There is some need for theoretical clarification in the therapeutic field. This chapter discusses two major oppositions frequently put forward among therapists. The first is the reestablishment versus reorganizational opposition; the second is the "top-down" or "bottom-up" approach.

REESTABLISHMENT OR REORGANIZATIONAL STRATEGIES

In most of the critical reviews concerned with the logic of reeducational strategies, opposition is generally presented between those for which the disturbance is conceived as "loss of function" and those for which it reflects a difficulty of access to knowledge still stocked in the central nervous system. It is in these terms, for example, that Albert et al. (1) present the problems of reeducation of aphasics when they suggest:

> if we view dysphasia as a loss of language then we have a rationale for replacing lost information through teaching techniques. If we view dysphasia not as a loss of language but as a reduction of efficiency in gaining access to linguistic knowledge, then we have a rationale for stimulating the patient to improve his accessing or retrieval strategies.

In the same way, Sarno (29) established a link between the "stimulation-facilitation" approach of reeducation and the impaired access theory on the one hand, and, on the other hand, pedagogic approaches and the loss theory. If such a partition has the advantage of permitting a general classification of the therapeutic practices, taken in isolation, it neglects other differences on the level of description and comprehension of the disturbances to which one should refer before commencing therapy. The information provided by neuropsychologic research indicates that definition and comprehension of the disturbances cannot be grouped under the simple opposition of loss of access versus loss of knowledge. For the sake of convenience, however, I use this subdivision here.

We first consider some of the major problems raised by the loss of function theory, in which the therapeutic course seems to run in two directions: it either attempts to rebuild or reteach what has been lost, or it tries to implant a different behavioral repertoire that is capable of analogously achieving the objectives. It is in the attempts at reconstruction and, more precisely, in the attempts to establish the chronology of the reeducational exercises that this therapeutic path encounters the most difficulty. Indeed, a theoretical framework must be devised that is able to determine the merits of the proposed successions. A rapid survey of the literature reveals the existence of four different hierarchies in the organization of such teaching exercises: (a) developmental, (b) structural, (c) psychometric, and (d) neuropsychologic hierarchies. Even though overlappings occur, none is satisfactory, in that none can guarantee that the proposed progressions have any psychologic significance for the patient.

The developmental hierarchy presupposes a sort of reverse parallelism between the acquired pathologic condition and the progressive process of function acquisition during childhood. Such a presupposition may have some local validity but is globally inadequate. Furthermore, if there is some degree of parallelism between the semiology of an acquired disorder in adulthood and a developmental stage, this parallelism is only phenomenologic, and numerous experimental studies have cast doubt on the existence of any parallelism at all between the defective functional subprocesses responsible for the disorders and those underlying the normal acquisition of specific behavior (see ref. 9). Therefore, there is no good reason to retrace the developmental stages with a cerebral patient.

Another limitation of the developmental hierarchy is that it defines only the content of the successive exercises and gives no indication about the training procedures to be used. With respect to the acquisition of language, for example, we are beginning to find out what is acquired and in what order, but we know much less about the endogenous and exogenous mechanisms responsible for the acquisitions. Examples of such developmental strategies in neuropsychology are given by Crystal et al. (11) and Lecours and Lhermitte (24) for the treatment of agrammatism and by Froschels (18) for the treatment of global aphasic patients.

The hierarchies based on the structure of overt behavior are hardly more convincing. These strategies are used in the treatment of disordered expressive speech skills with a precise succession of exercises: first, the vowels and consonants, then syllables (bilabial first), and finally words and sentences (see, for example, refs. 10 and 12). For the treatment of agrammatism, the work of Naeser (28) aims at establishing the hierarchy of descriptive linguistic theories of grammatic complexity. The difficulty with such an approach is that data indicate that these step-by-step strategies violate well-known clinical facts that suggest that the structural complexity of stimuli and responses are not the only factors responsible for the patients' difficulties. In fact, the structural hierarchies erroneously transfer the notion of complexity from observable units to mental subprocesses. What is difficult for the patient is not the structural complexity of the stimuli to be treated or the response to be emitted, but rather the processes he actually uses in treatment. Furthermore, several arguments presented in the literature dealing with language acquisition or adult second language acquisition indicate that such acquisition never follows hierarchical lines (for a similar position, see ref. 26).

We need not give much attention to the psychometric hierarchies. They have rarely been used in neuropsychologic therapy and are basically the most atheoretical. Such hierarchies intervene only indirectly in that they indicate, for some schools of therapy, the objectives to be attained. In this sense, the psychometric approaches influence therapies that are viewed as attempts to return to the norm.

The last and probably most pertinent model is the one that proposes a hierarchy based on observation of spontaneous recovery. It is important to distinguish between the studies devoted to the analysis of recovery from a medical, etiologic, or diagnostic point of view and those that examine recovery as a foundation for treatment. The former are numerous and useful and provide some insight into the prediction of the temporal pattern of recovery and the possible changes in the semiology or type of aphasia on the basis of the initial clinical picture and numerous other variables (3,4,19,23,27,30).

More serious is the lack of studies on the nature of the pathologic evolution and, particularly, on the logic of the so-called spontaneous evolution. There are undoubtedly cases in which the evolution of the clinical picture can be described as "simply the recovery of a mode of functioning already used before the cerebral attack." In these relatively simple cases, it would be useful to provide detailed descriptions of the order in which functions are recovered.

There are more numerous cases in which the reestablishment of adequate mental functioning means the reorganization of the processes underlying these functions. This second possibility is more difficult to analyze. Little useful information is available because of the synchronic nature of most neurolinguistic investigations, as they are geared to the description and interpretation of abnormal behavior at one particular point in the evolution or to the description of abnormal clinical pictures that are essentially unchanging. Longitudinal studies would be useful in some areas of neurolinguistic research, especially if these investigations are aimed at the elaboration of a model of the operations underlying the observed difficulties. One example is the evolution of neologic jargon found in sensory aphasia. The hypotheses of Buckingham and Kertesz (7) and of Butterworth (8) could be tested over time, as Green (20) attempted to do some years ago. Longitudinal analysis would, in effect, allow us to examine how the three or four different operations suggested could account for the neologisms that arise in different degrees during the course of the evolution of the semiologic picture.

In agreement with the theoretical considerations stressing the difficulty of establishing hierarchies with psychologic validity, the empirical data indicate that the teaching strategies centered on the apparent disorders are hardly effective. For example, this is clearly the case in the reeducation of global aphasics with the step-by-step retraining method for oral articulation disorders and also in the attempts to provide reeducation for agrammatic individuals. Furthermore, in the rare cases in which some success has been observed, first, the progress did not follow a classic progressive curve, as would be the case in a relearning paradigm; second, a learning plateau always developed; and third, most authors have reported only a slight transfer of learning (22,31).

These theoretical problems need not lead us to reject the recovery strategies. Indeed, it is possible that they constitute the most adequate approach in some pathologic contexts. This is probably the case for cerebral contusions without a macroscopic lesion of the CNS. It may be presumed that the postlesional picture in these cases is essentially due to a transitory inhibition of normal functioning, although one that could last for several years. Here a legitimate objective would be the progressive retraining of the disturbed mental functions, but the difficulties encountered by the patient are not very specific. For example, with respect to language, there are problems in following group conversations, discrete lacks of words, and low scores on verbal fluency and verbal memory tests—all problems that must be placed in the context of attentional disorders of greater import.

In such cases, the most efficacious reeducational strategy consists of involving the patient in activities that become progressively longer and more demanding in the area of attention. It is then essentially a matter of stimulating the patient by means of progressively lengthening the therapy sessions and increasing the demands placed on his concentration.

Progress recently has been made in this area, as shown by the work of Trexler et al. (34a), who have anlayzed the different components of attention disorders: alertness, selectivity, and capacity. With such distinction, these authors have constructed sensitive rehabilitation programs by using microprocessor technology.

Another area of pathology where the objective of recovery could be accepted is that of infantile aphasia. Rapid and clinically complete recovery has been reported for children with a cerebral lesion (see refs. 2 and 25), but this affirmation must be qualified, because recent clinical studies seem to indicate that this recovery may not be a simple reestablishment of former capacities or be as perfect as suggested (14,41).

There is a dearth of longitudinal studies of children that are sufficiently analytic and capable of describing the nature of the reorganization of the spontaneous recovery in order to determine the extent to which it is a matter of reestablishment or reorganization or, what is more likely, what part is played by each of these two mechanisms in the spontaneous recovery. At this level, developmental hierarchies may be of interest to determine the level of development attained at the time of the cerebral accident and the content of the reeducational exercises.

We now examine the other major theoretical approach: the reduction of access to knowledge and the classic therapeutic strategy of stimulation-facilitation. The context in which such a dichotomy seems particularly clear-cut is the reeducation of anomia. For example, one can contrast those therapeutic attempts that are intended to achieve the relearning of an extensive lexicon and those that view anomia as a difficulty of retrieving words already in the lexical store. In this latter orientation, some empirical studies indicate that there is also a transfer effect that brings out nondrilled words when the patient is working on one part of the lexicon (see, for example, refs. 33 and 39). This would indicate that, at least in some cases, anomia probably is a retrieval problem.

The presentation of this second therapeutic approach as a stimulation-facilitation strategy does not clarify the therapeutic debate. In fact, all rehabilitation strategies could agree with such a general proposition, and all therapists dealing with teaching or relearning use all possible facilitation procedures. Indeed, the essential difference seems to be linked more with the specific character of the hypothesis in relation to the nature of the disorder.

In the studies of Wiegel-Crump and Koenigsknecht (39) and Seron et al. (33), the dichotomy is global, and the effects are observed in groups of patients. Because of the lack of precision of these studies, they can only indicate global positive effects and cannot explain precisely with what patients or under what conditions these results were obtained. This imprecision in relation to therapeutic effects seems to be due to the poverty of our theoretical models and to the persistence of group-based analysis.

Much of the recent neuropsychologic research centered on individual cases and conducted in the framework of an information processing theory indicates that our classic semiology is probably too crude and insufficiently discriminatory.

In the context of the cognitive approach to mental functioning, as proposed by Luria (25a) (and also after him), most of the neuropsychologic entities move toward fragmentation into numerous subunits. This considerable fragmentation corresponds to differential disorganization of the mental processes sustaining treatment and interpretation of information on different levels. Ultimately, it makes little sense to speak about reeducation in Broca's, Wernicke's, conduction, anomic, or agrammatic aphasia, or any other neuropsychologic entity derived from an anatomoclinical model, because their unity is questionable.

The essential problem that must be overcome for anomia reeducation is not that of the loss-of-language theory versus the loss-of-access theory but the identification of the disordered operations in the search for words and the specification of what has been lost from the lexical store(s). In the same way that we now have different kinds of dyslexia and different kinds of conduction aphasia, we shall have in the near future different kinds of agrammatism, different kinds of prosopagnoses, and so on.

The clinician's idea that each patient is unique must be taken seriously. For example, the work being done in our laboratory on anomic patients examines for each patient in detail the influence of frequently cited variables in anomic studies, such as the dichotomies of abstract/concrete, figurative/operative, word length, functional/lexical contrast, frequency of usage, syllabic complexity, and so on. What presently appears is a contrasted picture for virtually every subject. Thus there is no reason to assume that general strategies may be efficacious for every anomic case.

If we accept the point of view that a cerebral lesion may affect some relatively independent subprocesses in certain cases, only more analytic strategies will be effective in our attempts to achieve reorganization. These efforts will be made easier with a single-subject paradigm, but, as we indicated elsewhere (32), this involves several prerequisites. First, to effect a reorganization of the processes that underly behavioral deficiencies, it is necessary that there be a sufficiently clear picture of these processes and of the manner in which they coalesce to produce the function observed. Second, it is necessary within the context of the pathology to be able to put forward plausible hypotheses aimed at identifying both the defective and the intact processes that could aid the whole functional ensemble. Third, it is necessary in any event that the intact processes to which one proposes to have recourse in order to reorganize the functioning should, on the whole, have a certain efficacy.

There are presently few therapeutic projects that meet the requirements and the logic of such an approach. Notable exceptions are the work of Hatfield (21) at Cambridge on surface and deep dysgraphia syndromes and the work of Beauvois and Dérouesné (6) on specific and selective disorders, such as optic aphasia and phonologic dyslexia. It has yet to be determined, however, what proportion such selective semiologic cases represent.

TOP-DOWN AND BOTTOM-UP OPPOSITION

Another opposition has been put forward recently between strategies focused on modality-specific delineated disorders [(the so-called "direct" approach of Wepman (38)] and, on the other hand, those that underline the necessity of exercises focusing on more global cognitive and communicative processes. In aphasiology, such an opposition exists between the psycholinguistic-modality approach and the pragmatic contextual approach. The debate may be summarized as follows: The opponents of the specific disorders oriented approach underline, first, the frequent absence of transfer of learning to daily life situations and, second, the artificial character of the exercises, which raises motivational difficulties during therapy. For their part, the opponents of the pragmatic approaches indicate that it is far more complex to analyze what changes occur in complex natural settings and to identify the variable responsible for changes that occur.

Presently, the debate cannot be resolved on the basis of empirical data. In each orientation, therapists have generally evaluated the progress they have obtained by scoring systems designed to fit their objectives. In the pragmatic approaches, functional tests of communication are generally used, such as the functional communication profile (28b), the Porch index of communicative ability (28a), and communicative abilities in daily living (22a). In modality-specific approaches, the tests used focus on the specific verbal behavior. Thus the validations are in some ways circular.

On a theoretical level, the psycholinguistic-modality approach is based on linguistically oriented models of language distinguishing lexical, syntactic, and phonologic components and their corresponding cognitive processes; pragmatic-oriented therapies are closer to models considering verbal activity in a more extended framework that includes the cognitive processes sustaining the communicatory functions of language. Such theoretical frameworks need not necessarily determine our therapeutic choices. Although there is more evidence in favor of the thesis that aphasia is predominantly a disorder situated on the level of the grammatic and lexical components of the verbal activity, it does not logically follow that the pragmatic approach has no value in reeducation. As Feyereisen (15) has noted, there is no evidence that aphasic disorders may be more adequately explained in a pragmatic framework. On the contrary, the author stresses that most studies indicate better preservation of the pragmatic level than what Bates et al. (5) have called the "more conversationally neutral" levels. This is evidenced in several studies on the receptive level by Wilcox et al. (40), Stachiowiak et al. (34), and Waller and Darley (37), as well as on the productive level by Ulatowska et al. (35,36) and Bates et al. (5). For nonverbal communication, which has some pragmatic pertinence, although the data at our disposal are still too limited (16,17), I share the general opinion of Davis and Wilcox (13) that if aphasic patients present some difficulties in producing and comprehending nonverbal messages in comparison with normals, their nonverbal competence is generally still better than their linguistic capacity.

If, as I suggest, there is a sort of dissociation in aphasia between relatively intact pragmatic competence and grammatical and lexical disorders, one may question the pertinence of designing therapy to deal with the pragmatic level, which is relatively well preserved. The main reason for doing so is that most aphasics must discover that their communicational abilities cannot be equated with their language disorders; in other words, they must know that they can communicate better than they can speak. Moreover, if we postulate a dissociation between the pragmatic and the linguistic components of language, such a dissociation is only relative, and we still must explore the interactions existing between the different levels. Thus there is a possibility that training communication efficiency has some secondary effects on lexical and grammatic components. Finally, certain kinds of aphasia, notably, the jargon aphasia at the onset of the disorder and dynamic aphasia, may present some pragmatic primary disorders.

In our opinion, there is no good reason to present the debate in terms of all or nothing, as though it were necessary to choose between these two orientations.

REFERENCES

1. Albert, M. L., Goodglass, H., Helm, N. A., Rubens, A. B., and Alexander, M. P. (1981): *Clinical Aspects of Dysphasia*. Springer Verlag, New York.
2. Basser, L. S. (1962): Hemiplegia of early onset and the faculty of speech with special reference to the effects of hemispherectomy. *Brain*, 85:427–460.
3. Basso, A., Capitani, E., and Vignolo, L. A. (1979): Influence of rehabilitation on language skills in aphasic patients. *Arch. Neurol.*, 36:190–196.

4. Basso, A., Fagnoli, P., and Vignolo, L. A. (1975): Etude contrôlée de la rééducation du langage dans l'aphasie: comparaison entre aphasiques traités et non traités. *Rev. Neurol.* (*Paris*), 131:607–614.
5. Bates, E., Hamby, S., and Zurif, E. (1983): The effects of focal brain damage on pragmatic expression. *Can. J. Psychol.*, 37:59–84.
6. Beauvois, M. F., and Dérouesné, J. (1981): Recherche en neuropsychologie et rééducation: Quels rapports? In: *Rééduquer le Cerveau, Logopédie, Psychologie, Neurologie*, edited by X. Seron and C. Laterre, pp. 163–189. Mardaga, Bruxelles.
7. Buckingham, H. W., and Kertesz, A. (1976): *Neologistic Jargon Aphasia*. Swets and Zeitlinger, Amsterdam.
8. Butterworth, B. (1979): Hesitation and the production of verbal paraphasias and neologisms in jargon aphasia. *Brain Lang.*, 8:133–161.
9. Caramazza, L., and Zurif, E. B., editors (1978): *Language Acquisition and Language Breakdown, Parallels and Divergencies*. The Johns Hopkins University Press, Baltimore.
10. Corbin, M. L. (1951): Group speech therapy for motor aphasia and dysarthria. *J. Speech Hear. Disord.*, 16:21–34.
11. Crystal, D., Fletcher, P., and Garman, M. (1976): *The Grammatical Analysis of Language Disabilities*. Elsevier, New York.
12. Dabul, B., and Bollier, B. (1976): Therapeutic approaches to apraxia. *J. Speech Hear. Disord.*, 41:268–273.
13. Davis, G. A., and Wilcox, J. (1981): Incorporating parameters of natural conversation in aphasia treatment. In: *Language Intervention Strategies in Adult Aphasia*, edited by R. Chapey, pp. 169–193. Williams & Wilkins, Baltimore.
14. Dennis, M., and Whitaker, H. A. (1977): Hemispheric equipotentiality and language acquisition. In: *Language Development and Neurological Theory*, edited by S. Segalowitz and F. Grueber, pp. 93–106. Academic Press, New York.
15. Feyereisen, P. (1983): Les troubles de l'expression et les niveaux de production verbale. In: *Pathologie de l'Expression Orale*, edited by P. Messerli, P. Lavorel, and J. L. Nespoulous, pp. 131–159. Monographies Françaises de Psychologie, CNRS, Paris.
16. Feyereisen, P., and Seron, X. (1982): Non verbal communication and aphasia. Part I, comprehension. *Brain Lang.*, 16:191–212.
17. Feyereisen, P., and Seron, X. (1982): Non verbal communication and aphasia. Part II: Production. *Brain Lang.*, 16:213–236.
18. Froschels, E. (1933): *Speech Therapy*. Expression CO, Boston.
19. Gloning, K., Trappl, R., Wolf-Dieter, H., and Quatember, R. (1976): Prognosis and speech therapy in aphasia. In: *Recovery in Aphasics*, edited by Y. Lebrun and R. Hoops, pp. 57–64. Swets and Zeitlinger, Amsterdam.
20. Green, E. (1969): Phonological and grammatical aspects of jargon in an aphasic patient: A case study. *Lang. Speech*, 12:103–118.
21. Hatfield, F. M. (1981): Diverses formes de désintégration du langage écrit et implications pour la rééducation. In: *Rééduquer le Cerveau, Logopédie, Psychologie, Neurologie*, edited by X. Seron and C. Laterre, pp. 135–156. Mardaga, Bruxelles.
22. Helm-Estabrooks, N., Fitzpatrick, P. M., and Barresi, B. (1981): Response of an agrammatic patient to a syntax facilitation program for aphasia. *J. Speech Hear. Disord.*, 46:422–427.
22a. Holland, A. (1980): *Communicative Abilities in Daily Living*. University Park Press, Baltimore.
23. Kertesz, A., and McCabe, P. (1977): Recovery patterns and prognosis in aphasia. *Brain*, 100:1–18.
24. Lecours, A. R., and Lhermitte, F., editors (1979): *L'Aphasie*. Flammarion, Paris.
25. Lenneberg, E. H. (1967): *Biological Foundations of Language*. Wiley, New York.
25a. Luria, A. R. (1973): *The Working Brain, an Introduction to Neuropsychology*. Allen Lane, London.
26. Martin, A. D. (1977): Processing strategies in aphasia rehabilitation. Paper presented at American Speech and Hearing Association Meeting, Chicago.
27. Messerli, P., Tissot, A., and Rodriquez, J. (1976): Recovery from aphasia: Some factors of prognosis. In: *Recovery in Aphasics*, edited by Y. Lebrun and R. Hoops, pp. 124–135. Swets and Zeitlinger, Amsterdam.
28. Naeser, M. A. (1974): A structured approach teaching aphasic basic sentence types. *Br. J. Commun.*, 10:70–76.
28a. Porch, B. E. (1967): *Porch Index of Communicative Ability*. Consulting Psychologist Press, Palo Alto, Calif.

28b. Sarno, M. T. (1969): The functional communication profile. Rehabilitation Monograph, 42, Institute of Rehabilitation Medicine, New York University, Medical Center, New York.
29. Sarno, M. T., editor (1981): Recovery and rehabilitation in aphasia. In: *Acquired Aphasia*, pp. 485–530. Academic Press, New York.
30. Sarno, M. T., and Levita, E. (1971): Natural course of recovery in severe aphasia. *Arch. Phys. Med.*, 52:175–178.
31. Sarno, M. T., Silverman, M., and Sands, E. (1970): Speech therapy and language recovery in severe aphasia. *J. Speech Hear. Res.*, 13:607–623.
32. Seron, X. (1982): The reeducation of aphasics: The problem of the reeducation strategies. *Intern. J. Psychol.*, 17:299–317.
33. Seron, X., Deloche, G., Bastard, V., Chassin, G., and Hermand, N. (1979): Word-findings difficulties and learning transfer in aphasic patients. *Cortex*, 15:149–155.
34. Stachowiak, F. J., Huber, W., Poeck, K., and Kerschenstein, M. (1977): Text comprehension in aphasia. *Brain Lang.*, 4:179–195.
34a. Trexler, L. E., Potter, S. L., Schmidt, M. S., and Thomas, J. D. (1982): Cognitive Rehabilitation program, Rehabilitation Monograph, August F. Hook Physical Rehabilitation Center, Community Hospital of Indianapolis.
35. Ulatowska, H. K., Doyel, A. W., Stern, R. F., and Haynes, S. M. (1983): Production of procedural discourse aphasia. *Brain Lang.*, 18:315–341.
36. Ulatowska, H. K., North, A. J., and Macaluno-Haynes, S. (1981): Production of narrative and procedural discourse in aphasia. *Brain Lang.*, 13:345–371.
37. Waller, M. R., and Darley, F. L. (1978): Effect of prestimulation in sentence comprehension by aphasic subjects. *J. Speech Hear. Res.*, 21:732–745.
38. Wepman, J. (1972): Aphasia therapy: A new look. *J. Speech Hear. Disord.*, 37:203–214.
39. Wiegel-Crump, C., and Koenigsknecht, R. A. (1973): Tapping the lexical score of the adult aphasic: Analysis of the improvement made in word retrieval skills. *Cortex*, 9:410–418.
40. Wilcox, M. J., Davis, G. A., and Leonard, L. B. (1978): Aphasic's comprehension of contextually conveyed meaning. *Brain Lang.*, 6:362–377.
41. Woods, B. T., and Carey, S. (1979): Language deficits after apparent clinical recovery from childhood aphasia. *Ann. Neurol.*, 6:405–409.

Advances in Neurology, Vol. 42: Progress in Aphasiology, edited by F. C. Rose.
Raven Press, New York © 1984.

Advances in the Evaluation and Treatment of Speech Apraxia

John C. Rosenbek

William S. Middleton Memorial Veterans Administration Hospital, Madison, Wisconsin 53705

A SHORT HISTORY

Considerable energy has been expended (much of it unnecessarily) since 1861, and especially since 1969, in arguments about whether apraxia of speech is a disorder distinct from the major forms of aphasia. The 19th century polemic was inevitable; seminal ideas are almost always assailed. The acrimonious debate of more recent times has been ignited by quite different tinder.

First is the label itself. Apraxia was borrowed from the neurologic literature, and such words as "verbal," "articulatory," or "of speech" were attached. As used in the neurologic literature, apraxia referred to particular kinds of disturbed limb movements. A close reading of a variety of texts shows that clinical researchers disagree about what the disorder is and how many forms it can take. It is predictable, therefore, that the term's transfer to speech movements would not have occurred without incident.

A larger problem was created by the uses and interpretations of data from the early descriptive studies of apraxic speech. The first studies were primarily perceptual, using broad phonetic transcription. Shankweiler and Harris (36) tried to put such studies in perspective. They emphasized that broad transcription could highlight the gross features of a disorder that was feckless at revealing the underlying physiology. The usual finding from broad transcription (18,24) was that substitution errors predominated in apraxic speech. Apostles for apraxia concluded that those errors differentiated the disorder from the dysarthrias and the aphasias and that they resulted from apraxic movements of the speech structures.

Some researchers, Martin (29) among them, argued that substitution errors proved that apraxia was a phonologic disorder and therefore one of the aphasias. Others (8,12) demonstrated that apraxic speech was influenced by "linguistic" variables, such as part of speech, frequency of occurrence, and meaningfulness. Still others (23,28) reported being able to predict apraxic errors using distinctive feature and markedness analyses. These data, too, were used to bolster arguments about whether or not apraxia of speech is an aphasia.

NEW INTERPRETATIONS

Speech scientists are now being lured into apraxia of speech research. New interpretations of existing data and new data are resulting.

Kent and Rosenbek (20) claim that the linguistic and motoric interactions used by some to deny apraxia its separateness from the aphasias is normal and inevitable. One sees it in all normal speakers and in a variety of abnormal ones, including stutterers. Nothing substantive is gained by calling stuttering, aphasia. As part of their evaluation of the distinctive feature and markedness studies, these same authors warn against confusing one's method of analysis with the results of that analysis. That apraxic errors are reported to be predictable from what are primarily linguistically oriented systems does not support the interpretation that apraxia of speech is a linguistic disorder. In addition, the apraxic speaker's tendency to use unmarked sounds may simply be one more example of entropy or movement toward the most natural or predictable. Even apraxic substitutions are being reinterpreted in light of modern motor theories of speech movements; the old idea that linguistic notions are the only ones capable of coping with substitutions is deteriorating (33).

NEW DATA

By far the greatest changes in attitudes about apraxia of speech, however, are resulting from acoustic and physiologic analyses. Such analyses have not and will not supplant that of the ear. They will, however, complement perceptual analyses and lead to further revisions of what apraxia of speech is and why the symptoms are what they are. They eventually may even make clinicians better listeners and more efficient teachers.

Acoustic Studies

Acoustic studies have been of two overlapping types. The first was primarily descriptive. Researchers were interested in quantifying features such as apraxic rate, intonation, and speech sound production, including voice onset time (VOT). The second was to examine the ability of the apraxic speaker to follow certain phonologic rules.

Speaking Rate

The general finding is that apraxic talkers are slower than normal (3,20,21). Studies reporting they are faster (6) have either measured something other than rate or have used relatively simple consonant-vowel-consonant (CVC) utterances (7).

Kent and Rosenbek (21) have identified two forms of slowness: articulatory prolongation and syllable segregation. Articulatory prolongation is defined as "a lengthening of steady-state segments and the intervening transitions" (p. 233). As but one example of the magnitude of such slowness, the authors report that for a group of apraxic talkers, the syllable nuclei in the utterance "In the summer they sell vegetables" were four or more times longer than those of normal speakers. Syllable segregation is defined as "a pattern of temporally separated or isolated syllables" (p. 233). Voicing sometimes, but not usually, continues through the breaks between syllables. These authors identified similar patterns of slowness in imitative speech, spontaneous speaking, and reading but were careful to underline the variability of rate disturbance, even for an individual speaker.

Other Prosodic Dimensions

Kent and Rosenbek (21) also studied aspects of loudness and fundamental frequency contour. The apraxic speakers "showed less variation in relative peak intensity across syllables" (p. 237), and they produced unstressed syllables with relatively greater intensity than did normal controls. These results were interpreted as showing "a flattening of the intensity envelope across a syllabic sequence" (p. 237). All utterances, even by individual patients, however, did not show this flattening, a finding that once again confirms the variability of apraxia of speech. Sentence terminal fall in the fundamental frequency, on the other hand, was preserved in apraxic utterances, leading the authors to suggest that this feature is "robust." Large variability made further conclusions about intonation contour impossible. At least one other study (19) has reported a constriction in the fundamental frequency contour similar to that reported for the intensity envelope.

Segmental or Speech Sound Errors

VOT analysis

Analysis of VOT is presently one of the most popular ways of analyzing apraxic productions of voiced and voiceless cognates. Blumstein et al. (1) describe VOT "as the timing relation between release of the burst in a stop consonant and the onset of glottal pulsing" (p. 155). Normal, average VOTs differ for voiced and voiceless cognates in predictable ways, depending on place of articulation and phonetic environment. Several studies (10,16,21) have documented abnormalities in the VOTs of apraxic talkers. Others (1,39) have demonstrated similar abnormalities in production by patients with Broca's aphasia. Both groups produce overlapping distributions of VOT that suggest the blurring of boundaries between voiced and voiceless cognates.

These abnormalities have been interpreted in two ways. Blumstein et al. (1) and Shewan et al. (39) have divided VOT abnormalities into phonetic and phonemic errors, depending on the amount of VOT error and the number of times these occur. Errors of certain magnitudes are classified as phonemic; errors of other magnitudes are classified as phonetic. These authors have identified both types in apraxic speech. Other authors (16) question the validity of the phonetic/phonemic dichotomy. They prefer to interpret most VOT errors as "indicative of the existence of a difficulty in the temporal programming of the laryngeal and supralaryngeal articulatory adjustments" (p. 209).

The peculiar status of productions by conduction aphasic individuals, which in some cases resemble those of apraxic talkers (1), highlights an increasingly important diagnostic and therapeutic issue: whether conduction aphasic and apraxic talkers can be differentiated and whether different mechanisms account for their symptomatology. A similar issue is raised by the apparent emergence of two apraxic types in the VOT literature. The possibility of at least two types is not new; it has been suggested by other authors (5,27) using other data.

Vowel errors

With few exceptions (26,37) early studies featured consonant errors and suggested that vowels were produced more or less normally. Recent research is confirming what some clinicians have long recognized: apraxic speakers also have difficulty with some vowels. The data of Kent and Rosenbek (21), for example, show that apraxic vowels are not only prolonged but often are distorted, sometimes by quite complex diphthong-like movements. They claim that to describe these as simple substitutions would be a misrepresentation.

Other segmental errors

Spectrographic analysis has also confirmed the presence of the traditional substitution and sequencing errors identified in the perceptual literature. Kent and Rosenbek (21), for example, identified /l/ and /r/ as especially difficult for some apraxic talkers. The traditional clinical litany held that apraxic talkers have difficulty initiating speech; this difficulty has been confirmed by acoustic analysis, as has the long-recognized ability to move closer to a target with repeated attempts.

Conformity To Phonologic Rules

In order to test whether apraxia of speech is linguistic or motoric, studies are being done of apraxic speaker's conformity to phonologic rules. Collins et al. (3) showed that apraxic talkers, like normal ones, reduce the length of vowel nuclei as utterances increase in length. They also documented the apraxic talker's ubiquitous slowness and variability. Duffy and Gawle (7) studied vowel durations preceding voiced and voiceless consonants in imitated CVC words. These authors tested whether apraxic speakers followed the rule that in normal speech, vowels preceding voiced consonants average 40 to 50% greater duration than those same vowels before voiceless consonants. They studied apraxic ($N = 5$), aphasic ($N = 4$), and normal ($N = 5$) speakers. In general, their data show that the apraxic and aphasic patients were variable but followed the rule. Some patients in both groups were more variable than normal. The authors explain the variability of aphasics by a thorough analysis of individual patient histories and symptoms. They conclude that their data do not support a linguistic explanation for apraxic errors.

Of greatest interest is the finding that apraxic talkers produced shorter than normal vowels (7). The authors admit the limitation of this finding, which was based on vowels in six CVC words. The CVCs indeed may be a special case. Increased vowel lengths in apraxic speech may be compensatory. Apraxic talkers may lengthen vowels as a way of preparing themselves for more difficult consonant productions; CVCs may not be difficult enough to require the compensation.

Physiologic Studies

Physiologic studies have used the X-ray microbeam, fiberscopic observation, electromyography (EMG), and movement transducers. The clinical importance of such measures was established years ago when, for example, Shankweiler et al. (37) said, "Precise information regarding which gestures of speech are defective and the physiological basis of the defects are requirements for rational therapy" (p. 1).

X-Ray Microbeam Research

Itoh and his group (15) were apparently the first to use an X-ray microbeam system to make physiologic measurements of an apraxic speaker. They confirmed the reduced velocity of apraxic speech movements that had been abundantly documented by acoustic analysis. They also concluded, by simultaneous analysis of palatal and tongue movements, that their "pure" apraxic talker suffered from an "apparent disorganization of timing among the several articulators" (p. 69). The authors further offered that apraxic errors are more often distortions than substitutions. Finally, because they also studied dysarthric speakers, one with amyotrophic lateral sclerosis and one with ataxic dysarthria, they were able to confirm that apraxic and selected dysarthric movement abnormalities are different.

Fiberscopic Observation

In an earlier study, Itoh et al. (14) used fiberscopic observation of apraxic velar movements. Their subject is reported to have preserved the general pattern of velar movements but to have been variable and to have produced many movements that resulted in speech sound distortion, with an occasional outright substitution, which they nonetheless call a "phonetic" change. The authors claim that the disturbed velar movements were not suggestive of phoneme selection or retrieval errors. To confirm this interpretation, Itoh's group (17) then made fiberscopic analyses of velar movements by two patients with Wernicke's aphasia. The patterns were different and less variable than those seen in apraxic talkers. Error movements (substitutions) were nearly identical to movements for the same sound when it appeared correctly.

EMG and Movement Analysis

Fromm et al. (11) report movement and EMG data from three relatively pure apraxic speakers, expanding on earlier EMG measurements reported by Shankweiler et al. (37). Fromm's group identified several movement abnormalities: (a) antagonistic muscle cocontractions, (b) continuous, undifferentiated EMG activity, (c) muscle activity shutdown, (d) movement without voice, (e) movement dyscoordination, (f) addition, and (g) groping. They suggest four implications for these data. First, they point up the substantial degree of dyscoordination characteristic of apraxia of speech and observe that it is different from that seen in ataxic dysarthria. Next, they claim that apraxic speakers have a high proportion of distortion errors. Third, they interpret the errors as representing motor execution and programing abnormalities rather than abnormal phonologic selection. Finally, they echo a common theme: disorders characterized by impaired movement and muscle control should be studied by direct observations of physiologic variables if they are to be adequately understood.

Revisionism

Quantification of apraxic abnormalities is increasing. Evidence that a high proportion of apraxic errors are distortions rather than substitutions, that apraxic movements differ from aphasic and dysarthric ones, and that apraxic talkers obey certain kinds of linguistic rules, despite being slow talkers, lend credence to the argument that apraxia of speech is a nonaphasic, nondysarthric syndrome. This is not to imply that it is a phonetic disorder. Indeed, a distinction between phonetic and phonemic may be artificial; certainly it is a hard distinction to make except by fiat.

Alternatives for Subsequent Research

Other constructs may be better guides for subsequent research. Candidates include recent models of neural organization and contemporary theories and models of motor programing. Models of neural organization include concepts about centers, coalitions, and stages (2,33). Models of motor programing include Lashley's (25) hierarchical model of serial ordering and more recent models, such as that by Sternberg and colleagues (40), that hypothesize the contributions to movement of advanced planning and feedback. Both models predict subtypes of apraxia secondary to cortical lesions and the possibility that speech apraxia may result from both cortical and subcortical lesions. Researchers using these and other models are already describing two apraxic syndromes resulting from cortical lesions (5,27) and a subcortical form of the disorder (22).

ADVANCES IN TREATMENT

Several surveys of apraxia treatment have been published (32,38,42) and are not summarized here. The problem, however, is that methods are abundant but criteria for case selection and data on treatment efficacy are few. People who believe in the label seem to believe in its treatment as well; but this belief is inadequate and may even be stultifying. As a result, this section highlights what seems to be necessary if future practice is to be more systematic and data based than present practice.

Better Candidate Selection

Better candidate selection is crucial. Distinctions between Broca's aphasia and apraxia of speech, between both these conditions and global and conduction aphasia, and between types of apraxia must come to be reflected in treatment differences as well. While a certain number of common principles may influence treatments of both neuromotor and linguistic disorders (33,42), many principles and most stimulus and methods selection are different. Diagnosticians have the obligation to separate their patients by label whenever possible and to tailor treatments to that label and to the patient's idiosyncracies.

Even when labeling is impossible (and it often is), focused treatment is not. The goals of treatment with the difficult to dissect patient are to improve communication and to be structured so that patients' responses reveal something about what they have. The process, called *diagnosis ex juvantibus*, is not new; in the United States, for example, Wepman and Van Pelt (41) discussed it years ago.

Better Structure

Treatments can profitably be organized according to the structures and restraints of single case design technology (31). The three most popular are (a) withdrawal, (b) multiple baseline, and (c) alternating treatments. General guidelines about specifying and limiting the treatment approach, amount and type of testing, data analysis, tester, test environment, and so on are similar for all three. If obeyed, these guidelines improve the rigor of the treatment. Rigor is increased even further by conducting treatment within the specific structures of one of these three designs. Apraxia of speech treatment demands this because professionals in all countries have had to rely for too long on each other's declamations rather than on their data. These data need not—indeed should not—be group data. Group studies will be appropriate after individual techniques have been tested and organized into treatment packages (13).

Regardless of whether treatment is to be conducted as an experiment or merely as a matter of clinical necessity, six other influences shape its structure: (a) nature of apraxia of speech, (b) relationship of physiologic and linguistic processes, (c) nonspeech residuals of brain damage, (d) data and heuristic notions about skill learning, (e) the clinician's education and experience, and (f) the patient's abilities, attitudes, and expectations. Time and space restrict our discussion of these; the last two are so idiosyncratic as to be of no use in a general discussion under any conditions. The first four have been discussed in detail elsewhere (42).

Only discussion of the first, the nature of apraxia of speech, is included here. Apraxia of speech is a nondysarthric, nonaphasic movement disorder or loss of skill. Primary symptoms are substitutions, distortions, and dysprosody. A major physiologic symptom, dyscoordination, responds predictably to a variety of stimulus conditions. This view has several advantages: it highlights the therapeutic targets, justifies the search for patterns during evaluation and their manipulation during treatment, reminds clinicians that treatment is the structured relearning of skilled speech movements, and provides the rationale for certain kinds of specific techniques.

Improved Methods

Behavioral Techniques

There has been no revolution—just evolution—in techniques. Newer methods are less strictly "articulation" and more strictly speech and communication oriented. Among the newer techniques are contrastive stress drills (9) in the form of question and answer dialogues requiring the apraxic talker to systematically vary stress and rhythm in ways that seem to facilitate speech sound production as well as improve prosody. Guidelines for constructing the drills and steps for executing them have been published (42). Another fairly recent development is gestural reorganization based on Luria's (27) concept of intersystemic reorganization. In this method, the apraxic talker is taught to pace speech by pairing limb or head and speech gestures. Rationale, guidelines for organizing the treatment, and specific treatment steps are appearing in the literature (42).

Instrumental Techniques

Instrumental techniques are also being described in the treatment literature because they are increasingly available and because characteristics of apraxia and the apraxic talker make certain of them logical. The EMG-assisted biofeedback (30) has promise. Apraxic talkers are often tense. McNeil et al. (30) examined the pre- and postrelaxation speech-language performance of three such patients. They were better communicators after the treatment than before, even though they had not received any specific speech-language treatment. Rubow et al. (35) compared the influence of imitation plus vibrotactile stimulation against that of simple imitation on the single word performance of one apraxic speaker. Words in the imitation plus vibrotactile condition improved significantly more than did words in simple imitation.

Imitation

Imitation, which has been the heart of much apraxia treatment (4,34), is being reevaluated. Its parsimony, if nothing else, has made it popular. It may be, however, that neuromotor controls for imitation and for spontaneous speech are different enough, so that responses elicited imitatively are difficult for patients to carry over into spontaneous speech. As a result, imitative paradigms are being evaluated against other approaches and are being expanded with specific carry over steps so that talking in treatment is more like talking outside of it.

CONCLUSION

It is difficult to exaggerate how rapidly data on apraxia of speech are accumulating. Revision of the traditional symptom profile and of historic attitudes about locus of lesion, existence of subtypes, and proper management is pandemic. Speech scientists are contributing models, experimental techniques and instrumentation, new data, and new interpretations. Clinicians are benefiting from and contributing to the change. Indeed, hopefully, this chapter will be outdated soon after it appears.

REFERENCES

1. Blumstein, S. E., Cooper, W. E., Goodglass, H., Statlender, S., and Gottlieb, J. (1980): Production deficits in aphasia: A voice-onset time analysis. *Brain Lang.*, 9:153–170.
2. Buckingham, H., Jr. (1979): Explanation in apraxia with consequences for the concept of apraxia of speech. *Brain Lang.*, 8:202–226.
3. Collins, M. J., Rosenbek, J. C., and Wertz, R. T. (1983): Spectrographic analysis of vowel and word duration in apraxia of speech. *J. Speech Hear. Res.*, 26:224–230.
4. Deal, J. L., and Florance, C. L. (1978): Modification of the eight-step continuum for treatment of apraxia of speech in adults. *J. Speech Hear. Disord.*, 43:89–95.
5. Deutsch, S. E. (1984): Prediction of site of lesion from speech apraxic error patterns. In: *Apraxia of Speech: Physiology-Acoustics-Linguistics-Management*, edited by J. C. Rosenbek, M. McNeil, and A. Aronson, pp. 113–134. College-Hill Press, San Diego.
6. DiSimoni, F. G., and Darley, F. L. (1977): Effect on phoneme duration control of three utterance-length conditions in an apractic patient. *J. Speech Hear. Disord.*, 42:257–264.
7. Duffy, J. R., and Gawle, C. A. (1984): Apraxic speaker's vowel durations in CVC syllables. In: *Apraxia of Speech: Physiology-Acoustics-Linguistics-Management*, edited by J. C. Rosenbek, M. McNeil, and A. Aronson, pp. 167–196. College-Hill Press, San Diego.
8. Dunlop, J. M., and Marquardt, T. P. (1977): Linguistic and articulatory aspects of single word production in apraxia of speech. *Cortex*, 13:17–29.
9. Fairbanks, G. (1960): *Voice and Articulation Drillbook*. Harper & Row, New York.
10. Freeman, F., Sands, E., and Harris, K. (1978): Temporal coordination of phonation and articulation in a case of verbal apraxia: A voice onset time study. *Brain Lang.*, 6:106–111.
11. Fromm, D., Abbs, J., McNeil, M., and Rosenbek, J. (1982): Simultaneous perceptual-physiological method for studying apraxia of speech. In: *Clinical Aphasiology*, edited by R. H. Brookshire, pp. 251–262. BRK Press, Minneapolis.
12. Hardison, D., Marquardt, T. P., and Peterson, H. A. (1977): Effects of selected linguistic variables on apraxia of speech. *J. Speech Hear. Res.*, 20:334–343.
13. Hersen, M., and Barlow, D. H. (1976): *Single Case Experimental Designs—Strategies for Studying Behavior Change*. Pergamon, New York.
14. Itoh, M., Sasanuma, S., and Ushijima, T. (1979): Velar movements during speech in a patient with apraxia of speech. *Brain Lang.*, 7:227–239.
15. Itoh, M., Sasanuma, S., Hirose, H., Yoshioka, H., and Ushijima, T. (1980): Abnormal articulatory dynamics in a patient with apraxia of speech: X-ray microbeam observation. *Brain Lang.*, 11:66–75.
16. Itoh, M., Sasanuma, S., Tatsumi, I. F., Murakami, S., Fukusako, Y., and Suzuki, T. (1982): Voice onset time characteristics in apraxia of speech. *Brain Lang.*, 17:193–210.
17. Itoh, M., Sasanuma, S., Hirose, H., Yoshioka, H., and Sawashima, M. (1983): Velar movements during speech in two Wernicke aphasic patients. *Brain Lang.*, 19:283–292.
18. Johns, D. F., and Darley, F. L. (1970): Phonemic variability in apraxia of speech. *J. Speech Hear. Res.*, 13:556–583.
19. Keatley, M. A. (1979): A comparison of intonational contours in subjects with apraxia of speech and normals. *Aphasia, Apraxia, Agnosia*, 1:30–42.
20. Kent, R. D., and Rosenbek, J. C. (1982): Prosodic disturbance and neurologic lesion. *Brain Lang.*, 15:259–291.
21. Kent, R. D., and Rosenbek, J. C. (1983): Acoustic patterns of apraxia of speech. *J. Speech Hear. Res.*, 26:231–249.
22. Kertesz, A. (1984): Subcortical lesions and verbal apraxia. In: *Apraxia of Speech: Physiology-Acoustics-Linguistics-Management*, edited by J. C. Rosenbek, M. McNeil, and A. Aronson, pp. 73–90. College-Hill Press, San Diego.
23. Klich, R. J., Ireland, J. V., and Weidner, W. E. (1979): Articulatory and phonological aspects of consonant substitutions in apraxia of speech. *Cortex*, 15:451–470.
24. LaPointe, L. L., and Johns, D. F. (1975): Some phonemic characteristics in apraxia of speech. *J. Commun. Dis.*, 8:259–269.
25. Lashley, K. S. (1951): The problem of serial order in behavior. In: *Cerebral Mechanisms in Behavior*, edited by L. S. Jeffress, pp. 112–136. Wiley, New York.
26. Lebrun, Y., Buyssens, E., and Henneaux, J. (1973): Phonetic aspects of anarthria. *Cortex*, 9:126–135.
27. Luria, A. R. (1970): *Traumatic Aphasia: Its Syndromes, Psychology and Treatment*. Mouton, Paris.

28. Marquardt, T. P., Reinhart, J. B., and Peterson, H. A. (1979): Markedness analysis of phonemic substitution errors in apraxia of speech. *J. Commun. Dis.*, 12:481–494.
29. Martin, A. D. (1974): Some objections to the term "apraxia of speech." *J. Speech Hear. Disord.*, 39:53–64.
30. McNeil, M. R., Prescott, T. E., and Lemme, M. L. (1976): An application of electromyographic biofeedback to aphasia/apraxia treatment. In: *Clinical Aphasiology*, edited by R. H. Brookshire, pp. 151–171. BRK Press, Minneapolis.
31. McReynolds, L., and Kearns, K. (1983): *Single-Subject Experimental Designs in Communicative Disorders*. University Park Press, Baltimore.
32. Rosenbek, J. C. (1978): Treating apraxia of speech. In: *Clinical Management of Neurogenic Communicative Disorders*, edited by D. F. Johns, pp. 191–250. Little, Brown, Boston.
33. Rosenbek, J. C., Kent, R. D., and LaPointe, L. L. (1984): Apraxia of speech; an overview and some perspectives. In: *Apraxia of Speech: Physiology-Acoustics-Linguistics-Management*, edited by J. C. Rosenbek, M. McNeil, and A. Aronson, pp. 1–72. College-Hill Press, San Diego.
34. Rosenbek, J. C., Lemme, M. L., Ahern, M. B., Harris, E. H., and Wertz, R. T. (1973): A treatment for apraxia of speech in adults. *J. Speech Hear. Disord.*, 38:462–472.
35. Rubow, R., Rosenbek, J. C., Collins, M. J., and Longstreth, D. (1982): Vibrotactile stimulation for intersystemic reorganization in the treatment of apraxia of speech. *Arch. Phys. Med. Rehabil.*, 63:150–153.
36. Shankweiler, D., and Harris, K. S. (1966): An experimental approach to the problem of articulation in aphasia. *Cortex*, 2:277–292.
37. Shankweiler, D., Harris, K. S., and Taylor, M. L. (1968): Electromyographic studies of articulation in aphasia. *Arch. Phys. Med. Rehabil.*, 49:1–8.
38. Shewan, C. (1980): Verbal dyspraxia and its treatment. *Hum. Commun.*, 5:3–12.
39. Shewan, C. M., Leeper, H. A., and Booth, J. C. (1984): An analysis of voice onset time (VOT) in aphasic and normal subjects. In: *Apraxia of Speech: Physiology-Acoustics-Linguistics-Management*, edited by J. C. Rosenbek, M. McNeil, and A. Aronson, pp. 197–220. College-Hill Press, San Diego.
40. Sternberg, S., Monsell, S., Knoll, R. L., and Wright, C. E. (1978): The latency and duration of rapid movement sequences: Comparisons of speech and typewriting. In: *Information Processing in Motor Control and Learning*, edited by G. E. Stelmach, pp. 118–152. Academic Press, New York.
41. Wepman, J. M., and Van Pelt, D. (1955): A theory of cerebral language disorders based on therapy. *Folia Phoniatr. (Basel)*, 7:233–235.
42. Wertz, R. T., LaPointe, L. L., and Rosenbek, J. C. (1984): *Apraxia of Speech: The Disorder and Its Management*. Grune & Stratton, New York.

Advances in Neurology, Vol. 42: Progress in Aphasiology, edited by F. C. Rose.
Raven Press, New York © 1984.

A Psychomotor Approach to Improving Speech by Modulating Suprasegmental Control in Motor Dysphasia and Articulatory Apraxia

U. Hadar, R. Twiston Davies, T. J. Steiner, and F. Clifford Rose

Department of Neurology, Charing Cross Hospital, London W6 8RF, England

This chapter presents a technique of working with dysphasic patients, treating those of their speech problems that directly involve disturbed suprasegmental control, such as decreased speech rate, arrest of speech onset, lexical and phonemic perseveration, improper application of stress, and impaired intonation. These aspects of speech affect linguistic operations, and their improvement may entail a considerable gain in language performance. The origins of the present technique lie in (a) the ecologic approach to perception and action and the conception of motor and linguistic operations as interdependent (7,19), (b) the close relationship between head movement (HM) and the regulation of suprasegmental features (Hadar et al. *this volume*), and (c) the Feldenkrais (4,5) approach to motor functioning in everyday life and the importance of awareness of self in action and perception. We deal extensively with the first two elsewhere (Hadar et al., *this volume*); other than a brief account, we concentrate here on the third.

Ecologic theories of action and perception argue that, because of the nature of musculoskeletal structures and forces in their immediate environment, organs are constrained to oscillate around zero positions. Thus the regulation of behavioral cyclicities underlies motor performance. Such cyclicities are essential to speech production, inasmuch as speech implies motor operations, thus offering a possible route through which speech disturbances may be approached.

Although a full account of the cyclicities involved in speech production is beyond the scope of this chapter, its basic principles are as follows: (a) Cyclicities of low frequency tend to be more fundamental than those of higher frequencies in that they are more stable or more resistant to change. This creates a weak hierarchy of motor organization, such that the restoration of an impaired faculty may best be approached from the behavioral cyclicities immediately under it. (b) In the domain of voluntary action, movements of the articulators are at the top of the motor hierarchy, being of the highest frequencies. (c) In the context of speech, the respiratory cycle is of the lowest frequency. Although other, slower cyclicities probably are involved in speaking (1), these are not strictly motor. (d) Intermediate frequencies are seen, in rising order, in intonation cycles, stress cycles, and speech rhythms, created by combinations of the first two (17). We suggest that speech rhythms are displayed in their pure forms in poetic verse. These principles provide the most general framework for the psychomotor training scheme.

Research in normal subjects has established the close relationship between HM and suprasegmental features of speech (Hadar et al., *this volume*). Specifically, smoothly varying contours, as toward a speech pause, correlated with smooth HM at an ordinary speed; short, sharp movements correlated with stress; and wide, linear movements accompanied speech onset after long pauses. It was inferred that the intermediate frequencies, i.e., those of intonation cycles, stress cycles, and speech rhythms, had originated from a common source (2), so that rehabilitation of these faculties may benefit from exercising coordinated HM.

Movement of the head also establishes the link with the theories and practice of Feldenkrais (4,5) both in its direct relationship to the rehabilitation of speech (5) and in its broader effects on cognition via visual and vestibular systems (4).

The importance of HM for visual perception has long been recognized, especially in the context of depth perception (11,20) and in adaptation to transformed optical conditions, as when the visual field is distorted by means of optical devices, such as prisms (10,15), or when a shift in the scale and magnitude of the visual events requires tuning of the visual system (18). Because HM directly affects the vestibular system, it is important in every aspect of eighth nerve function, e.g., auditory perception (14), sea sickness and nausea (12), and maintenance of balance and erect posture (4). This results in an intimate relationship between HM and integrative, cognitive functions that bear on voluntary, goal-directed action in general. The quality of execution of HM both affects and reflects the ability to plan and perform visually, or auditorily, guided motor sequences (5). Although HM is unique in this respect, it has a more general application in Feldenkrais' (4) conception of mature motor functioning, where each action strikes a unique balance between general and particular elements, and attention must be paid to both for improving any skill. The general, integrative aspect of action is achieved through a systematic awareness of the grain components of a specific movement and its effects on neighboring organs (4). In this sense, a properly executed movement is a lesson in anatomy.

These ideas were developed hand in hand with a technique for improving motor performances in everyday life, referred to as awareness through movement (6). The main constituents may be construed, in a prescriptive order, as follows: (a) A preliminary stage of reduced action, with little peripheral involvement, comprises the fine grain, imaginary depiction of the target movements. (b) This imaginary design is continued or amplified at the peripheral level, where amplification and continuation are conceptually opposed to the execution of central commands and are indicated by smoothness and ease of transition from imaginary to actual movement. (c) Close attention should accompany movement, created by continually transforming kinesthetic perceptions to visual images, and vice versa. The performing subject should develop an awareness of the motor space created by effects of the moving organ on

TABLE 1. *Subjects*

Parameter	B	E	W
Age (years)	76	69	55
Sex	M	F	M
Clinical diagnosis	Acute cerebral infarction	Acute cerebral infarction, left middle artery	Acute cerebral infarction
Motor disturbances	None	Right hemiparesis	None
Nature of speech disturbance	Expressive dysphasia, good comprehension	Severe expressive dysphasia or apraxia of speech	Expressive dysphasia, good comprehension
Time from onset (months)	12	24	20
Duration of previous speech therapy (months)	7	6	3

neighboring areas, and invariant, phase relationships between organs moving at the same time. (d) Awareness is generalized to an experience of self, emerging as that which is ever behind awareness in the sense of never confronting it as an object. In this respect, Feldenkrais' self is similar to Gibson's (8), for whom the self is that which is behind all seeing but never an object of vision: its most concrete manifestation is the flow of the optical array created by eye and head movements, which are the only sources of this exproprioceptive information (13).

The basic exercises of the psychomotor training program were inspired by the Feldenkrais technique. We describe and discuss work with three dysphasic patients on the psychomotor program, offering tentative ideas integrated into a relatively unitary approach with no attempt to prove its success or make other tested therapeutic claims.

METHOD

Subjects

Subjects were three right-handed stroke patients, two men and one woman aged 76, 69, and 55 years, referred to as B, E, and W (Table 1). They were chosen on the following grounds: (a) having an expressive speech disorder, (b) having relatively well-preserved comprehension, (c) being at least 6 months past onset of speech problems, and (d) being discharged from individual speech therapy, following stabilization of their language performance. Both E and W participated in a once-weekly speech group after ending their individual therapy; this continued during the psychomotor training.

Language Assessment

Language assessment consisted of: (a) the Boston Diagnostic Aphasia Examination (BDAE), (b) tests for the control of phonation, pitch, volume, and stress placement adapted from the Frenchay and Robertson dysarthria tests, and the Darley et al. (3) motor speech profile, and (c) analysis of continuous speech for rate, length of utterances, stutters, and pauses. This assessment was conducted prior to and after the beginning of the training program (pre- and posttraining, respectively) by a member of our team. Results of a BDAE conducted earlier in the Speech Therapy Department of the Charing Cross Hospital by a senior speech therapist were also available.

Procedure

The patients were initially approached by explaining to them the nature of the work with which they were asked to cooperate. Language assessment was followed by immediate introduction to the training program, conducted at the hospital on a twice-weekly basis. Training lasted 3.5 months; each subject missed occasional sessions (between two and five) during this period.

Table 2 presents an outline of the exercises comprising the training program, divided into three main groups: (a) elementary coordination, (b) advanced coordination, and (c) real speech exercises. Elementary coordination exercises were based on a one-to-one relationship between head and breathing or articulatory gestures, while the advanced exercises gradually increased the load on the exhalation phase of breathing in both duration and complexity. Real speech exercises incorporated HM in regulating stress, intonation, and rhythms of simple verse. The training program was considered complete with the achievement of good performance in real speech exercises.

The progress of each subject was recorded on a control sheet (Table 3), but no rigid, linear order was imposed. Frequent returns were made to elementary exercises, even if a satisfactory performance had been achieved months earlier, in an attempt to improve performance further. Moreover, the exercises in Table 2 formed the basis of many variations and improvisations. For instance, the coordination stage with subject E, who made very slow progress, consisted of approximately 15 different exercises, all based on a one-to-one relationship between articulatory and head gestures.

Each session began with exercises 1 or 2 in order to regulate proper breathing, achieve relaxation, and warm up the neck muscles. In these, movement was to be performed as slowly and as smoothly as possible, attempting the fine phasing of breathing with head gestures. All exercises were performed repetitively for 5 to 10 min, with eyes closed to enhance concentration and relaxation. During a preparatory phase, the patient was asked to visualize the target movement as accurately as possible; a terminal phase consisted of close attention to bodily sensations, elicited, initially, by asking the patient to report them to the therapist. Following exercise 1 or 2, the session concentrated on one or a few related exercises, repeated with variations until a good performance was reached, often enhanced by various psy-

TABLE 2. *Outline of exercises comprising the psychomotor treatment program for speech disturbances*

Index	HM task	Articulatory task	Coordinative task	Remarks
I. Elementary coordination of HM with breathing and phonation				
1	Rhythmic rolling of the head aside and back, lying supine	Rhythmic breathing with long phases of inhalation and exhalation	Transitions from inhaling to exhaling and vice versa are to coincide with transitions in linear direction of movement; turning with exhalation, returning with inhalation	Control of breathing may improve when the patient imagines that HM actually "drive" the breathing gestures
2	Rhythmic head raising and lowering in long movements; patient sitting upright on a chair	As above	As above; exhalation with head lowering, inhalation with raising	It is important for the patient to associate away movement with exhaling: the "work" phase of speech
3	As above	Production of constant sound during exhalation; repeated with all vowels and fricatives	As above	/f/ and /z/ proved most difficult to perform
4	Repeated slow head raising and very rapid, short lowering with and without extensive abdominal movements	Serial alternation between smooth breathing and sporadic, short production of intense phonation with open glottis ("ha") and with sharp glottal release ("ah")	Even phase with slow raising; intense phonation with rapid lowering	This mechanism of stress production is integrated into structured speech in exercise 10
II. Advanced coordination of head movement, breathing, and phonation				
5	Long raising, then rhythmic, cyclic, half-range movement, terminated by long lowering	Long, controlled phase of exhalation	Substantial intake with initial head raising; cyclic HM during exhalation; terminal lowering prior to exhaustion	Preparation for "siren" exercise (6); this breaks the one-to-one relationship between breathing and HM gestures, preparing for real speech exercises
6	Rhythmic raising and lowering	Serial, continuous transitions between top and bottom pitch (like a siren)	High pitch with head raising, low with lowering.	Performance of the "siren" task is often accompanied by spontaneous HM, even without an explicit instruction
7	Rhythmic tilting to one side and back, then to the other	Rhythmic, serial, rapid production of various phonemes	As above; 2–5 tilts on each phase of breathing; production of each phoneme with a separate movement	Head tilting is naturally a narrow movement, and so it is used for exercising sharp performances
8	Wide and even circular movement, in a serial alternation between clockwise and counterclockwise orientation	Rhythmic breathing	Inhalation during raising phase; exhalation during lowering	*Smooth* transition from raising to lowering renders it difficult to phase the shift from inhaling to exhaling with top position of the head
9	As above; head is to be allowed to *fall* with gravity on its way down	Arrhythmic breathing; production of arhythmic, continuous sound	Exhalation, during head lowering, should "accelerate" with the head, as should sound, with pitch and loudness "glides"	Learning to make use of inert and gravitational impacts on the articulators is an important aspect of normal speech (7).

(*continued*)

TABLE 2. (*continued*)

Index	HM task	Articulatory task	Coordinative task	Remarks
III. Integrating HM into real speech				
10	Arrhythmic lowering and raising	Regulation of stress in simple phonemic clauses (only one primary stress); example: "*John* went home", "John *went* home"	Head raising with inhalation; lowering during first two words, raising with last word; accelerate sharply with primary stress	Initially, it is important that performance of this is preceded and followed by the regulation of breathing rhythm
11	Combination of horizontal and vertical arrhythmic movements	Inflecting simple phrases by only manipulating the tone contour	Hold head still until first primary stress; sharp movement with primary stress; head raising with rising pitch	Patient to be allowed his own preferred patterns, apart from obligatory sharp movement with primary stress and terminal raising
12	As above	Answering a question only by proper placing of stress; example: "Who went home?" "*John* went home"; "Where did John go?" "John went *home*"	Any movement, as long as stress is accompanied by sharp, and smooth contour by smooth movement	This excercise starts a sequence of tasks, emphasizing the syntactic and semantic functions of stress and intonation
13	As above	Rephrasing a question using only stress and intonation; example: "Was it home John went?" "John went *home*??"	As above	
14	Circular movement with gravity effects, as in exercise 9; increasing speed gradually	Reciting a well-known verse with exagerated stress: "*Jack* and *Jill* went *up* the *hill*"; increase speed gradually	Stressed words are to coincide with acceleration phases	

chomotor "tricks." For instance, a short, rapid, cyclic HM was invariably found extremely difficult to achieve. Performance was significantly advanced when that type of movement was first produced by pronation and supination of the arm with extended pointing finger, the head joining in once performance with the arm was firmly regulated.

In the stress exercise (no. 11) the patient was required to answer different questions presented by the therapist, with only one target sentence. For instance, given the target sentence "The table is red," the question "What is red?" should have been answered by "The *table* is red," while "What color is the table?" should have been answered by "The table is *red*," and "Which table is red?" by "*The* table is red." A similar technique was employed in the inflectional intonation exercise (12).

Observations on Performance During Training

As mentioned above, patients' progress was diverse. Both B and W almost completed their program within 4 months, while E could only achieve a fair performance of the most elementary exercises, and none of the second phase. Patient E displayed overall poor control of voluntary action, with both breathing gestures and HM being jerky, hesitant, and almost impossible to coordinate. Although her spontaneous speech was markedly loud, performance of constant sound was initially inaudible

TABLE 3. *Example of patient control sheet*

Exercises	Quality of Performance			
	Nonexistent	Poor	Fair	Good
Elementary coordination				
1				
2				
3				
4				
Advanced coordination				
5				
6				
7				
8				
9				
Speech and movement				
10				
11				
12				
13				
14				

and, even when finally acquired, of uncontrollably low volume, with occasional lapses into soundlessness. Initially, she could not shout at will but learned to produce some kind of sharp and loud vocalization by coordinating it with a sharp and intense head nod. Most progress was achieved by utilizing her instinctive echoing responses: the production of a loud, constant sound by the therapist was invariably echoed by some sound production, although often of very short duration. Coordination of breathing with HM was impossible to achieve with exercise 1. Only in exercise 2, when she was asked to perform extensive movements of the trunk and abdomen with external pressure applied on her diaphragm, did she make eventual progress. Once a fair performance of exercise 2 was achieved, after about 2 months of work, emphasis was placed on the targeting of vowels. Initially, she showed poor or no targeting at all, responding to the target stimulus with any vowel or none, and with severe perseveration. Moreover, her performance was dyspraxic, with phenomena such as lip rounding for the production of /a/ or tongue protrusion for /f/ occurring during exercises but seldom in spontaneous speech. Later, it was found that she was only vaguely aware of her mistargeting and was often unable to indicate the vowel she had actually produced. Although her perception of the therapist's enunciation was much better, she often could not indicate the vowel performed or failed to recognize that two successive performances were of nonidentical vowels. In recent sessions, her targeting improved by asking her after each trial to indicate the vowel she had produced.

Subject B had poor control of breathing, which was of very short phases, but his speech was relatively effortless and fluent. His main speech problems seemed to be connected with his attempts to squeeze many words into short efforts of phonation, with frequent failure to retrieve long words, resulting in a stutter. Breathing phases were instinctively coordinated with vertical HM, as required in exercise 2. He generally made rapid progress within the range of medium amplitudes and frequencies but needed to pay special attention in order to extend this range to higher or lower amplitudes and frequencies. He displayed the most obvious asymmetric biases in performance. While head tilting to the left was fair, he failed to tilt to the right, turning his head instead. He had great difficulties in shifting from clockwise to counterclockwise circular movement, carried out along different trajectories. His vertical movements diverged from the central axis, with a top-left/bottom-right bias.

During the first stage of training, most work with B concentrated on the ability to maintain long breathing phases and smooth transitions between phases. He tended to produce these transitions with sharp glottal release, which had two main results: first, his prosodic phrases became longer and, second, it was found that the articulation of words that he failed to retrieve improved dramatically by coordinating them with one long HM. Despite his tendency to short and hasty phonations, B's control of sharp articulatory performances was poor, and so a considerable amount of training was required for satisfactory production of short, rapid movements or sounds. Once this was achieved, however, B found no problem in attaining the advanced coordination exercises. Furthermore, after relatively short training, he mastered the placement of stress in real speech exercises (10). Speedy progress was also achieved with the verse exercises (12), where significant differences in difficulty were shown between verses with short lines, such as "Jack and Jill," and those with longer lines, such as "Humpty Dumpty." Yet where stress was more than one syllable away from the beginning of lines, as in "There *was* a little girl/ And she *had* a little curl," performance was extremely poor, requiring at least five times more exercising. Like W, B required an extremely long time to understand inflections through intonation (exercise 11), and both have not yet been able to master this task fully.

Subject W was the opposite of B in his prosodic, suprasegmental style, having very effortful, slow speech and infrequent retrieval problems or stutter. He quickly acquired good control of breathing, and his performance of HM tasks was invariably good. His progress was rapid, reaching stage 3 of the program within 2 months, and few of the difficulties he met until then were greater than normal. Acquisition of the placement of stress was good in short sentences of three to four words but much disturbed in long ones. In the verse exercises, he displayed great difficulties of an agrammatic nature. Like B, he tended to place the stress on the first syllable in each line and lost his rhythm when this was not the natural placement. He found it most difficult to move negation to a noninitial position. Thus he repeatedly replaced "All the king's horses, and all the king's men/ couldn't put Humpty together again" with "None of the king's . . . ," at which point his speech was usually arrested.

Language Performance

For present purposes, we adapted the Z-score profile of the BDAE by weighting each subscore in a given category of the test according to a scale of 1 to 10 and then computing the mean score in each category. For instance, the "naming" category consists of 1, responsive naming; 2, confrontation naming; 3, animal naming; and 4, body part naming. These are scored, respectively, 0–30, 5–105, 0–23, and 0–30. Given the mark X in "responsive naming," its weighting through our 1 to 10 scale would produce an X/3 subscore, and the final rating of "naming" represented the mean of all four weighted subscores.

Similar conversions were applied to the motor control tasks, giving rise to four categories, reflected in the control of phonation, pitch, volume, and stress, each consisting of four to six subscores. We referred to this group of results as "prosody control."

Finally, we computed a variety of statistic features of a passage of continuous speech, which represent the basic correlates of fluency (9). Speech in this passage was elicited by asking the subject to describe in detail the preparation of a cup of tea.

Table 4 presents the language performance of subject E in three separate tests: during speech therapy (column a), immediately prior to training (column b), and after 3.5 months of therapeutic training (column c). It is evident from the BDAE summary (section A, columns a and b) that in the last year prior to beginning her training program, E's performance was stable, with little change in any of the available results. Her posttraining test (column c), however, reveals a 37.2% improvement in fluency ratings, a 6.2% improvement in oral reading ratings, and a 10.8% increase in paraphasias, of which more than 90% were literal. All other variations in her BDAE were negligible, being less than 5%. Subject E displayed distinct improvements in the control of phonation (27.5%) and pitch (18.4%) but none in the control of volume and stress (Table 4B). The improvement in fluency indicated in the BDAE was fully sustained in the analysis of the tea passage (Table 4C). Thus the mean duration of her pauses was 20.3% less in her posttraining assessment, and she produced 72.7% more syllables per unit time. Although the mean duration of her prosodic phrases, defined as periods of phonation enclosed by pauses, did not change significantly, she produced 36.3% more syllables in these phrases in her posttraining test. Moreover, the maximum number of syllables produced in a single prosodic phrase increased by 77.7%. This amounted to a consistent, overall improvement in fluency of approximately 50% (Table 4C).

Subject B's assessment during speech therapy was not based on the BDAE; thus we were unable to assess the stability of his language performance between speech therapy and the beginning of the training program. The main features shown in a comparison of his pre- and posttraining BDAE summary (Table 5A) are distinctly poorer repetition score (−32.8%) and an increase in paraphasias of 29.6%. Both were attributable, in more than 90% of cases, to literal repetitions and substitutions. However, B displayed marked improvement in oral reading (26.7%) and a dramatic

TABLE 4. *Language performance of subject E*

Parameter	a. During speech therapy[a]	b. Prior to beginning psychomotor training[b]	c. After 3.5 months of training[c]
A. From the BDAE			
Severity	—	3	3–4
Fluency	—	5.1	7.0
Comprehension	—	9.4	10
Naming	7.6	7.9	7.9
Oral reading	8.0	8.0	8.5
Repetition	6.0	6.5	6.3
Paraphasia	8.2	8.3	7.4
Serial speech	6.3	6.3	6.3
Music	—	2.5	2.5
B. Prosodic control			
Phonation	—	4.0	5.1
Pitch	—	3.8	4.5
Volume	—	5.2	5.2
Stress placement	—	7.7	7.7
C. Analysis of the description of the preparation of a cup of tea			
Total duration (sec)	—	68.5	56.5
Share of pauses (%)	—	63.0	62.0
Longest pause (sec)	—	6.6	2.8
Mean duration of pauses (sec)		1.28	1.02
Total number of syllables		78	109
Mean syllables per second		1.1	1.9
Total of prosodic phrases		35	36
Syllables per prosodic phrase		2.2	3.0
Maximum syllables per prosodic phrase		9	16
Maximum duration of prosodic phrase (sec)		2.2	1.9
Mean duration of prosodic phrase (sec)		0.7	0.6
Stutters		5	6

[a] April 28, 1982.
[b] May 6, 1983.
[c] August 8, 1983.

improvement in music ratings. No other variations in his BDAE were greater than 5% (Table 5A).

The BDAE indications of improvement in B's prosodic control were reinforced in section B of the tests, where he displayed distinct improvements in control of pitch (11.1%), volume (9.4%), and stress (16.6%). Based on observations during training, his lesser posttraining rating of phonation (– 10.9%) seemed to indicate an idiosyncrasy in specific test performance, but had actually improved as well.

Analysis of B's tea passage revealed a consistent, overall improvement in fluency of 10 to 20% (Table 5C). Although on average his pauses were only 6.3% shorter, his prosodic phrases were clearly longer (by a mean of 14.3%) and his rate of production greater, with a 13.3% increase in syllables per unit time. Furthermore, B

TABLE 5. *Language performance of subject B*

Parameter		a. Prior to beginning psychomotor training[a]	b. After 3.5 months of training[b]
A. From the BDAE			
Severity	—	3.5	4
Fluency	—	8.4	8.7
Comprehension	—	9.5	9.4
Naming	—	8.0	7.9
Oral reading	—	7.1	9.0
Repetition	—	7.0	4.7
Paraphasia	—	8.1	5.7
Serial speech	—	7.5	7.0
Music	—	2.5	10.0
B. Prosodic control			
Phonation	—	9.1	8.1
Pitch	—	9.0	10.0
Volume	—	6.4	7.0
Stress placement	—	6.6	7.7
C. Analysis of the description of the preparation of a cup of tea			
Total duration (sec)	—	83.0	89.0
Share of pauses (%)	—	54.0	51.0
Longest pause (sec)	—	3.3	2.0
Mean duration of pauses (sec)		0.83	0.78
Total number of syllables		127	155
Mean syllables per second		1.5	1.7
Total of prosodic phrases		55	58
Syllables per prosodic phrase		2.3	2.7
Maximum syllables per prosodic phrase		15	23
Maximum duration of prosodic phrase (sec)		2.1	1.4
Mean duration of prosodic phrase (sec)		0.7	0.8
Stutters		14	9

[a] May 9, 1983.
[b] August 23, 1983.

produced a mean of 17.4% more syllables in his posttraining prosodic phrases, and his maximum number of syllables per prosodic phrase was 53.3% greater. Finally, the number of stutters B produced fell by 35.7% (Table 5C).

Subject W was often inconsistent in his language performance, as in his pretraining oral reading (Table 6A, column b) or the poor repetition rating in his speech therapy assessment (column a). Although this may have been a result of his language pathology, we believe it arose from characteristic lapses of concentration, displayed in various aspects of his behavior. Apart from these inconsistencies, his language performance was fairly stable between speech therapy and pretraining assessments (columns a and b), but his fluency seemed to improve continuously, with an 11.7% increase in his posttraining ratings. He displayed some improvement in comprehension (~5.5%) and a marked improvement in music ratings. Patient W's control of

TABLE 6. *Language performance of subject W*

Parameter	a. During speech therapy[a]	b. Prior to beginning psychomotor training[b]	c. After 3.5 months of training[c]
A. From the BDAE			
Severity	4.	4	4
Fluency	7.7	8.5	9.5
Comprehension	9.3	9.1	9.8
Naming	8.8	8.7	8.5
Oral reading	10.0	8.3	10.0
Repetition	5.7	8.5	8.8
Paraphasia	9.3	9.1	9.3
Serial speech	7.5	7.5	7.5
Music	—	5.0	10.0
B. Prosodic control			
Phonation	—	6.3	8.3
Pitch	—	9.0	9.0
Volume	—	8.1	9.4
Stress placement	—	8.8	10.0
C. Analysis of the description of the preparation of a cup of tea			
Total duration (sec)	—	36.0	62.0
Share of pauses (%)	—	63.0	71.0
Longest pause (sec)	—	4.1	7.7
Mean duration of pauses (sec)		1.28	1.58
Total number of syllables		64	84
Mean syllables per second		1.7	1.4
Total of prosodic phrases		18	29
Syllables per prosodic phrase		3.5	2.9
Maximum syllables per prosodic phrase		10	15
Maximum duration of prosodic phrase (sec)		1.3	2.3
Mean duration of prosodic phrase (sec)		0.7	0.6
Stutters		0	3

[a] February 9, 1982.
[b] May 3, 1983.
[c] August 19, 1983.

prosody underwent a marked (10–30%) overall improvement (Table 6C), with 31.7% better ratings in phonation control, 16.1% better in volume control, and 13.3% better in stress placement. These, however, contributed only marginally to his performance in the tea passage.

As shown in Table 6C, there were increases in W's share of pauses (12.7%) and their maximum and mean durations (23.4%). This was accompanied by a lower speech rate, with a decrease in mean syllables per unit time (−17.6%) and mean syllables per prosodic phrase (−11.4%). However, it seemed that W's relatively poor posttraining performance of the tea passage emanated from a preoccupation with his personal problems throughout his assessment, with consequent failure to concentrate. Indeed, he performed consistently better on more mechanical tasks that required no taxing cognitive involvement. Even in the tea passage, he occasionally spoke very fluently, which was reflected in the maximum ratings: the longest prosodic phrase in the posttraining assessment contained 50% more syllables than the maximum of his pretraining assessment, at a high rate of 6.5/sec.

DISCUSSION

The above analysis of language performance of the subjects who underwent the psychomotor program indicates that two of them (E and B) made substantial progress, especially in speech fluency, which they also communicated to us from their personal experience. The more remarkable progress was made by E, who made the slowest progress in her motor performance of the exercises. In contradistinction, W, who progressed most impressively in his training program, had the least remarkable results in his posttraining assessment. Patient B's results, with an intermediate rate of progress in both his training and language performance, were in line with these observations. Together with the overall correlation between absolute levels of performance of the training exercises and the language assessments, they generally support our introductory line of reasoning concerning the relationships between motor and linguistic operations. Thus in our subjects, linguistic performance correlated with motor coordination, and overcoming a motor difficulty in the course of training seemed to result in overcoming a speech (fluency) problem.

Of the various aspects of language analyzed above, the most consistent increases in posttraining ratings were shown in the prosody control tasks, reflected in the ratings of all three subjects. This is not surprising, as the training program tackled these tasks directly. It is our belief that the improvement in speech fluency was a result of the improved control of prosody, especially of its continuous, rhythmic regulation. Moreover, we think that suprasegmentals provide the link between pure prosodic control and speech fluency. A number of our results support this, underlining claims that prosodic disturbances are an integral part of the aphasic speech disturbance (Weniger, *this volume*).

First, improvement in posttraining ratings was most distinct in prolonged, continuous performances, such as oral reading or spontaneous speech, where the task allowed the subject to regulate rhythm and cyclic action. Indeed, where the linguistic task required a short, well-targeted linguistic production, as in naming, repetition, and serial speech categories of the BDAE, performance slightly regressed in all three subjects. Second, in the prime indicator of segmental control, i.e., literal paraphasia, posttraining performance remained unchanged in W, who also displayed the least improvement in fluency, and actually regressed in E and B, whose fluency clearly had improved. This suggests that the improvement in the suprasegmental control of speech might have been achieved, at least temporarily, at the expense of segmental control. This most interesting phenomenon suggests that segmental and suprasegmental control of speech are relatively independent and possibly complementary.

During speech, the functional distinction between the left and right hemispheres is commonly associated with the conceptual distinction between linguistic and emotional processes, respectively. As Weniger (*this volume*) shows, there is mounting evidence against this, and so association of cerebral functional asymmetry with segmental and suprasegmental control may provide a more adequate basis for explaining the role of prosody in speech production. Association of segmental and suprasegmental control with the left and right hemispheres, respectively, may account for the observed compensatory relationships between segmental and suprasegmental performance of our subjects. It is possible that, in the course of training, they developed a greater dependence on the right hemisphere in their linguistic production. This requires further evidence.

We do not aim to evaluate here the success of our therapeutic methods, as we have insufficient evidence. We do note, however, that spontaneous speech in general and fluency in particular are some of the aspects of dysphasic communication that have been most resistant to intervention (16). In view of this, our preliminary results are more than encouraging.

ACKNOWLEDGMENT

The project reported here is supported by a grant made to U. Hadar by the Northwest Thames Regional Health Authority. We thank Ms. Perry, Chief Speech Therapist at the Charing Cross Hospital, and Ms. G. Edelman, Chief Speech Therapist at the Hammersmith Hospital, for their help with our project.

REFERENCES

1. Butterworth, B. (1980): Evidence from pauses in speech. In: *Language Production, Vol. 1*, edited by B. Butterworth, pp. 155–176. Academic Press, London.
2. Condon, W. (1980): The relation of interactional synchrony to cognitive and emotional processes. In: *The Relation of Verbal and Nonverbal Communication*, edited by M. R. Key, pp. 49–66. Mouton, The Hague.
3. Darley, F. L., Aronson, A. E., and Brown, J. R. (1975): *Motor Speech Disorders*. Saunders, Philadelphia.
4. Feldenkrais, M. (1966): *Body and Mature Behaviour*. International Universities Press, New York.
5. Feldenkrais, M. (1977): *The Case of Nora*. Harper & Row, London.
6. Feldenkrais, M. (1980): *Awareness Through Movement*. Penguin, Harmondsworth.
7. Fowler, C. A., Rubin, P., Remez, R. E., and Turvey, M. T. (1980): Implications for speech production of a general theory of action. In: *Language Production, Vol 1*, edited by B. Butterworth, pp. 373–420. Academic Press, London.
8. Gibson, J. J. (1979): *The Ecological Approach to Visual Perception*. Houghton Miflin, Boston.
9. Goldman Eisler, F. (1968): *Psycholinguistics: Experiments in Spontaneous Speech*. Academic Press, New York.
10. Held, R. (1964): The role of movement in the origin and maintenance of visual perception. *Acta Psychol.*, 23:308–309.
11. Helmholtz, H. von (1866): *Treatise on Physiological Optics, Vol. III*. Dover, New York.
12. Johnson, W. H., and Taylor, N. B. G. (1961): The importance of head movement in studies involving stimulation of the organ of balance. *Acta Otolaryngol.* 53:211–218.
13. Lee, D. N. (1980): Visuo-motor coordination in space-time. In: *Tutorials in Motor Behavior*, edited by G. E. Stelmach and J. Requin, pp. 281–296. North Holland, Amsterdam.
14. Marks, L. E. (1978): *The Unity of the Senses*. Academic Press, New York.
15. McCarter, A., and Mikielian, H. H. (1978): The role of acceleration information in prism adaptation. *Percept. Psychophys.*, 23:21–26.
16. Prins, R., Snow, C., and Wagnaar, E. (1978): Recovery from aphasia: Spontaneous speech versus language comprehension. *Brain Lang.*, 6:192–211.

17. Shaffer, L. H. (1982): Rhythm and timing in skill. *Psychol. Rev.*, 89:109–122.
18. Turvey, M. T. (1977): Preliminaries to a theory of action with reference to vision. In: *Perceiving Acting and Knowing*, edited by R. E. Shaw and J. Bransford, pp. 211–266. Lawrence Erlbaum, Hillsdale, N.J.
19. Turvey, M. T. (1980): Clues from the organisation of motor systems. In: *Signed and Spoken Language: Biological Constraints on Linguistic Form*, edited by U. Bellugi and M. Studdert Kennedy, pp. 41–56. Verlag Chemie, Weinheim.
20. Wallach, H., and O'Leary, A. (1979): Adaptation in distance perception with head movement parallax serving as the veridical cue. *Percept. Psychophys.*, 25:42–46.

SUBJECT INDEX

Subject Index